Clinical Companion for Maternity and Newborn Health

Clinical Companion for Maternity and Newborn Health

Edited by Nicole McConnell

AMERICAN
MEDICAL PUBLISHERS
www.americanmedicalpublishers.com

American Medical Publishers,
41 Flatbush Avenue,
1st Floor, New York,
NY 11217, USA

Visit us on the World Wide Web at:
www.americanmedicalpublishers.com

ISBN: 978-1-63927-152-8

Cataloging-in-Publication Data

Clinical companion for maternity and newborn health / edited by Nicole McConnell.
p. cm.
Includes bibliographical references and index.
ISBN 978-1-63927-152-8
1. Maternal health services. 2. Newborn infants--Health and hygiene. 3. Maternal and infant welfare.
4. Obstetrics. 5. Neonatology. I. McConnell, Nicole.

RG940 .C55 2022

618.24--dc23

Table of Contents

Preface

A number of complications can arise during pregnancy, childbirth and in the postpartum period. Most pregnant women experience at least one health problem in the immediate postpartum period. Women also report long-term health problems after pregnancy. Maternal mortality is associated with the occurrence of maternal bleeding, obstructed labor, hypertensive diseases of pregnancy, etc. Pregnant women are more susceptible to developing infections. This is due to an increased immune tolerance of the body during pregnancy to prevent an immune response against the fetus. Certain infections are also vertically transmissible, thus affecting the child as well. Gestational diabetes, anemia, hypothyroidism, peripartum cardiomyopathy, etc. can also occur in a pregnant woman. These need to be managed as these are considered risk factors for the development and safety of the child and the health of the mother. Ectopic pregnancy, miscarriage, placenta accreta, placental abruption, etc. are fetal and placental problems with considerable consequences for the mother. This book covers in detail some existent theories and innovative concepts revolving around maternal-newborn health. In this book, using case studies and examples, constant effort has been made to make the understanding of the difficult concepts of obstetrics, as easy and informative as possible, for the readers. It will serve as a source of reference to a broad spectrum of readers.

This book unites the global concepts and researches in an organized manner for a comprehensive understanding of the subject. It is a ripe text for all researchers, students, scientists or anyone else who is interested in acquiring a better knowledge of this dynamic field.

I extend my sincere thanks to the contributors for such eloquent research chapters. Finally, I thank my family for being a source of support and help.

Editor

1

Associations between social capital and maternal depression: results from a follow-up study in China

Chi Zhou[1], Weijun Zheng[2], Qi Yuan[3], Baodan Zhang[1], Hao Chen[1], Weijue Wang[1], Liu Huang[1], Liangwen Xu[1*] and Lei Yang[1*]

Abstract

Background: This study aims to investigate the association between social capital (SC) and depressive symptoms among Chinese primiparas at different time-points from their late pregnancy to postpartum.

Methods: A total of 450 primiparas were recruited for the current study. The assessments were conducted at three different time-points: T1 – while the participants were recruited at their 30–36 weeks of pregnancy in the antenatal clinic in the maternity hospital in Zhejiang, China; T2 – at their 2nd or 3rd days in the wards after delivery; T3 – at week 6 to 8 after the delivery in the postpartum examination clinic. SC was measured by the 29-item SC scale; while depressive symptoms were measured by the Edinburgh Postnatal Depression Scale. The relationships between SC and depressive symptoms were explored separately at each of the three time-points.

Results: The prevalence of depression among the primiparas was 25% at T1, 13.5% at T2 and 20.8% at T3, respectively. However, the score of SC and its components at three time-points followed an opposite 'V' direction, with the highest score at T2, following by T3 and T1. At T1, the analysis suggested that depressive symptoms among the primiparas were negatively correlated with their social trust and social network levels. At T2, only social trust was negatively associated with depression. While at T3, it is social trust and social participations that were significantly negatively associated with depression.

Conclusions: SC was associated with depression at all three time-points during and after pregnancy. More attention should be given to SC in the maternal health promotion programs of community pregnancy health care management.

Keywords: Antenatal and postpartum depression, Cognitive SC, Structural SC, The Edinburgh postnatal depression scale, Follow-up study

Background

Maternal depression is a serious public health issue [1]. Depressive symptoms are marked by an extended sense of sad mood, loss of interest, tearfulness, sleep problem, restlessness, irritability, appetite disturbance, and even suicidal ideation or attempt [2]. Previous studies suggested that depressive symptoms were found among about 10% to 20% of mothers, and such symptoms can last for several months or even a year [3]. Depression can happen at any time throughout the whole pregnancy process, from early pregnancy to even after delivery [4]. Antenatal depression itself is an important risk factor for maternal depression at other time-points for pregnant women as well [4]. Furthermore, due to the unique role of mothers in caring their babies, previous studies suggested that children of depressive mothers are three times more likely to develop serious emotional problems [5, 6].

A lot of studies have been done to explore the risk factors of maternal depression [7–9]. Recent reviews suggested that SC is a protective factor for individuals' mental health status and it could also significantly reduce the risk of antenatal and postpartum depression [10–12]. SC is defined as

* Correspondence: lwxu2006@163.com; yanglei62@hznu.edu.cn
[1]Medical School, Hangzhou Normal University, 16 Xuelin Rd., Xiasha District, Hangzhou 310036, China
Full list of author information is available at the end of the article

"features of social organization, such as trust, norms and networks that can improve the efficacy of society by facilitating coordinated actions" [13]. It comprises two components, namely the cognitive SC and the structural SC [14]. The cognitive component refers to the internally subjective aspects of SC that reflect people's perceptions on the level of interpersonal trust, sharing, reciprocity and other norms [15, 16]. The structural capital is more about the externally objective dimension and is featured by behavioral expression of social network and individual participation or community activities [17]. Till date, most studies on SC are cross-sectional in nature. In order to further explore the relationship between SC and maternal depression, a follow-up study design was used in the current study with both cognitive and structural SC being measured at the individual level.

The fourth baby boom period in China is approaching, as a result the number of women at their reproductive age is increasing rapidly, with an increment of about 2 million per year [18]; and a majority of them are the first generation of babies after the one-child policy was implemented [18, 19]. This group is very special, in the sense that they are the only child in their family and as a result most of them are 'spoiled'. Moreover, a majority of them will be parents for the first time. In the traditional Chinese culture, parturients should practice "sitting the month" after their delivery, a period where they should stay at home for about one or two months to recover after they discharge from the hospital [20, 21]. This practice could bring huge changes on the life style and social environment of the parturients during this period. On one hand, primiparas need to adjust to get used to their new roles as mothers; meanwhile, the focus of the whole family will suddenly move towards the baby. These changes could result in a sudden drop of emotional support perceived by the primiparas [22]. On the other hand, "sitting the month" will limit their social activities, which will ultimately lower their perceived social support levels [19, 22]. Other than the above-mentioned issues, a lot of families nowadays also need older generations' input (e.g. grandparents of the baby) while taking care of the babies. This arrangement has a high potential to cause cross-generation conflicts, which poses another potential risk towards the primiparas. Thus it is not surprising that about 50% to 75% of primiparas in China had reported experiences of unstable mood, accompanying by different level of physical symptoms in China [19].

To the best of our knowledge, there are very few studies had explored the relationships between SC and maternal depression at different time-points throughout the pregnancy progress. Using a sample of Chinese primiparas, the current study aims to answer the above question through a follow-up study design. We hypothesized that SC level of primiparas will be negatively correlated with depression among Chinese primiparas [10–12].

Methods

Study design

This study was conducted from March to December 2016 in the largest maternity hospital in Zhejiang Province, China. New mothers admitted to the hospital during the recruitment period were approached by the study team. Those who were willing to join the study were then assessed for their eligibility. To be included in the study, the primiparas should meet the following criteria: 1) in the hospital for the prenatal checkup, 2) 18 years old and above, 3) being pregnant for 30–36 weeks pregnant, 4) planning to give birth and attend postpartum follow up at the hospital, 5) willing to participate in the study, 6) literate in Chinese, and 7) not suffering from cognitive deficit. A total of 450 subjects were recruited for the current study and following informed voluntary written consent. The participation was voluntary, and they were informed that 'refusal to participate will not affect the care they are going to receive from the hospital'. This study was approved by the Ethics Board of the Hangzhou Normal on 4th March 2016 (reference no.: ISRCTN2016014).

Data were collected at three different time-points: 1) T1 - while the participants were recruited at their 30–36 weeks of pregnancy in the antenatal clinical; T2 - at their 2nd or 3rd days in the wards after the delivery; T3 - at week 6 to 8 after the delivery in the postpartum examination clinic. To enable easier administration, the survey was built using an e-platform, and a QR code was generated. By scanning this QR code using their mobile phones, individuals could access to the full questionnaire including the socio-demographics and scales to evaluate primiparas' SC and depressive symptoms. And they could choose the time point (i.e. T1, T2 and T3) and completed the survey on their mobile phones. This QR code was stuck onto the casebook of each participant, enabling the data collectors to easily identify the participants while they were in the hospital. In the case that the primiparas forgot to fill in the survey, phone calls were made by the investigators to remind them to scan that QR code to fill in the e-questionnaire. More detailed information regarding the measurement scales were included as the following.

Measurements

SC was measured by the Chinese version of SC Assessment Questionnaire (C-SCAQ) [23]. This questionnaire was developed by Zhou and colleagues among Chinese primiparas based on the World Bank's SC Assessment Tool and Bian's Chinese position Table [24, 25]. More details of the C-SCAQ and tis development and validation could be found in Zhou et al. [23]. The C-SCAQ can be used to measure primipraras' SC on both the cognitive and structural domains. Cognitive SC includes the social trust (ST) and social reciprocity (SR) sub-scales. The ST sub-scale has 8 items in total, and it measures the generalized trust among colleagues, neighbors and strangers. The SR consists of 7 items, and assesses the reciprocity among colleagues, neighbors and strangers. The score for each item varies from 1 to 5. The structural SC domain covers social network (SN) and social participation (SP). SN is assessed using Bian's Chinese position Table [25], which considers Chinese social characteristics by position generator method. SN includes network diversity (the sum of occupations of the social network members) score ranging from 0 to 20, upper reach ability (the highest prestige occupation scores of social network members) score ranging from 0 to 95, and network range (the highest prestige occupation scores minus the lowest score of social network members) score ranging from 0 to 94. The SP has 11 items, covering the activity types, motivation and involvement. The items of activity types and motivation were graded using a 5-point Likert scale, while involvement was coded with 0 (nonparticipation) and 1 (participation). Since the internal measurement units are not uniform, the standardized score of SN and SP were used. Higher score represents higher SC level. The Cronbach' α of cognitive and structural SC dimensions of C-SCAQ were 0.773 and 0.902 respectively in the previous study [26].

Depressive symptoms were measured by the Chinese version of Edinburgh Postnatal Depression Scale (C-EPDS). The scale consists of 10 items with 4 alternative answers for each item. The score for each item varies from 0 to 3, with a maximum score of 30 [27]. C-EPDS has been tested and validated among Chinese pregnant women before [28]. Compared to the Diagnostic and Statistical Manual of Mental Disorder-IV diagnosis of major depression as reference, C-EPDS demonstrated good reliability with a cutoff point score of 9 and above (sensitivity 0.72, specificity 0.88) [27]. This scale has also been used in other Chinese studies and showed high reliability in measuring prenatal and postnatal women's depression [29, 30]. In the current study following the evidences, a cut-off of 9 was used to indicate the status of having depressive symptoms.

Statistical analyses

Data were entered through EpiData 3.1 and analyzed by SPSS 20.0 (SPSS Inc., Chicago, IL, USA). We firstly described the socio-demographic characteristics of the sample. The participants were divided into two groups based on EPDS scores: the Depression group (score ≥ 9) and the Non-depression group (score < 9). The SC was compared between these two groups using T tests. Separate binary logistic regressions were conducted to assess the relationships between SC and depression at each of the three time-points, with the C-EPDS score being the dependent variable, and SC factors being the independent variables. The covariates in every regression included: age, district, education level, character, planned pregnancy, incoming per month, delivery by cesarean section, relationship with husband, relationship with parents-in-law, and sleep. In all regressions, a two-side p-value below 0.05 was treated as statistically significant.

Results

Sample characteristics

A total of 450 primiparas were eligible to participate in the study at T1, and 41 were excluded from the study representing a response rate of 91.1%. Of the 41 primiparas who were excluded, 25 (60.9%) refused to participate, and 16 (39.0%) intended to give birth in other hospitals. At T2 and T3, 376 (91.9%) and 288 (70.4%) primiparas completed the follow-up assessment, respectively. In the end, 288 primiparas who completed all the three interviews were chosen as research subjects in this study.

The demographic characteristics of primiparas are presented in Table 1. More than half of the subjects aged between 18 and 29 years old (68.4%), and 61.1% were from urban areas. More than half of the subjects had undergraduate college degrees and above (69.8%), and 63.5% described themselves as introverted. Most of the subjects had a planned to pregnancy (85.8%), and 58.3% had a monthly income of more than 4500 CNY. One third of participants were delivered by cesarean section (30.9%). After delivery, most of the subjects reported good relationships with husband (92.0%), and parents-in-law (74.7%). 15.3% of them suffered from poor sleep after delivery.

Prevalence, timing of depression and SC

Figure 1 shows 25% the prevalence of depressive symptoms of the participants. 25% of the primiparas were found to have antenatal depression at T1. 13.5% and 20.8% showed symptoms of postpartum depression at T2 and T3 after delivery, respectively. The mean scores of the EPDS were higher at T1 and T3, and lowest at T2.

The scores of cognitive and structural SC at three different time-points are presented in Figs. 2 and 3, and the curves had opposite directions comparing to that of the EPDS in Fig. 1. The mean scores of SC at different time-points are presented in Table 2. The cognitive and structural SC levels were lower at T1 and T3, and highest at T2.

Association between SC and depression

The association between SC and maternal depression are presented in Table 3. The ST, SR and SP mean scores of Depression group were significantly lower than those

Table 1 Sample characteristics

Variate	Category	Frequency	Percent
Age	18–29	197	68.4
	30–45	91	31.6
District	urban	176	61.1
	rural	112	38.9
Education level	secondary school and below	2	0.7
	senior high school	24	8.3
	junior college	61	21.2
	undergraduate college	160	55.6
	master degree and above	41	14.2
Character	extrovert	105	36.5
	introvert	183	63.5
Planned pregnancy	yes	247	85.8
	no	41	14.2
Incoming per month	less than 1500 RMB	11	3.8
	1500–3000 RMB	18	6.3
	3001–4500 RMB	91	31.6
	more than 4500 RMB	168	58.3
Delivery by cesarean section	yes	89	30.9
	no	199	69.1
Relationship with husband	good	265	92.0
	general	20	6.9
	poor	3	1.1
Relationship with parents-in-law	good	215	74.7
	general	66	22.9
	poor	7	2.4
Sleep	good	104	36.1
	general	140	48.6
	poor	44	15.3

of the Non-depression group at all three assessments ($p < 0.05$). The mean SN score of the Depression group was significantly lower than that of the Non-depression group at T1 ($p < 0.01$).

After controlling for the exogenous variables, adjusted associations between antenatal depression and SC are displayed in Table 4. The model at T1 shows that ST ($\beta = -0.90$, $p < 0.01$) and SN ($\beta = -0.83$, $p < 0.01$) were significantly negatively correlated with antenatal depression. The model at T2 shows that ST ($\beta = -0.76$, $p = 0.04$) was significantly negatively correlated with postpartum depression. The model at T3 shows that ST ($\beta = -0.85$, $p = 0.04$) and SP ($\beta = -0.74$, $p = 0.04$) were significantly negatively correlated with postpartum depression.

Discussion

Depression status of primiparas

This study showed that the prevalence of depressive symptoms of Chinese primiparas throughout the pregnancy process following a "V" shape, and this is similar to findings from a previous study in Greece [27]. The highest prevalence of EPDS was at T1, and the lowest one at T2. EPDS scores at T1 were higher than T3. However, studies in China tended to pay more attention to the period of 6–8 weeks postpartum among the primiparas [31–33]. We observed that the prevalence of depression was highest at the late pregnancy among our primiparas sample. This suggested a potential high cost-effectiveness if timely interventions could be implemented at this time-point.

In the literature, one cohort study by Milgrom et al. in UK showed that depression scores were 6.72 at 32 weeks of pregnancy, and higher than 5.84 at 8 weeks postpartum [34]. Rich-Edwards et al. found that the prevalence of depressive symptoms was 9% at mid-pregnancy and 8% at postpartum [35]. These are similar to our study,

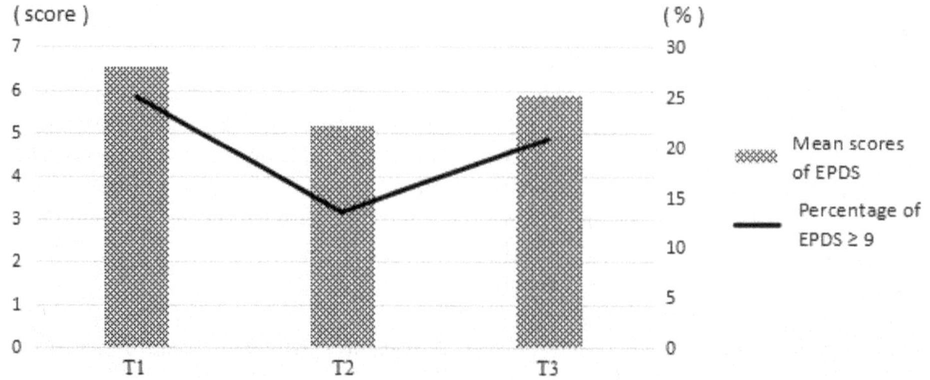

Fig. 1 Timing of maternal depression. Mean scores of Edinburgh Postnatal Depression Scale and percentage of Edinburgh Postnatal Depression Scale ≥9 among Chinese primiparas at different time-points

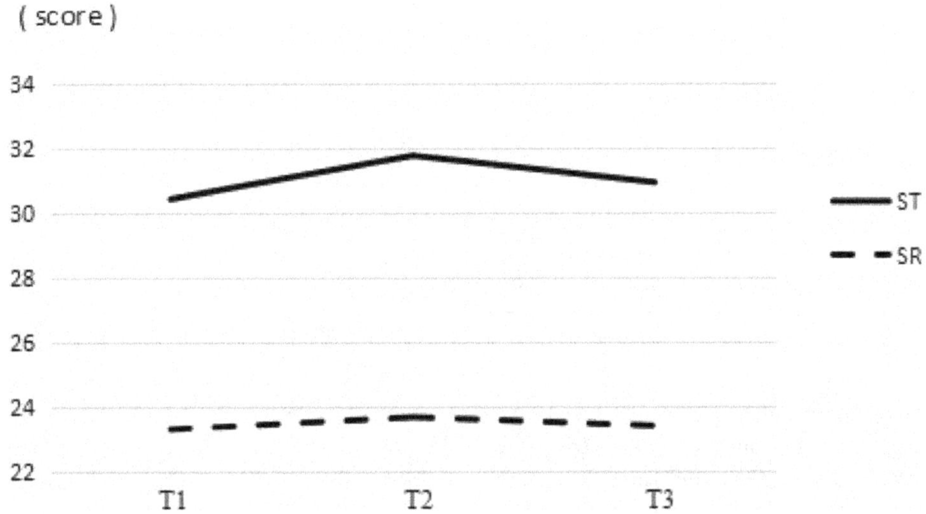

Fig. 2 Timing of cognitive SC. The scores of social trust and social reciprocity at three different time-points. ST: social trust; SR: social reciprocity

but some other studies in the literature have different findings. O'Hara et al. found that the highest depression rate was 12% at 9 weeks postpartum, and 9% at the second trimester pregnancy [36]. A 6-month follow-up study indicated that 6.8% women were found to have postpartum depression at the end of first week after delivery, and the prevalence were 12.5%, 9.0%, and 4.9% at the end of the first, third, and sixth month respectively [27]. Josefsson et al. showed that the prevalence of depressive symptoms during late pregnancy was 17%; in the maternity ward 18%; 6–8 weeks postnatally 13%; and 6 months postnatally 13% in Sweden [37].

SC status of primiparas

Results from the current study suggested that the SC scores throughout the pregnancy process followed an upside-down "V" shape. The curve is opposite to that of the EDPS scores, and consistent with our hypothesis. Firstly, the highest social capital level was at T2. Usually, primiparas will leave the hospital 3 to 5 days after delivery, thus they were still in the hospital at the 2nd to 3rd days after delivery. During this period, their husband or parents will carefully take care of them, and their relatives, friends and colleagues will visit them and give red envelopes or newborn gifts [38]. Those social interactions

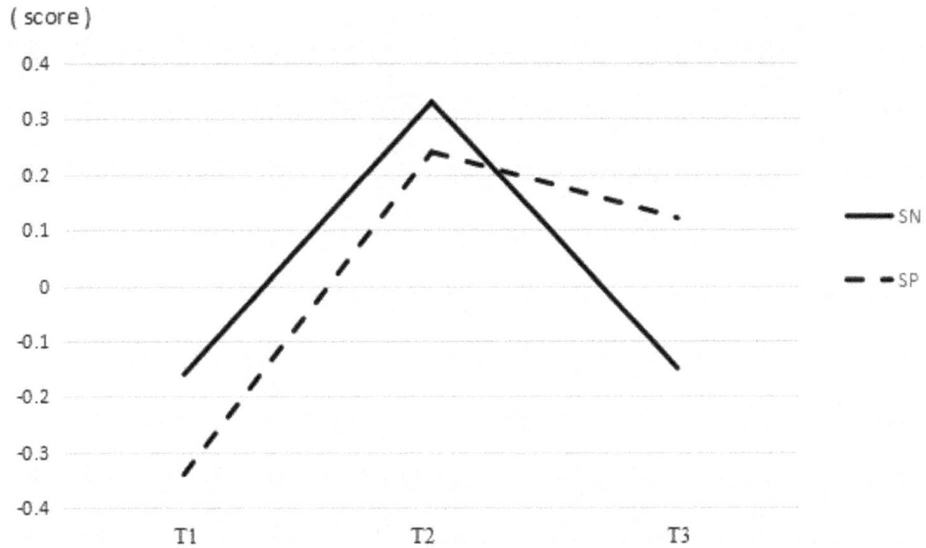

Fig. 3 Timing of structural SC. The scores of social network and social participation at three different time-points. SN: social network; SP: social participation

Table 2 The mean scores of SC at three different time-points

Variable	T1		T2		T3	
	Mean	SD	Mean	SD	Mean	SD
Cognitive SC						
Social trust	30.44	4.21	31.77	4.61	30.93	5.02
Social reciprocity	23.20	4.36	23.68	4.65	23.40	5.03
Structural SC						
Social network	− 0.16	2.35	0.33	2.53	−0.15	2.51
Social participation	−0.34	2.22	0.24	2.54	0.12	2.88

and gifts might give them with greater support and comfort. Moreover, the happiness levels for new mothers are normally very high at this time-point due to the joyfulness they would experience in the sense of having a baby.

Secondly, the results shows that SC level went down after they discharged from hospital, and moved to a relatively low level at T3. In China, primiparas should be confined at home for one full month of convalescence after discharge from the hospital [39]. This practice might change their normal social environment. Moreover, their psychological status might be largely affected by the attitude of family caregivers [38]. Similar finding was reported by another study in China, suggesting that pregnant women had the highest level of social support level at 1 week postpartum, and decreased afterwards [38]. The government needs to encourage regularly postpartum visits to improve the primary maternal health management, and doctors can provide them with more professional supports.

Table 4 Adjusted associations between SC and depression

Variables	*β*	SE	*df*	*P*
T1 model				
Social trust	−0.90	0.34	1	< 0.01
Social reciprocity	−0.41	0.34	1	0.24
Social network	−0.83	0.29	1	< 0.01
Social participation	−0.38	0.33	1	0.24
T2 model				
Social trust	−0.76	0.41	1	0.04
Social reciprocity	−0.76	0.46	1	0.10
Social network	−0.17	0.36	1	0.65
Social participation	−0.72	0.40	1	0.05
T3 model				
Social trust	−0.85	0.41	1	0.04
Social reciprocity	−0.46	0.40	1	0.25
Social network	−0.26	0.31	1	0.42
Social participation	−0.74	0.36	1	0.04

Thirdly, it was beyond our expectation that the lowest SC level was at T1. It may be the case that pregnant women at this time-point are too clumsy to move around [40, 41]. This will limit their social activities, and result in loss of face-to-face contacts with friends and acquaintances [40, 41].

Another important finding of our study is that, the two curves of structural SC had larger fluctuations than curves of cognitive SC. Through interviews with primiparas, we learnt that a lot of the primiparas took part in training such as parenting classes provided by the maternity hospital before delivery to better prepare for their

Table 3 SC comparison between depression and non-depression group

Variable	Depression group		Non-depression group		*t* test	
	Mean	SD	Mean	SD	*t*	*p*
Cognitive SC						
Social trust (T1)	28.72	4.17	31.01	4.07	4.11	< 0.01
Social trust (T2)	29.38	4.29	32.15	4.56	3.55	< 0.01
Social trust (T3)	28.62	3.87	31.54	5.12	4.13	< 0.01
Social reciprocity (T1)	21.79	3.80	23.67	4.44	3.22	< 0.01
Social reciprocity (T2)	22.00	3.64	23.95	4.74	2.97	< 0.01
Social reciprocity (T3)	20.85	4.22	24.07	5.02	4.56	< 0.01
Structural SC						
Social network (T1)	−0.86	2.39	0.08	2.30	2.97	< 0.01
Social network (T2)	− 0.42	2.60	0.44	2.51	1.98	0.05
Social network (T3)	−0.54	2.45	−0.04	2.52	1.39	0.17
Social participation (T1)	−0.82	2.13	−0.18	2.23	2.17	0.03
Social participation (T2)	−0.95	2.05	0.43	2.57	3.20	< 0.01
Social participation (T3)	−1.06	2.63	0.44	2.86	3.66	< 0.01

coming first-time delivery. Through these activities, they got the opportunities to meet doctors, nurses, and other new mothers; and make friends with others, as a result to expand their social networks [38]. Their activity levels and networks would decline rapidly during the confinement. However, ST and SR which require longer time to develop would stay. According to the blood relationship culture in China, they specifically trust their family members [42]. During the whole pregnancy and childbirth period, their family members will always be around with them. Although their cognitive SC level might be influenced by the confinement, it is still more stable than the structural SC.

Influence of SC on antenatal and postpartum depression among primiparas

This study examined the effect of SC on antenatal and postpartum depression among Chinese primiparas, and analyzed the relationship between SC and maternal depression. In previous review articles, few studies carried out follow up research on the association between SC factors and maternal depression among pregnant women [43, 44]. Our study includes four dimensions of SR, ST, SN, and SP from cognitive and structural SC at the individual level, and is also the first follow-up study in China with such a sample size.

The current study found that the Non-depression primiparas had higher SC levels (ST, SR, SN and SP) than Depression group at all three time-points. Similar findings were also reported in a longitudinal study by Lamarca et al. [43]. They investigated the associations between individual SC (social support and social networks) and consistent self-rated health in women between the first trimester of pregnancy and six months postpartum, and found that the good self-rated health group had higher scores of SC than the poorer group [43].

In our study, ST had strong association with depression at all the three time-points. This is consistent with previous studies. Fujiwara and Kawachi found that perceptions of higher levels of cognitive SC (social trust) were associated with lower risks of developing major depression among adults during the 2–3 year follow-up [44]. A prospective analysis also indicated that low interpersonal trust appears to be an independent risk factor for new-onset and long-term depression in South Korea [45]. A potential explanation could be that interpersonal trust can provide emotional support to help primiparas to deal with their stress [45, 46].

It is interesting that SN has a strong association with antenatal depression at T1, and SP was associated with postpartum depression at T3. It may be the case that primiparas will get to know new mothers and nurses and expand their networks through pregnant women school activities as mentioned above. These networks can provide emotional support for primiparas on delivery and parenting, and it might also be beneficial to reduce their depression level and needs to be further verified [34]. After delivery, appropriate participation is helpful to alleviate depression, but the traditional confinement seems to be an obstacle for SP. Armstrong and Edwards showed that mothers in the pram-walking intervention group improved their fitness levels and reduced their level of depressive symptomatology significantly more than the social support group [47]. Zhang also indicated that taking active parts in social activities if physical conditions permit can reduce postpartum anxiety [48].

There are a few limitations for the current study. Firstly, this study examines the relationship between SC and peripartum depression at only three time-points: 30–36 weeks of pregnancy, 2–3 days and 6–8 weeks postpartum. So we might miss the highest point of depression and the lowest point of SC level. If the survey can be extended to include the first trimester to 6 months after delivery, and the results of observation might be more intact. Secondly, EPDS is a self-report tool to measure mood, and there might overpathologising motherhood [49]. This phenomenon has a certain effect on the results. Thirdly, although a follow-up design was used, regression analyses to explore the relationships between SC and maternal depression were conducted separately at each time-point. Fourthly, given that the study participants were from Zhejiang province, this might limit the generalization of the study findings. Lastly, personality of primiparas was measured by a single question 'Would you describe yourself as extroverted or introverted?', without using a scale. More studies are still needed to confirm whether the findings from the current study will be applicable nation-wide.

Conclusions

We examined the association of SC and maternal depression among Chinese primiparas. The prevalence of EPDS had a "V" type distribution and SC form an upside-down "V". The two curves of structural SC had larger fluctuations than curves of cognitive SC. The SC level of Depression group was lower than Non-depression group at all three time-points. ST and SN were significantly associated with the depression of primiparas at T1, ST was associated at T2, and ST and SP were associated at T3. For future maternal health education and promotion programs, more attention could be given to SC improvement in the community pregnancy health care management.

Abbreviations
C-EPDS: Chinese version of Edinburgh postnatal depression scale; C-SCAQ: Chinese version of social capital assessment questionnaire; PPD: Postpartum depression; QR Code: Quick response code; SC: Social capital; SN: Social network; SP: Social participation; SR: Social reciprocity; ST: Social trust

Acknowledgements
We thank the help of clinic nurses from the Women's Hospital School of Medicine Zhejiang University Hangzhou, and research staffs during the surveys.

Funding
This study was supported by Grant 71503064 from the National Natural Science Foundation of China

Authors' contributions
CZ and WJZ designed the study and completed the first draft of this article. QY critically reviewed and edited the manuscript, and provided comments for its further improvements. BDZ, HC, WJW, and LH participated in data collection and analysis, and LWX、LY revised the manuscript and made valuable suggestions on scholarly writing. All authors contributed to and have approved the final manuscript.

Consent for publication
This study was obtained consent to publish from the participant to report individual patient data.

Competing interests
The authors declare that they have no competing interests.

Author details
[1]Medical School, Hangzhou Normal University, 16 Xuelin Rd., Xiasha District, Hangzhou 310036, China. [2]School of Basic Medical Science, Zhejiang Chinese Medical University, Hangzhou 310053, China. [3]Research Division, Institute of Mental Health, Singapore 539747, Singapore.

References
1. Wisner KL, Chambers CD, Sit D. Postpartum depression: a major public health. J. Am. Med. Assoc. 2007;296(21):2616–23.
2. Demissie Z, Maria Siega-Riz A, Evenson KR, Herring AH, Dole N, Gaynes BN. Associations between physical activity and postpartum depressive symptoms. J. Womens Health. 2011;20(7):1025–34.
3. Teissedre F, Chabrol H. A study of the Edinburgh postnatal depression scale (EPDS) on 859 mothers: detection of mothers at risk for postpartum depression. L'Encephale. 2004;30(4):376–81.
4. Shrivastava SR, Shrivastava PS, Ramasamy J. Antenatal and postnatal depression: a public health perspective. J. Neurosci. Rural Pract. 2015;6(1): 116–9.
5. Glasser S, Levinson D, Bina R, Munitz H, Horev Z, Kaplan G. Primary care physicians' attitudes toward postpartum depression: is it part of their job? J. Prim. Care Community Health. 2016;7(1):24–9.
6. Weissman MM, Feder A, Pilowsky D, Shea S. Depressed mothers coming to primary care: maternal reports of problems with their children. J. Affect. Disord. 2004;78(2):93–100.
7. Chaaya M, Campbell OMR, El Kak F, Shaar D, Harb H, Kaddour A. Postpartum depression: prevalence and determinants in Lebanon. Arch Women's Ment. Health. 2002;5(2):65–72.
8. Giri RK, Khatri RB, Mishra SR, Khanal V, Sharma VD, Gartoula RP. Prevalence and factors associated with depressive symptoms among post-partum mothers in Nepal. BMC Res. Notes. 2015;8:111–7.
9. Daley AJ, Foster L, Long G, Palmer C, Robinson O, Walmsley H, Ward R. The effectiveness of exercise for the prevention and treatment of antenatal depression: systematic review with meta-analysis. BJOG. 2015;122(1):57–62.
10. Kim THM, Connolly JA, Tamin H. The effect of social support around pregnancy on postpartum depression among Canadian teen mothers and adult mothers in the maternity experiences survey. BMC Pregnancy and Childbirth. 2014;14:162–71.
11. Senturk V, Abas M, Berksun O, Stewart R. Social support and antenatal depression in extended and nuclear family environments in Turkey: a cross-sectional survey. BMC Psychiatry. 2011;11:48–58.
12. Wind TR, Komproe IH. The mechanisms that associate community social capital with post-disaster mental health: a multilevel model. Soc. Sci. Med. 2012;75(9):1715–35.
13. Putnam RD. The prosperous community: social capital and public life. Am. Prospect. 1993;13:35–42.
14. Putnam RD, Leonardi R, Nanetti RY. Making democracy work: civic traditions in modern Italy. New Jersey: Princeton University Press; 1993.
15. Murayama H, Fujiwara Y, Kawachi I. Social capital and health: a review of prospective multilevel studies. J. Epidemiol. 2012;22(3):179–87.
16. Harpham T, Grant E, Thomas E. Measuring social capital within health surveys: key issues. Health Policy Plan. 2002;17(1):106–11.
17. Bassett E, Moore S. Social capital and depressive symptoms: the association of psychosocial and network dimensions of social capital with depressive symptoms in Montreal, Canada. Soc. Sci. Med. 2013;6(86):96–102.
18. Ding X. Promote natural birth and reduce the cesarean rate. Beijing Med. J. 2015;37(7):613–5. In Chinese
19. Lu H, Zheng XX. Social support and postpartum depression among primiparas. Chin. J. Nurs. 2001;36(10):44–7. In Chinese
20. Pillsbury BLK. 'Doing the month': confinement and convalescence of Chinese women after childbirth. Soc. Sci. Med. 1978;12:11–22.
21. Wong J, Fisher J. The role of traditional confinement practices in determining postpartum depression in women in Chinese cultures: a systematic review of the English language evidence. J. Affect. Disord. 2009; 116(3):161–9.
22. Sun Y, Li HH. Influence of psychological intervention on role adaption of mother in primipara. Chin. Nurs. Res. 2004;18(11B):2023–4. In Chinese
23. Zhou C, Lai RN, Zhang XN, Chen H, Wang WJ, Zhang BD. Development and evaluation on the primipara social capital scale. Chin. J. Prev. Med. 2017; 51(4):313–8. [In Chinese]
24. Grootaert C, Bastelaer TV. Understanding and measuring social capital. Washington, DC: The World Bank Publishing; 2002.
25. Bian YJ. Source and functions of urbanites' social capital: a network approach. Soc. Sci. China. 2004;3:136–46. In Chinese
26. Cao WM, Li L, Zhou XD, Zhou C. Social capital and depression: evidence from urban elderly in China. Aging Ment. Health. 2015;19(5):418–29.
27. Gonidakis F, Rabavilas AD, Varsou E, Kreatsas G, Christodoulou GN. A 6-month study of postpartum depression and related factors in Athens Greece. Compr Psychiatry. 2008;49:275–82.
28. Zhao Y, Kane I, Wang J, Shen BB, Luo JF, Shi SX. Combined use of the postpartum depression screening scale (PDSS) and Edinburgh postnatal depression scale (EPDS) to identify antenatal depression among Chinese pregnant women with obstetric complications. Psychiatry Res. 2015;226(1): 113–9.
29. Lau Y, Wong DF, Chan KS. The utility of screening for perinatal depression in the second trimester among Chinese: a three-wave prospective longitudinal study. Arch. Womens Ment. Health. 2010;13:153–64.
30. Lau Y, Yin L, Wang Y. Antenatal depressive symptomatology, family conflict and social support among Chengdu Chinese women. Matern. Child Health J. 2011;15:1416–26.
31. You H, Chen JH, Bogg L, Wu Y, Duan SN, Ye CY, Liu XF, Yu H, Diwan V, Dong HJ. Study on the factors associated with postpartum visits in rural China. PLoS One. 2013;8(2):1–6.

32. Chen X, He LK, He HY, Chen XL, Lin XD. Application of foot reflexology with traditional Chinese medicine combined with ear acupoint therapy in promoting postpartum rehabilitation of parturients. Mod. Clin. Nurs. 2013;4: 8–11. In Chinese
33. Ai X. Therapeutic observation on acupuncture plus psychotherapy for postpartum depression. Shanghai J. Acupunct. Moxibustion. 2013;32(9):711–2. In Chinese
34. Milgrom J, Schembri C, Ericksen J, Ross J, Gemmill AW. Towards parenthood: an antenatal intervention to reduce depression, anxiety and parenting difficulties. J. Affect. Disord. 2011;130:385–94.
35. Rich-Edwards JW, Kleinman K, Abrams A, Harlow BL, Mclaughlin TJ, Joffe H, Gillman MW. Sociodemographic predictors of antenatal and postpartum depressive symptoms among women in a medical group practice. J. Epidemiol Community Health. 2006;60:221–7.
36. O'Hara MW, Neunaber DJ, Zekoski EM. Prospective study of postpartum depression: prevalence, course, and predictive factors. J. Abnorm. Psychol. 1984;93(2):158–71.
37. Josefsson A, Berg G, Nordin C, Sydsjö G. Prevalence of depressive symptoms in late pregnancy and postpartum. Acta. Obstet. Gynecol. Scand. 2001;80(3): 251–5.
38. Yang KG, Wang JJ. The review on social support of puerperal women. Chin. Gen. Nurs. 2015;13(16):1505–7. [In Chinese]
39. Du FY, Li L, Zhang XP, Gao LY, Zhou J, Zhu JM. Study on women's social support and quality of life within a year after delivery. Chin. J. Rehabil. Med. China. 2015;10:1107–9. [In Chinese]
40. Zhou C, Ogihara A, Chen H, Wang WJ, Huang L, Zhang BD, Zhang XN, Xu LW, Yang L. Social capital and antenatal depression among Chinese primiparas: a cross-sectional survey. Psychiatry Res. 2017;257:533–9.
41. Faramarzi M, Pasha H. The role of social support in prediction of stress during pregnancy. J. Babol Univ. Med. Sci. 2015;17(11):52–60.
42. Li WM, Liang YC. Special credit and generally credit: the Chinese structure and characteristics of credit. Social Study. 2002;3:11–22. [In Chinese]
43. Lamarca GA, MDC L, Sheiham A, Vettore MV. The association of neighborhood and individual social capital with consistent self-rated health: a longitudinal study in Brazilian pregnant and postpartum women. BMC Pregnancy Childbirth. 2013;13:1–17.
44. Fujiwara T, Kawachi I. A prospective study of individual-level social capital and major depression in the United States. J Epidemiol Community Health. 2008;62:627–33.
45. Kim SS, Chung Y, Perry MJ, Subramanian KI. Association between interpersonal trust, reciprocity, and depression in South Korea: a prospective analysis. PLoS One. 2012;7(1):1–8.
46. Yan YH, Xiong B. Relationship between psychological health and social support in primpara. China Med. Herald. 2010;16:119–23. [In Chinese]
47. Armstrong K, Edwards H. The effectiveness of a pram-walking exercise programme in reducing depressive symptomatology for postnatal women. Int. J. Nurs. Pract. 2004;10(4):177–94.
48. Zhang Y. Study of psychosocial factors for postpartum depression among 479 women. Wuhan: Huazhong University of Science and Technology Publishing; 2011. [In Chinese]
49. Matthey S. Are we overpathologising motherhood? J Affect Disord. 2010; 120:263–6.

2

Demand-side financing for maternal and newborn health: what do we know about factors that affect implementation of cash transfers and voucher programmes?

Benjamin M. Hunter* and Susan F. Murray

Abstract

Background: Demand-side financing (DSF) interventions, including cash transfers and vouchers, have been introduced to promote maternal and newborn health in a range of low- and middle-income countries. These interventions vary in design but have typically been used to increase health service utilisation by offsetting some financial costs for users, or increasing household income and incentivising 'healthy behaviours'. This article documents experiences and implementation factors associated with use of DSF in maternal and newborn health.

Methods: A secondary analysis (using an adapted Supporting the Use of Research Evidence framework – SURE) was performed on studies that had previously been identified in a systematic review of evidence on DSF interventions in maternal and newborn health.

Results: The article draws on findings from 49 quantitative and 49 qualitative studies. The studies give insights on difficulties with exclusion of migrants, young and multiparous women, with demands for informal fees at facilities, and with challenges maintaining quality of care under increasing demand. Schemes experienced difficulties if communities faced long distances to reach participating facilities and poor access to transport, and where there was inadequate health infrastructure and human resources, shortages of medicines and problems with corruption. Studies that documented improved care-seeking indicated the importance of adequate programme scope (in terms of programme eligibility, size and timing of payments and voucher entitlements) to address the issue of concern, concurrent investments in supply-side capacity to sustain and/or improve quality of care, and awareness generation using community-based workers, leaders and women's groups.

Conclusions: Evaluations spanning more than 15 years of implementation of DSF programmes reveal a complex picture of experiences that reflect the importance of financial and other social, geographical and health systems factors as barriers to accessing care. Careful design of DSF programmes as part of broader maternal and newborn health initiatives would need to take into account these barriers, the behaviours of staff and the quality of care in health facilities. Research is still needed on the policy context for DSF schemes in order to understand how they become sustainable and where they fit, or do not fit, with plans to achieve equitable universal health coverage.

Keywords: Demand-side financing, Vouchers, Cash transfers, Maternal health, Newborn health, Implementation

* Correspondence: benjamin.hunter@kcl.ac.uk
King's College London, Department of International Development, The Strand, London WC2R 2LS, UK

Background

Women and their families can face multiple barriers to accessing maternity care services, and financial barriers are a well-documented concern [1, 2]. In many countries there are demands for out-of-pocket formal fees and informal payments for care services or supplies such as medicines, sutures, gloves and diagnostic tests [3, 4]. There are the practical and financial difficulties of travel to health centres and the opportunity costs of being away from home or from work, or from dependents. For poor families, any such costs can cause severe financial hardship [5], and may result in delays or avoidance of care-seeking that increase health risks for mothers and newborns and further escalate costs. One approach to ameliorate these effects is the use of 'demand-side' financing (DSF) interventions that are designed to promote health by providing cash or vouchers to users to offset some of the financial costs of using or getting to maternity care services, or to increase household income and incentivise 'healthy behaviours'.

Within this overarching definition there are five types of DSF that have been used in the health sector and there are important differences in their intended mechanism of action [6, 7]. *Conditional cash transfers*, which have been widely used in Latin America, aim to increase utilisation of maternity care services by making regular payments to households linked to 'conditionalities' including attendance at community meetings and uptake of government health services. These are primarily focused on child health and development but some schemes include maternity care uptake. *Unconditional cash transfers* are similar regular payments but, in the absence of specific conditionalities for service utilisation, have the more general aim of alleviating the effect of poverty on a woman's health during pregnancy. *Short-term cash payments to offset costs* are typically retrospective payments made at government health facilities to those who attend for care. *Vouchers for maternity care services* aim to reduce the cost of maternity care services and *vouchers for 'merit' goods* aim to reduce the cost of merit goods (such as food or insecticide-treated nets) that promote maternal health. Vouchers may be distributed by community-based workers or at health facilities, and voucher schemes may be designed to incorporate services in the private sector as well as government facilities.

There have been seven systematic reviews of evidence on the impact of DSF mechanisms on maternal health during the period 2007–2012 [7–13]. Two of the reviews examined the impact of cash transfers [9, 11], three the impact of vouchers [8, 12, 13], and two the role of multiple types of DSF [7, 10]. The systematic reviews reported on a rapidly growing body of evidence that DSF can lead to a short-term increase in uptake of maternity care services, but could offer little evidence on longer-term effects on service uptake or maternal and neonatal morbidity and mortality. A recently published systematic review has confirmed these findings [14].

This article has been commissioned by the World Health Organization's Department of Maternal, Newborn, Child and Adolescent Health as part of a series of articles on health promotion interventions. The series aims to document factors that affect programme implementation in order to support policy-makers and decisions on how best to improve access to skilled care during pregnancy, childbirth and after birth. This article focuses on factors that have been found to affect implementation of DSF programmes in maternal and newborn health and has three components: a review of stakeholder perspectives and experiences of DSF interventions; information on the barriers and facilitators to implementation of the interventions, and a discussion on how these relate to the improvements in care-seeking outcomes reported elsewhere and what this means for programmatic initiatives [14].

Methods

This article is a secondary analysis of studies identified in a systematic review that was conducted in 2012 [6, 7] and repeated in 2015 [14]. The systematic review used the Joanna Briggs Institute approach, which incorporates both quantitative and qualitative data into reviews and has been used to review evidence on a range of policy and healthcare systems topics [15]. The population of interest in the review was economically poor women who were pregnant or within 42 days of end of pregnancy, in the context of low- and middle-income (both lower- and upper-middle) countries as defined by the World Bank at the time the study was published. The intervention of interest was DSF as a mechanism to increase consumption of goods and services intended to impact positively on maternal and newborn health. Outcomes of interest in the systematic review related to the effectiveness of DSF programmes to promote uptake of maternity care services and maternal and newborn health, and wider impact on quality of care. In addition to questions of effectiveness, the 2012 review also analysed qualitative research relating to barriers and facilitators for effective and sustainable programme implementation.

The systematic searches for the review used 30 terms in 19 medical, health and social policy databases and seven databases of unpublished research, and aimed to retrieve quantitative and qualitative studies that were published between January 1990 and June 2015. Retrieved studies were examined using Joanna Briggs Institute tools for critical appraisal of quantitative and qualitative research that include questions on study methods and the presentation of findings [15]. The review team assigned an overall quality rating to individual studies using a three-point rating system (low-, medium- or high-quality), similar to that used to assess study bias in the Effective Public Health Practice Project (EPHPP) quality assessment tool. The rating assigned to each study was based on assessments of study methods and reporting using critical appraisal tools produced by the Joanna Briggs Institute. The assessments are described in detail in a linked systematic review [14].

Data were extracted from included studies using standardised tools developed by the Joanna Briggs Institute, and the findings presented in this article have been analysed thematically using a comprehensive framework for factors affecting implementation of health promotion interventions, adapted from the SURE (Supporting the Use of Research Evidence) framework for preparing policy briefs [16]. The analytical framework, which is described in detail in a paper by Smith et al. in this series, includes five 'levels' of factors that affect policy implementation (main stakeholders in communities, healthcare providers, other stakeholders, health service delivery factors and social and political factors) and provides a list of types of barrier and enabler for each level. One of the authors, BMH, read through all included studies and extracted data relating to each level of the framework, then both authors examined the extracted data and re-organised them into themes based on the list of types of barrier and enabler.

Results

Range and quality of the body of literature

The article includes findings from 49 quantitative studies and from an additional 49 qualitative studies that contained information relevant to the quantitative studies (see Table 1 for details of included studies) that relate to the five types of DSF in 22 country programmes:

- conditional cash transfers (Brazil's Bolsa Familia [17, 18], El Salvador's Comunidades Solidarias Rurales [19], Guatemala's Mi Familia Progresa [20], Programa de Asignación Familia in Honduras [21], the Muthulakshmi Reddy Maternity Benefit Scheme in India [22, 23], Indonesia's Program Keluarga Harapan [24–26], Mexico's Oportunidades [27–34], and Plan de Atención Nacional a la Emergencia Social (PANES) in Uruguay [35]);
- unconditional cash transfers (Zambia's Child Grant Programme [36]);
- short-term cash payments to offset costs (CHIMACA in China [37], India's Janani Suraksha Yojana [38–74], the Safe Delivery Incentive Programme in Nepal [75–77] and the SURE-P programme in Nigeria [78]);
- vouchers for maternity care services (Bangladesh's Maternal Health Voucher Scheme [79–84], a pilot programme in Bangladesh [85], a voucher programme in Cambodia [86, 87], the Chiranjeevi Yojana in India [88–92], Kenya's Vouchers for Health programme [93–102], pilot programmes in Pakistan [103, 104], and the HealthyBaby vouchers [105, 106] and Mekerere University Voucher Scheme in Uganda [107, 108]), and vouchers for merit goods (the Tanzanian National Voucher Scheme [109–111]).

Programmes ranged from small-scale pilot voucher schemes in Pakistan and Bangladesh to large national programmes such as Janani Suraksha Yojana in India, Bangladesh's Maternal Health Voucher Scheme and multiple conditional cash transfer programmes in Latin American countries. Programme design varied from those that were purely demand-side to those that included supply-side incentives such as output-based payments to service providers (for example many of the voucher programmes), or incentives for community-based workers (such as in India's Janani Suraksha Yojana). Funding for programmes has come from national and state governments or from donor organisations such as the German Agency for International Cooperation (GIZ), the UK Department for International Development and the Bill and Melinda Gates Foundation.

The studies were generally of medium quality. Many of the quantitative studies were conducted early in the implementation of programmes and some made only limited efforts to account for confounding factors. Qualitative studies were often part of larger programme evaluations that focused primarily on quantitative outcomes and some of the articles reporting these findings lacked detailed descriptions of the methods used to collect and analyse data. Despite these limitations an overview of this literature does offer insights into the programmatic processes across a wide range of DSF initiatives and allows us to identify common features across programmes as well as some programme specific challenges.

Stakeholder perspectives and experiences

Three groups of stakeholders in DSF programmes have been studied in most detail: women service users, community-based workers, and staff in health facilities. Documented experiences from each of these groups are reviewed below and relate to awareness of programmes, cultural attitudes, perceptions of maternity care services, reasons for using or joining programmes and the challenges faced during participation. Many findings reflect wider issues in healthcare systems, however this section focuses on DSF implementation, and findings have been disaggregated by type of DSF where possible.

Table 1 Table of characteristics of included studies

Study	Study design	Setting	Description of intervention	Recommendation	Outcomes of interest reported
Conditional cash transfers					
Oportunidades, Mexico					
Barber and Gertler (2008)	Cross-sectional	Rural communities, Mexico	Oportunidades (conditional cash transfers)The programme was launched in 1997 as PROGRESA and later renamed Oportunidades. Monthly cash transfers are paid directly to mothers and are conditional on meeting health and education requirements. These included regular antenatal visits for pregnant women and attendance at health education meetings.	Conditional cash transfers	Perinatal morbidity, ANC
Barber and Gertler (2009)	Cross-sectional	Rural communities, Mexico		Conditional cash transfers	QoC
Barber (2010)	Cross-sectional	Rural communities, Mexico		Conditional cash transfers	C/I
Barham (2011)	Retrospective area study	Rural communities, Mexico		Programme less effective in areas that do not meet minimum level of sanitation	Infant mortality, NM
Hernandez Prado et al. (2004)	Retrospective area study	Rural, semi-urban and urban areas, Mexico		Conditional cash transfers	MM, infant mortality
Hernandez Prado et al. (2004)	Repeat cross-sectional	Rural, semi-urban and urban areas, Mexico		Conditional cash transfers	ANC, SBA, C/I, QoC, infant morbidity
Sosa-Rubai et al. (2011)	Cross-sectional	Rural communities, Mexico		Conditional cash transfers, but need better targeting to marginalised groups	ANC
Urquieta et al. (2009)	Repeat cross-sectional	Rural communities, Mexico		Conditional cash transfers, but need to include household members who influence decision-making on place of birth	SBA
Program Keluarga Harapan, Indonesia					
Alatas et al. (2011)	Repeat cross-sectional	Rural and urban districts in Indonesia	Program Keluarga Harapan (conditional cash transfers)The programme was introduced in 2007 and was targeted to five provinces. It was piloted in sub-districts that were felt had sufficient supply-side capacity to meet additional demand for services. Eligible households included those with pregnant or lactating women and women were expected to attend ANC, use a SBA and receive PN/PP. A cash transfer is paid quarterly to the women through a nearby post office. Facilitators are expected to verify that conditionalities are met.	Conditional cash transfers, but relax conditionalities in areas with weaker health systems	ANC, SBA, FB, PN, NM, infant mortality
Febriany et al. (2011)	Qualitative – interviews and focus groups	12 villages (mixed urban and rural) in 2 provinces, Indonesia		Conditional cash transfers, but need to reduce gaps in service provision and overcome social, economic and geographical barriers	Implementation
Triyana (2012)	Repeat cross-sectional	Rural and urban areas in Indonesia		Conditional cash transfers	MM, NM, infant mortality, SBA, QoC
Plan de Atención Nacional a la Emergencia Social (PANES), Uruguay					

Table 1 Table of characteristics of included studies *(Continued)*

Amarante et al. (2011)	Repeat cross-sectional	Uruguay	Plan de Atención Nacional a la Emergencia Social (PANES) (conditional cash transfers)Between April 2005 and December 2007, Plan de Atención Nacional a la Emergencia Social was implemented by the Uruguayan government. Monthly payments were made to eligible households. In homes with a pregnant woman, payments were conditional on her attendance at ANC.	Conditional cash transfers	Perinatal morbidity, maternal morbidity, ANC, SBA
Muthulakshmi Reddy Maternity Benefit Scheme, India					
Bala-subramanian and Ravindran (2012)	Cross-sectional	Tamil Nadu, India	Muthulakshmi Reddy Maternity Benefit Scheme (conditional cash transfers)The programme was launched in Tamil Nadu, India, in 1987 and provided unconditional payments (in two instalments) to pregnant women. Payments were increased in size over time and were made conditional on antenatal care attendance in 2012. The eligibility of women is determined by a village health nurse and includes those who meet criteria for poverty and who had previously had no more than two live births.	Conditional cash transfers, but shorter application process needed	FB
Public Health Resource Network (2010)	Qualitative – in-depth interviews	2 districts in Tamil Nadu, India		Conditional cash transfers, but with universal eligibility, timely payments, assistance from community-based workers, and supply-side investment so that maternity care services are universally available and are free	Implementation
Comunidades Solidarias Rurales, El Salvador					
De Brauw et al. (2011)	Repeat cross-sectional	Rural communities, El Salvador	Comunidades Solidarias Rurales (conditional cash transfers)The programme was introduced in 2005 and eligible households are identified from census data. Pregnant woman in eligible households must attend ANC and monthly local health education meetings are held. The programme coincided with health system strengthening programmes introduced by the government.	Conditional cash transfers, but should be conditional on ANC during first trimester, SBA and PNC	ANC, FB, SBA, PN
Bolsa Familia, Brazil					
Guanais (2013)	Retrospective area study	Brazil	Bolsa Familia (conditional cash transfers)Since 2003 Brazil has		Post-neonatal mortality

Table 1 Table of characteristics of included studies *(Continued)*

			paid monthly cash transfers to eligible households that meet conditionalities including that pregnant women attend ANC. Payments are made to women and are credited to electronic benefit cards.	Conditional cash transfers, but should be accompanied by supply-side interventions	
Shei (2013)	Retrospective area study	Brazil		Conditional cash transfer effective but need to meet increased demand for services and need to target vulnerable groups	NM, post-neonatal mortality, infant mortality
Mi Familia Progresa, Guatemala					
Gutierrez et al. (2011)	Repeat cross-sectional	Guatemala	Mi Familia Progresa (conditional cash transfers)Introduced by the Guatemalan government in 2008, Mi Familia Progresa payments are made to eligible households with a pregnant woman and are conditional on ANC attendance.	Conditional cash transfers	ANC, FB, PM
Programa de Asignación Familia, Honduras					
Morris et al. (2004)	Repeat cross-sectional	Rural municipalities, Honduras	Programa de Asignación Familia (conditional cash transfers)Vouchers with a cash value were distributed to eligible households on a regular basis. Distribution to households with a pregnant woman was conditional on her ANC attendance.	Conditional cash transfers	ANC, PN
Unconditional cash transfers					
Child Grant Programme, Zambia					
Handa et al. (2015)	Repeat cross-sectional	Three rural districts in Zambia	Child Grant Programme (conditional cash transfers)Launched in 2010, the programme operates in three districts with the highest rates of mortality and morbidity. Eligibility is universal within programme areas as long as there is a young child in the household. Payments are made directly to mothers.	Unconditional cash transfers, but need access to maternity services and may need complimentary short-term payments that are conditional on uptake of maternity care services	ANC, QoC, SBA
Short term cash payments to offset costs of access					
Janani Suraksha Yojana, India					
Amudhan et al. (2013)	Quasi-experimental pre- and post- comparative with control groups	Rural area in Haryana, India	Janani Suraksha Yojana (payments to offset costs of access)The programme was launched in 2005 as part of the National Rural Health Mission. A	Short-term payments, but followed by supply-side strengthening	FB
Carvalho et al. (2014)	Cross-sectional				PN, PP

Table 1 Table of characteristics of included studies *(Continued)*

		National sample of districts (mixed urban and rural), India	cadre of community-based workers (accredited social health activists) were created to promote the programme in communities. Women from low-income households could receive a cash payment if they give birth in a health facility (usually government, although some states also accredited private facilities). Accredited social health activists are salaried and expected to encourage ANC, facility-based births and PN/PP. They are eligible to receive a payment for accompanying a woman to a health facility to give birth.	Short-term payments, but need appropriate systems for payments	
Chaturvedi and Randive (2009)	Qualitative – semi-structured interviews and focus groups	Ahmednagar district in Maharashtra, India		Short-term payments, but ensure that private service providers are monitored and regulated	Implementation
Chaturvedi and Randive (2011)	Qualitative – semi-structured interviews and focus groups			Ensure sufficient government capacity to design and manage public-private partnerships	Implementation
Chaturvedi et al. (2015a)	Qualitative – observations and interviews	11 health facilities in Madhya Pradesh		Improve quality of care before introducing short-term payment programmes	Implementation
Chaturvedi et al. (2015b)	Qualitative – record reviews and interviews	73 health facilities in Madhya Pradesh		Train and support staff to use partographs	Implementation
Coffey (2014)	Qualitative – interviews and observations	Three villages in a rural district in Uttar Pradesh		Short-term payments, but need to incentivise health outcomes	Implementation
Dasgupta (2007)	Qualitative – maternal death investigations	7 districts in Uttar Pradesh, India		Invest in supply-side capacity, promote awareness of programme benefits, and develop systems to track each pregnancy	Implementation
Devadasan et al. (2008)	Qualitative - interviews	One district in each of four states, India		Short-term payments, but need to ensure quality of care, use streamlined processes for distribution of payments and monitor the programme	Implementation
Gopalan et al. (2012)	Qualitative – interviews and focus groups	Three districts in Orissa		Short-term payments, but with greater protection for families from costs of care	Implementation
Gupta (2007)	Qualitative – interviews and focus groups	Nalanda and West Champaran (rural) districts in Bihar, India		No recommendations made	Implementation
Hangmi and Kuki (2009)	Qualitative – interviews and focus groups	Churachandpur (rural) district in Manipur, India		Short-term payments, but need to invest in capacity of service providers, ensure fair selection of community-based workers, and streamline cash payments	Implementation
Human Rights Watch (2009)	Qualitative – individual and group interviews	Rural areas in Uttar Pradesh, India		Develop monitoring systems	Implementation
Joshi and Sivaram (2014)	Repeat cross-sectional	National sample of districts (mixed urban and rural), India		Concurrent supply-side strengthening and flexibility in guidelines	ANC, SBA, PN
Khan et al. (2010)	Qualitative – interviews				Implementation

Table 1 Table of characteristics of included studies *(Continued)*

		24 villages in Uttar Pradesh (rural), India	Short-term payments, but with adequate training and incentives for community-based workers, and inclusion of private service providers	
Krishna and Ananthpur (2011)	Qualitative – interviews and focus groups	Gulbarga and Raichur (rural) districts in Karnataka, India	No recommendations made	Implementation
Kumar et al. (2009)	Qualitative – focus groups	Una (predominantly rural) district in Himachal Pradesh, India	Short-term payments, but with streamlined distribution of cash payments and ensure community-based workers appropriately trained and that posts are filled	Implementation
Lim et al. (2010)	Repeat cross-sectional	National sample of districts (mixed urban and rural), India	Short-term payments, but need improved targeting and quality of care	ANC, FB, SBA, PM, NM
Lodh et al. (2009)	Qualitative – interviews and focus groups	Muzaffarpur district (predominantly rural) in Bihar, India	Short-term payments, but with streamlined distribution of cash payments	Implementation
Mazumdar et al. (2012)	Repeat cross-sectional	National sample of districts (mixed urban and rural), India	Short-term payments, but caution regarding unintended consequences	ANC, FB, SBA, C/I, NM
Nandan et al. (2008)	Qualitative – semi-structured and in-depth interviews and focus groups	3 districts in Orissa (predominantly rural), India	Short-term payments using streamlined payment systems, inclusion of private service providers, supply-side investment and awareness generation	Implementation
Nandan et al. (2008)	Qualitative – semi-structured and in-depth interviews and focus groups	3 districts in Orissa, India	Short-term payments using streamlined payment systems, supply-side investment and awareness generation	Implementation
Purohit et al. (2014)	Cross-sectional	Four districts in Rajasthan, India	Short-term payments	ANC, PN, QoC
Rai et al. (2012)	Qualitative – in-depth interviews and focus groups	12 villages in Jharkhand, India	Short-term payments alongside investment in supply-side capacity	Implementation
Randive et al. (2013)	Repeat cross-sectional	284 districts across nine Indian states	Short-term payments, but need to improve quality of care to impact on MM	FB
Santhya et al. (2011a)	Repeat cross-sectional	Alwar and Jodhpur districts (mixed rural and urban), India	Short-term payments, but improve awareness among communties, quality of services and administrative capacity	ANC, FB, SBA, PP, QoC, oxytocin
Santhya et al. (2011b)	Qualitative – in-depth interviews			Implementation

Table 1 Table of characteristics of included studies *(Continued)*

		Alwar and Jodhpur districts in Rajasthan, India	Short-term payments with trained community-based workers to raise awareness in communities	
Singh and Chaturvedi (2007)	Qualitative – focus groups and interviews	Five districts in Uttar Pradesh and three districts in Uttarakhand, India	Short-term payments using streamlined systems, inclusion of postpartum care and removal of formal and informal user fees	Implementation
Sri et al. (2012)	Qualitative – maternal death reviews	Barwani district, Uttar Pradesh, India	Investments must be made in supply-side strengthening and ensuring quality of care before short-term payments are considered	Implementation
Uttekar et al. (2007a)	Qualitative - interviews	3 districts in Himachal Pradesh, India	Short-term payments, but need to ensure quality of care by investing in supply-side capacity, use streamlined payments and raise awareness among hard-to-reach communities	Implementation
Uttekar et al. (2007b)	Qualitative - interviews	3 districts in West Bengal, India	Short-term payments, but need to ensure quality of care by investing in supply-side capacity, use streamlined payments and raise awareness among hard-to-reach communities	Implementation
Uttekar et al. (2007c)	Qualitative - interviews	3 districts in Orissa, India	Short-term payments, but need to ensure quality of care by investing in supply-side capacity, use streamlined payments and raise awareness among hard-to-reach communities	Implementation
Uttekar et al. (2007d)	Qualitative - interviews	3 districts in Rajasthan, India	Short-term payments, but need to ensure quality of care by investing in supply-side capacity, use streamlined payments and raise awareness among hard-to-reach communities	Implementation
Uttekar et al. (2007e)	Qualitative - interviews	3 districts in Assam, India	Short-term payments, but need to ensure quality of care by investing in supply-side capacity, use streamlined payments and raise awareness among hard-to-reach communities	Implementation
Uttekar et al. (2008a)	Qualitative - interviews	3 districts in Uttar Pradesh, India	Short-term payments, but need to ensure quality of care by investing in supply-side capacity, use streamlined payments and	Implementation

Table 1 Table of characteristics of included studies *(Continued)*

				raise awareness among hard-to-reach communities	
Uttekar et al. (2008b)	Qualitative - interviews	3 districts in Bihar, India		Short-term payments, but need to ensure quality of care by investing in supply-side capacity, use streamlined payments and raise awareness among hard-to-reach communities	Implementation
Vora et al. (2012)	Cross-sectional	Rural areas in Gujarat and Tamil Nadu, India		Short-term payments, but should expand availability of health facilities, develop referral networks, include public and/or private facilities depending on local health system, promote awareness generation, and divide payments across maternity care services to incentivise multiple services.	ANC, FB, C/I
CHIMACA project, China					
Hemminki et al. (2013)	Cross-sectional	One county in Anhui province, China	CHIMACA project (payments to offset costs of access)Women could claim a small cash payment from a health centre if they attended ANC between 2007 and 2009. The size of the payment was increased with the number of ANC visits. Village family planning workers distributed leaflets in communities to advertise the programme and midwives distributed the leaflets to women attending ANC.	Short-term payments, but need payments that are appropriately sized and relatively easy to obtain	ANC, C/I, PN, QoC
SURE-P, Nigeria					
Okoli et al. (2014)	Retrospective area study	Nine states, Nigeria	SURE-P (short term payments to offset costs of access)Cash payments were made to women who attended specific maternity care services (ANC, childbirth and PN/PP). Eligibilty was geographic and was based on the selection of health facilities participating in the wider SURE-P health programme. If a woman was referred to a higher level hospital, the hospital received a payment.	Short-term payments, but need to improve retention of programme recipients throughout pregnancy	ANC, SBA
Safe Delivery Incentive Programme, Nepal					

Table 1 Table of characteristics of included studies *(Continued)*

Powell-Jackson et al. (2009)	Retrospective area study	Makwanpur district (rural), Nepal	Safe Delivery Incentive Programme (payments to offset costs of access)The programme was launched in 2005 and provides a cash payment to women who give birth in a health facility, and to a health worker who attends her birth (either at home or in a health facility). Payments were initially only available to women who have had two or fewer previous live births, but this condition was later removed. The programme was initially limited to government health facilities but later expanded to include the private sector.	Short-term payments, but need to improve quality of care to impact on NM and need to ensure good communication to communities	ANC, FB, SBA, C/I, NM
Powell-Jackson et al. (2009)	Qualitative – interviews and focus groups	10 districts, Nepal		Attention to implementation challenges in countries with poor capacity to administer programmes and provide services, and careful planning	Implementation
Powell-Jackson and Hanson (2012)	Cross-sectional	National sample of districts (mixed urban and rural), India		Short-term payments, but need effective implementation	SBA, FB, C/I
Vouchers for maternity care services					
Pilot programmes, Pakistan					
Agha (2011a)	Repeat cross-sectional	Dera Ghazi Khan City (urban), Pakistan	Pilot voucher scheme (vouchers for maternal health services)12 month programme in which vouchers were sold to eligible families and local officials verified eligibility. Vouchers could be exchanged at participating Greenstar facilities for ANC, childbirth (including caesarean section if needed), PP and PN. Providers were reimbursed for each voucher accepted.	Vouchers for maternity care services	ANC, FB, PN
Agha (2011b)	Repeat cross-sectional	Jhang district (rural), Pakistan		Vouchers for maternity care services	ANC, FB, PN
Maternal Health Voucher Scheme, Bangladesh					
Ahmed and Khan (2011)	Cross-sectional	Sarishabari district (predominantly rural), Bangladesh	Maternal Health Voucher Scheme (vouchers for maternal health services) Since 2007 poor pregnant women received vouchers (some districts had universal distribution, some had targeted distribution) entitling them to free maternity care services (ANC, childbirth, PN/PP), transport subsidies, a cash incentive for delivery with a qualified provider (at home or in a designated facility) and a gift box. Providers received incentives to distribute vouchers	Vouchers for maternity care services	ANC, FB, SBA, PN
Ahmed and Khan (2011)	Qualitative – semi-structured interviews	Sarishabari district (predominantly rural), Bangladesh		Vouchers for maternity care services, but with significant expansion of service delivery capacity of health facilities	Implementation
Hatt et al. (2010)	Cross-sectional	Early implementation subdistricts (mainly rural), Bangladesh		Vouchers for maternity care services	ANC, FB, C/I, PN
	Qualitative – interviews and focus groups	Early implementation subdistricts (mainly rural), Bangladesh		Vouchers for maternity care services	Implementation
Koehlmoos et al. (2008)					Implementation

Table 1 Table of characteristics of included studies *(Continued)*

	Qualitative – structured and in-depth interviews and focus groups		and provide services that were covered by the vouchers.	Vouchers for maternity care services, but with investment in physical infrastructure at government facilities, appropriate human resources, and attention to incentives to conduct caesarean sections	
Nguyen et al. (2012)	Cross-sectional	Early implementation subdistricts (mainly rural), Bangladesh		Vouchers for maternity care services as part of a wider initiative that includes supply-side strengthening	ANC, FB, SBA, C/I, PN
Reproductive Health Vouchers Evaluation Team (2011)	Qualitative - interviews	22 sub-districts, Bangladesh		Vouchers for maternity care services	Implementation
Pilot voucher programme, Bangladesh					
Rob et al. (2009)	Repeat cross-sectional	Habiganj district (rural), Bangladesh	Pilot voucher scheme (vouchers for maternal health services)12 month programme in which fieldworkers identified a total of eligible women who were then validated as "poor" by a community support group Women could use vouchers for ANC, childbirth, PN and PP. Providers were reimbursed for vouchers accepted. Service providers and fieldworkers were trained and strengthened health facilities for providing ANC, delivery, and PNC services.	Vouchers for maternity care services	ANC, FB, SBA, PN
	Qualitative – semi-structured interviews	Habiganj district (rural), Bangladesh		Vouchers for maternity care services	Implementation
Makerere University Voucher Scheme, Uganda					
Alfonso et al. (2015)	Retrospective area study	Kamuli and Pallisa districts, Uganda	Makerere University Voucher Scheme (vouchers for maternal health services)Between June 2010 and May 2011, vouchers were distributed to women in two selected areas of two Ugandan districts during ANC visits. Vouchers could be exchanged at public facilities or participating private facilities for intrapartum care, transport to and from the hospital, and for PN/PP in case of complications. Transport vouchers' reimbursement covered the cost of the average distance in the treatment areas, and health	Vouchers for maternity care services	FB
Pariyo et al. (2011)	Qualitative – focus groups	Kamuli district, Uganda		Vouchers for maternity care services, but with inclusion of transport providers	Implementation

Table 1 Table of characteristics of included studies *(Continued)*

			facilities were reimbursed for services provided.		
HealthyBaby vouchers, Uganda					
Okal et al. (2013)	Qualitative - interviews	7 districts, Uganda	HealthyBaby vouchers (vouchers for maternal health services)Since 2008 vouchers for maternity care services have been sold to eligible women in 20 districts. Vouchers can be exchanged at accredited private providers for ANC, childbirth, PN. Community-based voucher distributors are responsible for targeting poor pregnant women using district-customized poverty grading tool.	Vouchers for maternity care services, but with public facilities included, greater awareness raising in communities and support for policy champions	Implementation
Reproductive Health Vouchers Evaluation Team (2012)	Repeat cross-sectional	6 districts, Uganda		Vouchers for maternity care services	ANC, FB, PN
	Qualitative - interviews	30 health facilities, Uganda		Vouchers for maternity care services	Implementation
Vouchers for Health, Kenya					
Abuya et al. (2012)	Qualitative – in-depth interviews	Three districts and two urban slums	Vouchers for Health (vouchers for maternal health services)Since 2006 vouchers have been sold to eligible women in three districts and two informal settlements in Kenya. Vouchers can be exchanged for ANC, childbirth (including caesarean section if needed) and PN. A facility was accredited if it met criteria set by the public authorities in terms of staffing and quality of care.	Vouchers for maternity care services, with strong partnerships between public and private sectors and leading role for government	Implementation
Amendah et al. (2013)	Repeat cross-sectional	Two urban slums in Nairobi, Kenya		Vouchers for maternity care services	FB for subsequent pregnancy
Arur et al. (2009)	Qualitative – semi-structured interviews	Kenya		Vouchers for maternity care services if financial issues are the main barrier to care-seeking	Implementation
Bellows et al. (2012)	Repeat cross-sectional	Informal settlements in Nairobi (urban), Kenya		Vouchers for maternity care services	ANC, FB, SBA
Njuki et al. (2013)	Qualitative – structured interviews and focus groups	Three districts in Kenya		Vouchers for maternity care services, but with adequate information and availability of voucher distributors	Implementation
Njuki et al. (2015)	Qualitative – in-depth interviews	Three districts in Kenya		Vouchers for maternity care services, but greater awareness of eligibility criteria and entitlements, and greater flexibility for public facilities to use income from vouchers	Implementation
Obare et al. (2012)	Cross-sectional	Six districts (all mixed urban and rural), Kenya		Vouchers for maternity care services	ANC, FB, SBA, PN
Obare et al. (2014)	Repeat cross-sectional				FB

Table 1 Table of characteristics of included studies *(Continued)*

		Six districts (all mixed urban and rural), Kenya		Vouchers for maternity care services, but transport costs should be included	
Reproductive Health Vouchers Evaluation Team (2011)	Qualitative - interviews	6 rural districts and 2 informal settlements, Kenya		Vouchers for maternity care services with awareness generation, monitoring of quality of care, and adequate provisions to overcome geographical (transports) issues	Implementation
Watt et al. (2015)	Repeat cross-sectional	Six districts (all mixed urban and rural), Kenya		Vouchers for maternity care services, and need to include PP before discharge from hospital within hospital agreements	QoC
Chiranjeevi Yojana, India					
Bhat et al. (2009)	Cross-sectional	Dahod district (mixed urban and rural), India	Chiranjeevi Scheme (vouchers for maternal health services)The programme was introduced in five districts in Gujarat, India, in 2005. Women with documentation that indicate eligibility can receive free maternity care services at participating private facilities. Facilities are reimbursed for every 100 women who they provide care to.	Vouchers for maternity care services	PN
De Costa et al. (2014)	Retrospective area study	Gujarat, India		Further research needed	FB
Ganguly et al. (2014)	Qualitative – interviews	Two districts in Gujarat, India		Vouchers for maternity care services, but with greater attention to developing trust between service providers and communities	Implementation
Jega (2007)	Qualitative – interviews	2 districts in Gujarat (mixed urban and rural), India		Vouchers for maternity care services, but with antenatal and postnatal care included, supply-side investment (to establish blood banks) and formal monitoring systems	Implementation
Mohanan et al. (2014)	Cross-sectional	Gujarat, India		Further research needed	ANC, FB, PN
Voucher programme, Cambodia					
Ir et al. (2010)	Qualitative – in-depth interviews and focus groups	3 districts in Kampong province, Cambodia	Voucher programme (vouchers for maternal health services)The programme was implemented in 22 districts between 2007 and 2010. Voucher distribution was universal in 14 districts and targeted in 8 districts. Eligible women were identified local volunteers and could use vouchers for free ANC, childbirth and PN/PP at public health facilities. Health centres were reimbursed for vouchers.	Vouchers for maternity care services alongside interventions to promote quality of care and to overcome non-financial barriers to demand	Implementation
Van de Poel et al. (2014)	Cross-sectional	Nationally representative sample, Cambodia		Vouchers for maternity care services, but universal distribution may be more effective than targeting	ANC, FB, C/I, PN
Vouchers for merit goods					
Tanzanian National Voucher Scheme, Tanzania					

Table 1 Table of characteristics of included studies *(Continued)*

Hanson et al. (2009)	Repeat cross-sectional	21 districts (mixed urban and rural), Tanzania	Tanzanian National Voucher Scheme (vouchers for merit goods)Women attending ANC were given a voucher that entitled them to a discounted insecticide-treated net (of any size) from an approved supplier. The programme began in 2004 and expanded globally over subsequent years.	Vouchers for merit goods	Ownership and use of insecticide-treated net
Koenker et al. (2013)	Qualitative – meetings, site visits and mathematical modelling	Five areas in Tanzania		Vouchers for merit goods, with voucher distribution in schools and at health clinics	Implementation
Mubyazi et al. (2010)	Qualitative – interviews and focus groups	Mkuranga and Mufindi districts (rural), Tanzania		No recommendation made	Implementation

ANC denotes antenatal care, SBA skilled birth attendance, FB births attended in healthcare facilities, PN postnatal care, PP postpartum care, C/I care-seeking for complications or illness in women and newborns, QoC quality of care, MM maternal mortality, PM perinatal mortality and NM neonatal mortality

Women who are potential DSF programme users

Target groups may be unaware of programme details [24, 25, 41, 46, 50, 58, 59, 61, 63, 64, 67, 71, 76, 77, 81, 85, 89, 91, 98, 101]. Women and their families may not realise that they are eligible for programmes (or incorrectly think that they are) and may not know which facilities they can use through the scheme [48, 63]. Remote areas may be less likely to receive promotional activities [93, 101]. Effective forms of awareness generation have included community dissemination of information [81], radio broadcasts [93], and networks of women's groups [19, 28, 29, 77].

Social and cultural attitudes towards women play an important role in utility of vouchers as well as in use of services. Some women reported not being able to use a voucher because their husband did not want to be labelled as poor [98, 105], because they were expected to return to a family home elsewhere to give birth [105], or because nobody was available to accompany them to a participating hospital [63, 71, 85]. Of those who did travel to facility for birth care, many sought early discharge in order to return to look after children [52].

Perceptions of the quality of care and behaviour of providers were important for utilisation of health services, and therefore the implementation of DSF schemes. Prospective users were discouraged by reputations that facilities had long waiting times [81, 85], were poorly equipped and unclean [39, 49, 58, 61, 63, 65, 71, 80, 85, 92], or were places where one encountered disrespectful and abusive care [33, 44, 49, 50, 52, 54, 56, 61, 63, 81, 86, 94, 101, 105]. Modesty rules made some women reluctant to be treated by male doctors [58] or to visit midwives where it is considered inappropriate to let someone else see one's genitals [25]. Other deterrents included fear of being subjected to unwanted procedures such as injections, surgical procedures and stitches [61, 71, 72] and of testing for HIV at a health facility and the attached stigma of HIV [98, 101]. Regular antenatal care visits may help women to become familiar and more relaxed with facilities and staff [52], and community visits by staff and women who were satisfied with their care could promote uptake [71, 73].

Community-based workers

Workers based in communities (including voucher distributors) can be important facilitators for DSF programmes. India's accredited social health activists (ASHA) were found to be have played an important role in raising the awareness of Janani Suraksha Yojana and assisting women to obtain payments [38, 39, 52, 56, 58, 63, 64, 68–70, 72, 112], as did workers for Program Keluarga Harapan in Indonesia [24, 25]. Community health workers were an important source of information on DSF programmes in India [64, 88] and Tanzania [109], and voucher distributors performed a similar role in Kenya [99], Pakistan [103, 104] and Cambodia [87].

Community-based workers occupy a challenging position between communities, DSF programmes and health facilities. In communities, they can face criticism and accusations of theft if cash transfer payments are delayed [23], or if women go to a facility to give birth but do not receive payments they had been told about, or receive a smaller amount than expected [49, 56, 58, 65]. When visiting facilities, community-based workers who are reimbursed for facilitating DSF programmes may be asked for informal payments by facility staff [50, 56]. They may be used as go-betweens to request money from families on behalf of service providers and service providers have reportedly punished those who resist by refusing to register the facilitator's subsequent service users, referring them to other facilities unnecessarily, or withholding DSF payments [44, 50, 56]. In some cases women have been reluctant to allow workers to accompany them to a facility because they feared money would be taken from them [48].

The potential of community-based workers to implement DSF programmes can also be undermined by geographically over-large operating areas that entail long distances for travel [25]. Some female workers were restricted by their family members in when they could accompany pregnant women to a facility [56]. Some workers' usefulness was limited by their poor knowledge of programme details [53] and others reported difficulties in applying eligibility criteria because their guidelines were not clear [23]. Financial issues included resistance to their continued work for the programme from their families if their payment was delayed [56], and having to pay for food and transport when accompanying a women for antenatal care yet not receiving any reimbursement if the woman later gave birth at home [47, 56, 58]. Other difficulties include the risks of co-option of schemes by community members for personal gain. Positions as programme workers are sometimes regarded by communities as 'lucrative' compared to other forms of work [44], and there have been reports of recruitment processes being hijacked by local politicians and community leaders to appoint family members even though they were unlikely to want to perform the necessary duties [48, 65].

Staff in health facilities

Experiences among service providers and managers at participating health facilities seem to be mixed. In evaluations of voucher schemes, government and private providers report gaining skills and experience, making investments in infrastructure, being able to hire more staff, and reduced absenteeism among existing staff [86, 106, 108]. However, staff at some facilities in voucher schemes felt that increased user-load and administrative work was not adequately compensated by provider payments [79, 82, 106]. Some felt that schemes designed to target specific groups created problems and complained that they had been threatened by women who were excluded by means-testing criteria [81], or subjected to pressure from local politicians to distribute vouchers to ineligible women [81].

In short-term cash payment programmes, service providers at government facilities reported a significant increase in their workload exacerbating the existing inadequacies of services [40, 46, 50, 54, 59, 61]. Knowledge of schemes varied. Some government providers in India admitted that they knew nothing about Janani Suraksha Yojana other than that they needed to give payments to women who gave birth in the facility [54, 59]. One study reported that women were treated with hostility by facility staff when they sought cash assistance [54]. On the other hand, delayed or irregular reimbursements by programmes could lead to difficulties distributing money to women and expose the service providers as targets for criticism from families [48, 76].

In programmes designed to allow opt-in of private providers, respondents reported that they joined to help the poor to access health services [81, 90, 91] and conversely to increase business [81, 90]. In one study some said they felt coerced, fearing that they would otherwise be subjected to unwarranted but damaging investigations [90]. Private providers reported subsequently dropping out of voucher schemes because they felt 'overwhelmed' by the number of voucher users [93], or were unhappy with inadequate and delayed payments [108]. Some private providers in the Chiranjeevi Scheme in India reported that revenue had fallen because there were too few voucher users, their facility had gained an unwanted reputation as a place for poor people, and that pregnant women who used to pay fees to be attended there were now using the voucher programme [90]. Providers in the Tanzanian National Voucher Scheme for insecticide-treated nets stated that they enjoyed participating but that the programme required substantial investment of money and storage space to stock slow-selling nets, at the expense of other more popular items such as soap [110].

Barriers and facilitators to successful implementation

Seven themes were identified regarding barriers and enabling factors for the implementation of DSF programmes: scope of the programme, supply-side capacity, contracting private providers, administrative processes and procedural considerations, information systems, fraudulent practices and their control, and sustainability issues.

Scope of the programme

A common barrier found across many DSF programmes was that they were insufficient in their scope to overcome continued financial, social and geographical barriers to accessing services. Vouchers for maternity care services typically cover treatment costs but many do not include other important 'demand-side' costs such as transport, which can be prohibitive for households [79, 85, 88, 92, 96, 98–101, 104–106]. There is also the opportunity cost for women and their families of spending time away from their home and children [86, 103]. In contexts where pregnant women are asked to buy vouchers, for example the Vouchers for Health programme in Kenya, women may be deterred by the price of vouchers [96, 100]. Experiences with vouchers for merit goods in Tanzania have been similar. Women highlighted the cost of travel to obtain a voucher from health facilities, the cost of travelling to an approved shop to use the voucher and the remaining cost of the insecticide-treated net (which was only part-subsidised by a voucher) [109, 111].

Possible options to increase the accessibility of voucher services include, inclusion of travel costs within voucher entitlements [80, 81, 85, 100, 107], community distribution of vouchers to reduce travel to *obtain* a voucher and accreditation of additional facilities and providers to reduce travel to *make use* of a voucher [105]. For example, the Maternal Health Voucher Scheme in Bangladesh included short-term cash payments to facilitate uptake by offsetting costs of access [79].

In short-term payment programmes and in cash transfer schemes, payments may simply be too small or too late to offset out-of-pocket costs that include transport, tests, medicines and sutures [23, 25, 33, 37, 44, 46–49, 54, 55, 58–61, 66, 67, 77]. The size of payments may need to be increased periodically to keep pace with inflation and the Muthulakshmi Reddy Maternity Benefit Scheme in India has repeatedly increased the amount paid to women during its 30 year implementation period [22]. The programme offered 300 rupees to eligible women when launched in 1987 and now offers 12,000 rupees (approximately USD 190).

Provisions for onward referral in the case of an obstetric complication have often not been included in DSF schemes yet should be considered (see also sections on supply-side capacity and on procedural considerations below). Some families reported having to pay for treatment costs after they were referred to a non-participating facility [101], and others returned home when faced with additional expenditure [54, 66]. Bangladesh's Maternal Health Voucher Scheme included 'seed funds' that could be used by health facilities for supply-side investments and to pay for emergency transport for voucher users [81].

Narrow eligibility criteria were highlighted as a barrier by studies of many DSF programmes. For example, schemes that exclude women who have more than a certain number of children are reported as unfair, difficult to enforce and completely counter-intuitive for programmes that aim to reduce maternal mortality [22, 76, 79, 82]. If a decision is made to design a targeted programme then use of locally appropriate poverty screening tools should be considered [94, 95, 98, 99, 101, 106]. Programmes in India have often used an existing system of 'below poverty line' cards however such programmes are constrained by any pitfalls in the existing system such as non-ownership of cards by those in need but lacking documentation, and leakage of cards to those least in need [88].

Supply-side capacity

The contextual evidence highlights that DSF cannot work well without adequate supply-side investment in public services and systems, and many of the findings in this sub-section are indicative of wider challenges in health-care systems. Many evaluations of DSF programmes described problems at health facilities as a key barrier. Poor availability of medicines and other medical supplies – sometimes linked to bureaucratic procedures for procurement that discourage restocking [48] – meant that women in Bangladesh and India needed to make considerable personal expenditure [81, 82, 85]. Bed shortages meant many women were discharged within 24 h of giving birth, which may not allow sufficient time for post-partum care [46, 48]. In Indonesia's Program Keluarga Harapan, cash transfers were contingent on using midwives however village midwife posts were reported to be unfilled in many areas [25]. Contracting private providers in voucher schemes does not remove the need for quality public sector provision as private providers often refer complicated cases to the public sector [105].

In India, where DSF schemes can be found in many states, there have been widespread reports of poor quality of care and improper practices, linked to increased workloads of staff in health facilities [40, 55, 60, 63]. It is important to monitor quality of care and adverse outcomes after childbirth, however DSF programmes were reported to lack adequate monitoring systems in this area [45, 46, 50] and women reported having no way to register and process their complaints at health facilities [50, 66]. Incidents included delays in starting treatment for women with serious conditions [66], chaotic delivery rooms [40], low utilisation of partographs [43], babies being left unmonitored in birth pans [44], physical abuse of women [44, 66], episiotomies conducted without permission and stitched without local anaesthesia [44], high incidence of oxytocin injections for labour induction [45], and pregnant women who have been diverted from a public to a private facility at the behest of an owner who worked on-call at the public facility [41].

Referrals from one facility to another are a key issue that may put the life of the woman and her baby at risk and are a cause of substantial expenditure for families who face additional costs for transport, food and accommodation [41, 45, 50, 53, 54, 66, 70, 76, 79]. Reported reasons for referral related to wider healthcare systems issues including absence of specialists at lower level facilities [42, 50, 59, 79], busy or absent doctors and midwives [49, 50, 58, 62, 66, 67], and a lack of functioning equipment for operations or blood transfusions (including faulty or stolen generators) [40, 48, 50, 65, 91]. In India, private practitioners in the Chiranjeevi Yojana were reluctant to provide care for clusters of women requiring care for complications due to the associated costs and the risk of adverse outcomes [90, 91].

There are two key enabling factors for programme designers and managers to support facilities and promote care-seeking. Firstly, designers need to realistically examine the capacity of local health systems to provide care to women who use DSF programmes. This needs to include emergency transport [62], round-the-clock opening hours [38, 60] and clearly stated guidelines for onward referrals [45, 50, 66, 69]. Procurement systems for essential medicines may need to be included within programme designs, at least until government procurement systems can be adequately strengthened [101].

Secondly, designers may consider how best to support participating facilities to maintain and improve the quality of care. Concurrent supply-side investments can improve working conditions for staff and expand service coverage, and 'seed funds' have reportedly been used to good effect in Bangladesh's Maternal Health Voucher Scheme [81]. El Salvador's Comunidades Solidarias Rurales and Guatemala's Mi Familia Progresa were reported to have been implemented successfully alongside investments in the infrastructure and human resources of health facilities [19, 20], and similar supply-side investments have been important in India [38, 60] and Nigeria [78]. Another approach that has been advocated is to link provider payments to uptake of services [77, 87, 94, 107]. For programmes using government facilities (including if they are used for onward referrals), it is important that government facilities receive any linked payments and are able to invest them in infrastructure and human resources [93, 101, 105]

Contracting private providers

For programmes that are designed to include the opt-in of private providers, there is a risk that programmes will struggle to maintain sufficient number of participating providers if revenue from service users is considered to be inadequate [90, 91, 93, 101]. Providers and programme managers have reported that attempts to contract private providers to implement Janani Suraksha Yojana in some Indian states struggled due to low provider payments [42] and lack of interested providers that meet accreditation criteria [68].

Four particular issues have been documented for the contracting of private providers in voucher programmes.

Firstly, providers may deliver differential treatment to voucher users compared to fee-paying pregnant women [93, 98]. Secondly, providers may seek to increase revenue by charging pregnant women for services that should be provided free according to the DSF scheme guidelines and agreements, including ultrasound scans, medicines and surgical care [88, 91, 92]. Thirdly, some providers may engage in the 'skimming' of voucher users requiring little intervention and referral of those requiring operations to avoid incurring costs [90, 91], or avoid the risk (and associated litigation) of being held responsible for any adverse outcomes [90]. Fourthly, providers may withdraw from a programme [89, 90, 93, 108].

Programme designers could consider how best to reimburse private facilities for childbirth. As noted above, private facilities may be reluctant to perform surgical interventions if reimbursements are the same regardless of level of intervention [90, 91], and programme officials in India suggested that provider contracts should include a clause stating that caesarean sections must be provided to any voucher user who needed one. Conversely, there are fears that differential reimbursement rates may provide an incentive for participating private facilities to perform high rates of caesarean sections, and that close monitoring may be an important deterrent [83].

Administrative processes and procedural considerations

Requirements for formal documents to be produced in order to prove eligibility should be carefully considered as in some cases the undocumented will be those most in need, including migrants, young and multiparous women [22, 41, 50, 53, 55, 58, 76, 94, 101]. In Kenya, for instance, young women were effectively excluded from a voucher scheme as the required government identification cards are only issued at 18 years of age [101]. It may be necessary to allow alternative forms of evidence (such as photos or letters signed by community leaders) [46], or to avoid restrictions and requirements for formal documents altogether [41, 46, 53].

For short-term cash payment programmes, rigid insistence on bureaucratic processes is a barrier to payment claims by women and some women did not travel to a facility for childbirth if they had heard reports other women had been denied money [48, 49]. The distribution of payments was considered to lack transparency [46, 58], and respondents reported being repeatedly sent away from facilities to obtain additional documents [41, 76]. Payments have been denied for reasons including because a seven-day claim period had passed, women were more than 12 weeks gestation at the time of registration, an official would not approve payments to women who gave birth before he took his post, a woman had given birth on the way to a facility and a woman was not accompanied by a community-based worker [41, 48, 68, 76].

It is important that payments to users and participating facilities in DSF programmes use streamlined and timely systems. For short-term cash payment programmes, women received payments as late as 12 months after giving birth [46], or not at all [76], and some families reported selling possessions or incurring debts to pay for transport and medicines for childbirth [47]. Service providers have suggested that such payments to women should be made before childbirth [71], however this may not be enough to overcome irregular disbursements of funding to local levels [41, 42, 58, 72].

The distribution of payments to users can be an administrative burden for officials and service providers, who may not fully understand the programme [58, 59]. Some service providers highlighted a need for more support to cope with paperwork [59, 67], while others had restricted payments to a specific desk at a certain time of day to cope with demand for payments [59]. Local officials suggested that community health workers who manage accounts and distribute payments should be trained accordingly [68, 69].

Payments to health facilities have reportedly been delayed due to bureaucratic procedures and a lack of understanding among facility staff regarding what supporting documentation must be submitted [82, 90, 93, 97, 101]. Stringent fraud detection systems may cause delays [106], but need to be balanced against the effects of fraud (see section on corruption). Providers can benefit from feedback mechanisms on how to make payment claims [93]. District officials reacted to unpredictability in funding by adopting first come, first served approaches, sharing smaller amounts among women, borrowing money from other sources, or using their own money [76].

Information systems

In targeted DSF programmes, information on target groups can help to inform locally appropriate poverty screening tools but may be difficult to obtain or use [94, 95, 98, 99, 101, 106]. Use of existing government systems for monitoring helps to reduce duplication [81, 82, 84], however these need to be functional – district officials in India and Nepal reported not having time, resources or guidelines to conduct monitoring visits [59, 76] and stated that they had to assume quality of care was good unless they heard otherwise [68]. An alternative approach advocated by studies in the review was for communities and non-governmental organisations to be supported to monitor quality of care, provision of free services and distribution of vouchers or cash transfers [45, 70]. Another suggested approach was to contract monitoring to an external organisation, although experiences with Kenya's Vouchers for Health programme indicated that close scrutiny was needed to ensure that the contracted organisation performed monitoring processes as mandated [95, 101]. Such external oversight will also require additional financial outlay and may cause tensions within health services and administrations.

Fraudulent practices and their control

Fraudulent practices (by users, community-based workers and providers) have been documented as occurring in many DSF programmes. Local government officials may attempt to use programmes to get care for ineligible family members and friends [90], and officials in India and Nepal are reported to have embezzled programme funds [44, 76]. A recurring complaint across many short-term cash payment and voucher schemes is that families have been exposed to demands for informal payments by staff in health facilities [39, 44, 45, 47, 48, 50, 56, 60, 63, 77, 86, 93, 101]. In short-term cash payment programmes, staff have been known to deduct money before giving the scheduled payments [44, 46, 53, 59, 63], and indeed one study in India reported that around half of the amount due to be paid to women through Janani Suraksha Yojana was deducted by service providers [44]. Suggestions from officials include using pre-printed cheques and tracking these using online financial reporting systems [58, 70].

Community-based workers have also been known to apply informal charges to women and their families [44, 86, 93, 101]. Commission-based (rather than salaried) payments for such workers may have unintended consequences including workers placing inappropriate pressure on women to travel to health centres to give birth [53], and issuing vouchers to ineligible women in order to achieve the requisite numbers [93]. Initiatives taken by programme managers in Kenya to reduce dishonest behaviour included putting up posters with the true cost of vouchers on market days to prevent informal fees, and switching from commission-based to stipend-based payments for voucher distributors [93].

Some studies have emphasised the importance of strong monitoring systems [106, 108]. If false claims are reported sufficient resources need to be allocated so that they can be adequately followed-up [76]. Similarly, it is important to be able to remove providers from a programme if they are found to be engaged in malpractice [106], although in practice this may be difficult in districts where there are few providers or little interest in joining a programme.

Sustainability issues

The experience with DSF programmes ranges from cash transfers that have been in operation for almost 30 years, to voucher programmes that have only been implemented as short pilot programmes. Thorough planning and political support seem important for the sustainability of DSF programmes and programme designers need to ensure that all organisations involved in the programme have sufficient capacity to perform mandated tasks [59, 78, 81, 95]. Research has emphasised the importance of good communication between the different levels and different organisations [68, 77, 93]. Planning may take several years as appropriate systems and expertise are developed, and this may be an expensive process [24, 78]. Data should be monitored during implementation to adjust programme design as needed [93, 95]. Local government officials, community leaders and community-based workers can play an important role raising awareness of programmes [55, 81, 84, 101], however regular communication is needed as turnover of officials and poor communication between levels may lead to confusion and distribution of misinformation [79, 81, 84, 106].

Policy champions in donor and governmental organisations proved helpful to ensure political and financial support for programmes in Kenya and Uganda [93, 101, 106]. In Kenya the Vouchers for Health programme reportedly received support from national policy-makers because it was seen as a useful model to prepare for a national social health insurance programme [93]. However, programmes may also become subject to specific political interests. In Nepal, the national government reportedly forced programme roll-out before planning was complete and created tensions with state governments [76].

Ministry of Health engagement is often sought in donor-initiated programmes [84, 101], but programmes may become an administrative burden for under-resourced departments and facilities [81, 84]. In Kenya, a planned transfer of ownership to the Ministry of Health was repeatedly delayed and eventually required the assistance of a contracted consultancy firm [93].

Discussion

This analysis has highlighted a series of well-documented challenges for the implementation of DSF schemes in maternal and newborn health. These include issues of programme scope (in terms of programme eligibility, size and timing of payments and voucher entitlements), wider problems in healthcare systems (including inadequate infrastructure and human resources, lack of medicines and problems with corruption) and the population's awareness and perceptions of programmes and health services. A recent systematic review concluded that despite evaluations spanning 15 years of implementation, DSF programmes have yet to demonstrate positive impact of programmes on quality of care or maternal and newborn health outcomes [14]. That finding may reflect insufficient attention during programme design and implementation to improving the quality of care being provided and to conditions of access to comprehensive emergency care [113]. Research highlighted in our analysis indicates that the implementation of DSF programmes may reinforce existing healthcare system problems including poor quality of care, demands for informal fees and the systematic exclusion of vulnerable groups. Vouchers for maternity care services are often proposed as a means to improve quality of care however experiences indicate private providers may find reimbursement rates to be unattractive and engage in practices such as providing differential quality of care or 'skimming' programme users who require minimal intervention. Taken together, these findings suggest a need for greater attention to issues of implementation in DSF programmes and to the context in which they are to be introduced. They indicate serious concerns for the use of DSF as a stand-alone interventions in maternal and newborn health in low- and middle-income countries, and raise questions regarding which (if any) maternal and newborn healthcare services are suited to modalities of DSF.

Where DSF programmes have improved care-seeking, the programmes have tended to include (or be accompanied by) additional investment in health facilities or staff, while those without such investment have struggled (see Tables 2 and 3). Other important factors that have enabled DSF programmes to improve care-seeking have included appropriate payment size and timing for short-term cash payments and cash transfer programmes, and an adequate package of entitlements (including transport costs) in voucher schemes. When well-supported and -supervised, community-based workers, leaders and women's groups have been important facilitators for programmes as they have raised awareness of programme details and helped to counter negative perceptions of programmes.

The longest-running DSF programmes included in this review have been cash transfer schemes that were introduced by national or state governments as part of wider social welfare programmes. Programmes since the launch of the Millennium Development Goals have tended to focus more narrowly on specific maternal health services with the aim to improve their coverage on indicators such as skilled attendants at birth or facility births. Most evaluations have shown quantitative improvements in coverage rates [14]. However, many have relied on funding from donors, and some were implemented for only short pilot periods. Studies have highlighted the high start-up costs of DSF programmes [24, 78], and those running in parallel to welfare systems are likely to have continued high overhead costs. Policy-makers need to consider whether DSF programmes that involve cash payments or vouchers are likely to be an optimal use of resources, or whether increased supply-side investment would be equally effective.

Limitations of the review

The scope of literature included systematic review may have been limited by use of English search terms and English language databases. Findings were incorporated from a range of studies, including some that were of low quality, in order to gain insights for implementation from a wide range of contexts. The most common methodological weaknesses of studies related to the length of time for follow-up after programme initiation (quantitative studies), and failure to address to role of the researcher on data generation and analysis (qualitative studies). By including studies with such weaknesses, there is a risk that findings reported in this review over-emphasise short-term factors affecting implementation, and that findings are subject to unknown biases based on the value systems and social positioning of researchers.

Conclusions

After quite widespread implementation and considerable policy enthusiasm in some quarters, evaluations have shed light on the importance of a number of detailed design and implementation issues as outlined above. The synthesis of findings reveals a complex picture of experiences DSF programmes in maternal and newborn health. While they indicate that cash payments and vouchers can be successful in improving service utilisation rates at least in the short term in an array of contexts, there are frequent concerns about inclusion criteria or distribution mechanisms that effectively exclude migrants, young and multiparous women, about staff charging informal fees once at the facilities, and about the struggle to maintain quality of care under greater demand. Unsurprisingly, the programmes that have successfully promoted uptake of specific maternity care services using cash or voucher incentives, such as Nepal's Safe Delivery Incentive Programme and Bangladesh's Maternal Health Voucher Scheme, are those which were carefully designed with adequate scope (in terms of programme eligibility, payment size and timing, or services and goods to which they provide entitlement) to properly address maternal and newborn health aims, were well-supported in communities and/or which operated within effective healthcare systems.

Table 2 Summary of key findings from quantitative studies on short-term cash payments and cash transfers

Programme	Effect on care-seeking outcomes[a]	Key findings from synthesis of factors influencing implementation	
		Enablers	Barriers
Conditional cash transfers			
Comunidades Solidarias Rurales, El Salvador	Increased skilled birth attendance and facility births. No effect on antenatal care and postnatal care	-Awareness generation during monthly meetings [19] -Concurrent investments in health facility infrastructure and recruitment of health workers [19] -Payments made to women (not their husbands) [19]	None stated
Mi Familia Progresa, Guatemala	Increased antenatal care. No effect on facility births	-Concurrent investments in health facility infrastructure and recruitment of health workers [20]	None stated
Programa de Asignación Familia, Honduras	Increased antenatal care. No effect on postnatal care	-Conditionalities to submit paperwork at health facilities [21]	-Poor awareness among women of programme conditionalities [21]
Muthulakshmi Reddy Maternity Benefit Scheme, India	Associated with use of public facilities for antenatal care and childbirth	-Increased total amount of payments [22]	-Delays in receipt of money for women [22] -Overly bureaucratic process for determining eligibility [22] -Eligibility criteria that restrict payments to women for her first or second live birth [22]
Program Keluarga Harapan, Indonesia	Increased antenatal and postnatal care. Mixed picture of positive and no effect on skilled birth attendance. No effect on facility births	-Awareness generation by community-based workers [24]	-Poor awareness of the programme among target groups [24] -Delays in receipt of money for women [24] -Failure to implement verification systems to penalise households that do not meet conditionalities [24] -Poor availability of midwives [26] -High start-up costs [24]
Oportunidades, Mexico	Mixed picture of positive and no effect on skilled birth attendance. No effect on antenatal care	-Awareness generation during monthly meetings [28, 29]	-Perceived poor behaviour of staff at participating hospitals [33] -Attitudes towards formal maternity care services of family members who do not attend monthly meetings [34] -Distance to participating facilities [33] -Cost of travel to health facilities [33] -Lack of concurrent investment in health facilities [28, 29]
Plan de Atención Nacional a la Emergencia Social (PANES), Uruguay	Increased antenatal care. No effect on skilled attendance at birth.	-Conditionalities for antenatal care were not enforced [35]	-Conditionalities for antenatal care were not enforced [35]
Unconditional cash transfers			
Child Grant Programme, Zambia	No effect on skilled birth attendance or antenatal care	None stated	-Lack of concurrent investment in health facilities [36]
Short-term cash payments			
CHIMACA programme, China	No effect on antenatal care or postnatal care	None stated	-Payment too small [37] -Overly difficult process for claiming money [37]
Janani Suraksha Yojana, India	Increased skilled birth attendance and facility births. Mixed picture of positive, negative and no	-Awareness generation by community-based workers [38, 39]	-Poor awareness of the programme among target groups [63]

Table 2 Summary of key findings from quantitative studies on short-term cash payments and cash transfers *(Continued)*

	effect on antenatal care and postnatal care	-Round-the-clock opening of health facilities [38, 60] -Emergency transport programmes [62] -Accreditation of remote health facilities to reduce travel distances [55] -Active involvement of state and district officials [55] -Detailed implementation plans [38]	-Distance and lack of transport to participating facilities [55, 60] -Payments not made until after childbirth, thereby reducing incentive for antenatal care [55, 62] -Delays in receipt of money for women [39, 51, 55, 60, 63] -Demands for additional or informal payments [39, 60, 63] -Perceived poor quality of care at participating facilities [39] -Overly bureaucratic process for determining eligibility [55] -Inappropriate proxy measures of poverty, such as caste [38] -Women who travel to another area to give birth [51] -Delays in recruitment of community-based workers [39] -Poor awareness of the existence of community-based workers [63] -Delays in payments for community-based workers [55] -Increased workloads and reduced quality of care at participating health facilities [55, 62, 63] -Lack of trained midwives [62] -Existence of a similar programme – the National Maternity Benefit Scheme [55]
Safe Delivery Incentive Programme, Nepal	Increased antenatal care. Mixed picture of positive or no effect on skilled birth attendance and facility births	-Awareness generation by women's groups in communities [77] -Lack of geographical barriers in the study district [77] -Universal eligibility [77] -Output-based reimbursements for providers [77]	-Poor awareness of the programme among target groups [77] -Delays in receipt of money for women [77] -Payments not sufficient to cover treatment costs [77] -Demands for additional or informal payments [77] -Overly difficult process for claiming money [77] -Confusion amongst health workers and officials regarding eligibility criteria, sharing of health worker incentives and payment mechanisms for women [77]
SURE-P programme, Nigeria	No effect on skilled birth attendance or antenatal care	-Prompt payments to pregnant women [78] -Defined roles and contracts for local banks and for organisations that will develop information systems [78] -Concurrent programmes to expand availability of maternity care services [78]	-Increased workload at participating health facilities [78] -High start-up costs including research, advocacy, development of information systems, recruitment of workers for data collection and the logistics and security of payments to pregnant women [78]

[a]See systematic review for further details of effect on care-seeking outcomes [14]

Research is still needed in a number of areas and the opportunity to update our original systematic review has reminded us of the narrow range of issues and indicators included in many evaluations of DSF programmes. Review papers on this topic are at risk of tunnel vision as a result. It is our considered view that after almost 15 years of evaluating DSF schemes there are some questions about the DSF approach which are important but rarely posed. For example, we found no evaluations that attempted to gauge the

Table 3 Summary of key findings from quantitative studies on vouchers

Programme	Effect on care-seeking outcomes [a]	Key findings from synthesis of factors influencing implementation	
		Enablers	Barriers
Vouchers for maternity care services			
Maternal Health Voucher Scheme, Bangladesh	Increased skilled birth attendance, facility births, antenatal care and postnatal care	-Activities by community workers and local leaders to raise awareness of the programme [81] -Inclusion of transport costs [80, 81] -'Seed' funds for participating facilities to promote investment in services and capacity [81]	-Perceived poor quality of care at participating facilities [81] -Pressure from local politicians to distribute vouchers to ineligible women [81]
Pilot vouchers, Bangladesh	Increased skilled birth attendance, facility births, antenatal care and postnatal care	-Inclusion of transport and medicine costs [85]	-Poor awareness of the programme among target groups [85] -Perceived poor quality of care at participating facilities [85]
Voucher programme, Cambodia	Increased skilled birth attendance and postnatal care. No effect on antenatal care.	-Awareness generation by voucher distributors [87] -Output-based reimbursements for providers [87]	None stated
Chiranjeevi Yojana, India	No effect on skilled birth attendance, antenatal care and postnatal care	-Community health workers provided information on the programme [88] -Use of an existing government system ('below poverty line' cards) as a targeting mechanism [88]	-Poor awareness of the programme among target groups [89] -Distance to participating facilities in rural areas [88] -Cost of transportation [92] -Demands for additional or informal payments [88, 92] -Providers not reimbursed for postnatal care [88] -Provider attrition in urban areas [89] -Waning political commitment [89]
Vouchers for Health, Kenya	Increased skilled birth attendance and facility births. No effect on antenatal care and postnatal care	-Awareness generation by voucher distributors and previous service users [99] -Locally appropriate tool for targeting pregnant women from low-income households [99] -Output-based reimbursements for providers [94]	-Perceived poor behaviour of staff at participating hospitals [94] -Distance and lack of transport to participating facilities [96, 100] -Cost of travel to health facilities [99, 100] -Cost of purchasing vouchers [96, 100] -Overly bureaucratic process for determining eligibility [94] -Delays in contract signing and voucher printing [99]
Pilot vouchers, Pakistan	Increased facility births. Mixed picture of positive and no effect on antenatal and postnatal care	-Awareness generation by voucher distributors [103, 104]	-Many women left the facility within 24 h after giving birth as there was no one to look after their homes and children [103] -Distance to participating facilities [104]
Makerere University Voucher Scheme, Uganda	Increased facility births	-Inclusion of transport costs [107] -Output-based reimbursements for providers [107]	None stated
HealthyBaby vouchers, Uganda	Increased facility births, antenatal care and postnatal care	-Locally appropriate tool for targeting pregnant women from low-income households [106]	-Turnover of staff in the Ministry of Health [106] -Cost of travel to health facilities [106] -Procedural burden of fraud detection system [106]

Table 3 Summary of key findings from quantitative studies on vouchers *(Continued)*

			-Inclusion (based on geographical needs) of facilities that did not meet minimum quality requirements [106]
Vouchers for merit goods			
Tanzanian National Voucher Scheme	Increased use of insecticide-treated nets	-Awareness generation by service providers [109]	-Distribution of vouchers during antenatal care visits misses women who do not seek formal antenatal care [109] -Cost of purchasing insecticide-treated net (even at a reduced rate) [109]

[a]See systematic review for further details of effect on care-seeking outcomes [14]

experience of coercion when birth in a health facility becomes a conditionality for women to receive state welfare payments. There is comparatively little evidence on the implementation of unconditional cash transfers as part of maternal and neonatal health programmes, despite growing interest in these within the international development community. Similarly, comparative research on alternative forms of financing, such as health equity funds, would provide useful insights. Furthermore, research on policy processes and the reasons for introducing DSF schemes rather than efforts to remove user fees or improve supply-side quality of care could also help to generate understanding of the role of these initiatives, how they become sustainable and where they fit (or do not fit) with plans to achieve equitable universal health coverage.

Abbreviations
ASHA: Accredited social health activists; DSF: Demand-side financing; EPHPP: Effective Public Health Practice Project; GIZ: German Agency for International Cooperation; HIV: Human immunodeficiency virus; PANES: Plan de Atención Nacional a la Emergencia Social; SURE: Supporting the Use of Research Evidence framework; USD: US dollars

Acknowledgements
We thank Helen Smith (Liverpool School of Tropical Medicine) and Anayda Portela (World Health Organization) for coordinating this series and for their feedback on this article. The linked systematic review was an update of an earlier review that was commissioned and funded by the Australian Agency for International Development and assisted by the Joanna Briggs Institute. We thank Debra Bick (King's College London), Ramila Bisht (Jawaharlal Nehru University) and Tim Ensor (University of Leeds) for their extensive work on that earlier review.

Funding
This article and the linked systematic review were funded by the World Health Organization's Department of Maternal, Newborn, Child and Adolescent Health as part of a series of reviews on health promotion interventions.

Authors' contributions
Both authors contributed equally to the study design and data analysis. BMH prepared the first draft and revised subsequent versions, and SFM contributed to the writing of all drafts. Both authors gave final approval for the paper to be published, and are accountable for all aspects of the work.

Consent for publication
Not applicable

Competing interests
The authors declare that they have no competing interests.

References
1. Bohren MA, Hunter EC, Munthe-Kaas HM, Souza JP, Vogel JP, Gulmezoglu AM. Facilitators and barriers to facility-based delivery in low- and middle-income countries: a qualitative evidence synthesis. Reprod Health. 2014;11:71.
2. Thaddeus S, Maine D. Too far to walk: maternal mortality in context. Soc Sci Med. 1994;38:1091–110.
3. Borghi J, Ensor T, Somanathan A, Lissner C, Mills A. Mobilising financial resources for maternal health. Lancet. 2006;368:1457–65.
4. Ensor T, Cooper S. Overcoming barriers to health service access: influencing the demand side. Health Policy Plan. 2004;19:69–79.
5. Krishna A. One illness away : why people become poor and how they escape poverty. Oxford: Oxford University Press; 2010.
6. Murray SF, Hunter B, Bisht R, Ensor T, Bick D. Demand-side financing measures to increase maternal health service utilisation and improve health outcomes: a systematic review of evidence from low- and middle-income countries. Joanna Briggs Institute Library of Systematic Reviews. 2012;10:4165–567.
7. Murray SF, Hunter BM, Bisht R, Ensor T, Bick D. Effects of demand-side financing on utilisation, experiences and outcomes of maternity care in low- and middle-income countries: a systematic review. BMC Pregnancy Childbirth. 2014;14:30.
8. Bellows NM, Bellows BW, Warren C. The use of vouchers for reproductive health services in developing countries: systematic review. Tropical Med Int Health. 2011;16:84–96.
9. Glassman A, Duran D, Fleisher L, Singer D, Sturke R, Angeles G, Charles J, Emrey B, Gleason J, Mwebsa W, Saldana K, Yarrow K, Koblinsky M. Impact of conditional cash transfers on maternal and newborn health. J Health Popul Nutr. 2013;31:48–66.

10. Gopalan SS, Mutasa R, Friedman J, Das A. Health sector demand-side financial incentives in low- and middle-income countries: a systematic review on demand- and supply-side effects. Soc Sci Med. 2014;100:72–83.
11. Lagarde M, Haines A, Palmer N. Conditional cash transfers for improving uptake of health interventions in low- and middle-income countries: a systematic review. JAMA. 2007;298:1900–10.
12. Meyer C, Bellows N, Campbell M, Potts M: The Impact of Vouchers on the Use and Quality of Health Goods and Services in Developing Countries: A systematic review 2011; 2011.
13. Brody CM, Bellows N, Campbell M, Potts M. The impact of vouchers on the use and quality of health care in developing countries: a systematic review. Glob Public Health. 2013;8:363–88.
14. Hunter BM, Portela A, Bick D. The effects of cash transfers and vouchers on the use and quality of maternity care services: a systematic review. PLoS One. 2017;12(3):e0173068.
15. Joanna Briggs Institute: JBI SUMARI. 2015.http://joannabriggs.org/sumari.html. Accessed 21 Jan 2015.
16. The SURE Collaboration. SURE Guides for Preparing and Using Evidence-Based Policy Briefs: identifying and addressing barriers to implementing policy options. Geneva: World Health Organization; 2011.
17. Guanais FC. The combined effects of the expansion of primary health care and conditional cash transfers on infant mortality in Brazil, 1998-2010. Am J Public Health. 2013;103:2000–6.
18. Shei A. Brazil's conditional cash transfer program associated with declines in infant mortality rates. Health Aff. 2013;32:1274–81.
19. De Brauw A, Peterman A: Can Conditional Cash Transfers Improve Maternal Health and Birth Outcomes? 2011. Washington D. C.: International Food Policy Research Institute (IFPRI); 2011.
20. Gutierrez JP: Evaluacion Externa de Impacto del Programa de Transferencias Monetarias Condicionadas: Mi Familia Progresa. 2011. Washington D.C.: Banco Interamericano de Desarrollo; 2011.
21. Morris SS, Flores R, Olinto P, Medina JM. Monetary incentives in primary health care and effects on use and coverage of preventive health care interventions in rural Honduras: cluster randomised trial. Lancet. 2004;364:2030–7.
22. Balasubramanian P, Ravindran TKS. Pro-poor maternity benefit schemes and rural women findings from Tamil Nadu. Econ Polit Wkly. 2012;47:19–22.
23. Public Health Resource Network: Towards Universalisation of Maternity Entitlements: An Exploratory Case Study of the Dr. Muthulakshmi Maternity Assistance Scheme, Tamil Nadu. 2010. New Delhi, India: Public Health Resource Network; 2010.
24. Alatas V, Cahyadi N, Ekasari E, Harmoun S, Hidayat B, Janz E, Jellema J, Tuhiman H, Wai-Poi M. Program Keluarga Harapan: main findings from the impact evaluation of Indonesia's pilot household conditional cash transfer program. 2011. New York: World Bank; 2011.
25. Febriany V, Toyamah N, Sodo J, Budiyati S: Qualitative Impact Study for PNPM-Generasi and PKH on the Provision and the Utilization of the Maternal and Child Health Services and Basic Education Services in the Provinces of West Java and East Nusa Tenggara. Jakarta, Indonesia: The SMERU Research Institute; 2011.
26. Triyana M: Do Health Care Providers Respond to Demand-Side Incentives? Evidence from Indonesia 2014. Chicago, IL: University of Chicago; 2014.
27. Barber SL. Mexico's conditional cash transfer programme increases cesarean section rates among the rural poor. Eur J Pub Health. 2010;20:383–8.
28. Barber SL, Gertler PJ. The impact of Mexico's conditional cash transfer programme, Oportunidades, on birthweight. Tropical Med Int Health. 2008;13:1405–14.
29. Barber SL, Gertler PJ. Empowering women to obtain high quality care: evidence from an evaluation of Mexico's conditional cash transfer programme. Health Policy Plan. 2009;24:18–25.
30. Barham T. A healthier start: the effect of conditional cash transfers on neonatal and infant mortality in rural Mexico. J Dev Econ. 2011;94:74–85.
31. Hernandez Prado B, Ramirez D, Moreno H, Laird N. In: Hernandez Prado B, Cuernavaca HAM, editors. Evaluación del impacto de Oportunidades en la mortalidad materna e infantil In Evaluación externa de impacto del Programa Oportunidades 2003. Mexico: Instituto Nacional de Salud Pública; 2004a.
32. Hernandez Prado B, Salomon JEU, Villalobos MDR, Figueroa JL. Impact of Oportunidades on the reproductive health of its beneficiary population. External Evaluation of the Impact of the Human Development Program Oportunidades 2004b. Cuernavaca, Mexico: Instituto Nacional de Salud Publica; 2004b.
33. Sosa-Rubâi SG, Walker D, Servâan E, Bautista-Arredondo S. Learning effect of a conditional cash transfer programme on poor rural women's selection of delivery care in Mexico. Health Policy Plan. 2011;26:496–507.
34. Urquieta J, Angeles G, Mroz T, Lamadrid-Figueroa H, Hernández B. Impact of oportunidades on skilled attendance at delivery in rural areas. Econ Dev Cult Chang. 2009;57:539–58.
35. Amarante V, Manacorda M, Miguel E, Vigorito A: Do Cash Transfers Improve Birth Outcomes? Evidence from Matched Vital Statistics, Social Security and Program Data 2011. Cambridge, MA: National Bureau of Economic Research; 2011.
36. Handa S, Peterman A, Seidenfeld D, Tembo G. Income transfers and maternal health: evidence from a national randomized social cash transfer program in Zambia. Health Econ. 2015;
37. Hemminki E, Long Q, Zhang W-H, Wu Z, Raven J, Tao F, Yan H, Wang Y, Klemetti R, Zhang T, Regushevskaya E, Tang S. Impact of financial and educational interventions on maternity care: results of cluster randomized trials in rural China, CHIMACA. Maternal & Child Health Journal. 2013;17:208–21.
38. Amudhan S, Mani K, Rai SK, Pandav CS, Krishnan A. Effectiveness of demand and supply side interventions in promoting institutional deliveries–a quasi-experimental trial from rural north India. Int J Epidemiol. 2013;42:769–80.
39. Carvalho N, Thacker N, Gupta SS, Salomon JA. More evidence on the impact of India's conditional cash transfer program, Janani Suraksha Yojana: quasi-experimental evaluation of the effects on childhood immunization and other reproductive and child health outcomes. PLoS One. 2014;9
40. Chaturvedi S, De Costa A, Raven J. Does the Janani Suraksha Yojana cash transfer programme to promote facility births in India ensure skilled birth attendance? A qualitative study of intrapartum care in Madhya Pradesh. Glob Health Action. 2015;8:27427–7.
41. Chaturvedi S, Randive B. In Reaching the Unreached: Rapid Assessment Studies of Health Programmes Implementation in India. In: Hagopian A, House P, Das A, editors. Are arrangements for public private partnerships for emergency obstetric care services adequate under JSY? A study in Ahmednagar District, Maharashtra. New Delhi: Nidhi Books; 2009.
42. Chaturvedi S, Randive B. Public private partnerships for emergency obstetric care: lessons from Maharashtra. Indian J Community Med. 2011;36:21–6.
43. Chaturvedi S, Upadhyay S, De Costa A, Raven J. Implementation of the partograph in India's JSY cash transfer programme for facility births: a mixed methods study in Madhya Pradesh province. BMJ Open. 2015;5:e006211–1.
44. Coffey D. Costs and consequences of a cash transfer for hospital births in a rural district of Uttar Pradesh, India. Soc Sci Med. 2014;114:89–96.
45. Dasgupta J. Experiences with Janani Suraksha Yojana in Uttar Pradesh: analysis of case studies by SAHAYOG and partners Reviewing Two Years of NRHM 2007. Centre for Health and Social Justice: New Delhi; 2007.
46. Devadasan N, Elias MA, John D, Grahacharya S, Ralte L. A conditional cash assistance programme for promoting institutional deliveries among the poor in India: process evaluation results. Health Services Organisation & Policy. 2008;24:257–73.
47. Gopalan SS, Durairaj V. Addressing maternal healthcare through demand side financial incentives: experience of Janani Suraksha Yojana program in India. BMC Health Serv Res. 2012;12:319–9.
48. Gupta A. Study of maternal health Care Services for the Rural Poor in Bihar Reviewing Two Years of NRHM 2007. New Delhi: Centre for Health and Social Justice; 2007.
49. Hangmi PZM, Kuki J. In Reaching the Unreached: Rapid Assessment Studies of Health Programmes Implementation in India. In: Hagopian A, House P, Das A, editors. Role of JSY in institutional delivery. A study in Churachandpur District, Manipur. New Delhi: Nidhi Books; 2009.
50. Human Rights Watch. No tally of the anguish: accountability in maternal health care in India. New York: Human Rights Watch; 2009.
51. Joshi S, Sivaram A. Does it pay to deliver? An evaluation of India's safe motherhood program. World Dev. 2014;64:434–47.
52. Khan ME, Hazra A, Bhatnagar I. Impact of Janani Suraksha Yojana on selected family health behaviours in rural Uttar Pradesh. J Fam Welf. 2010;56
53. Krishna A, Ananthpur K. Reasons for seeking (and not seeking) institutional health care: a qualitative examination in 12 villages of Karnataka. 2011. Durham, NC: Working Paper, Sanford School of Public Policy, Duke University; 2011.
54. Kumar D, Manisha Dwivedi A. In Reaching the Unreached: Rapid Assessment Studies of Health Programmes Implementation in India. In: Hagopian A, House P, Das A, editors. Has Janani Suraksha Yojana stimulated institutional delivery? A study in Una district of Himachal Pradesh. New Delhi: Nidhi Books; 2009.

55. Lim SS, Dandona L, Hoisington JA, James SL, Hogan MC, Gakidou E. India's Janani Suraksha Yojana, a conditional cash transfer programme to increase births in health facilities: an impact evaluation. Lancet. 2010;375:2009–23.
56. Lodh A, Haque M, Singh P, Singh Dipu D, Kumar S, Bhatia GP. In Reaching the Unreached: Rapid Assessment Studies of Health Programmes Implementation in India. In: Hagopian A, House P, Das A, editors. To what extent are ASHAs able to perform their assigned roles? A study of Muzaffarpur District in Bihar. New Delhi: Nidhi Books; 2009.
57. Mazumdar S, Powell-Jackson T, Mills A. Financial incentives in health: new evidence from India's Janani Suraksha Yojana. 2012. London: Working paper, London School of Hygiene & Tropical Medicine; 2012.
58. Nandan D, Malini S, Tripathy RM, Khatter P, Nair KS, Tekhre YL, Dhar N. A rapid appraisal on functioning of Janani Suraksha Yojana in South Orissa. 2008. New Delhi: National Institute of Health and Family Welfare; 2008.
59. Nandan D, Mohapatra B, Datta U, Gupta S, Tiwari VK, Nair KS, Adhish V. An assessment of functioning and impact of Janani Suraksha Yojana in Orissa. 2008. National Institute of Health and Family Welfare: New Delhi; 2008.
60. Purohit N, Mehra V, Govil D. Tracking benefits of Janani Suraksha Yojana-a maternal cash transfer scheme: evidence from Rajasthan, India. J Health Manag. 2014;16:289–302.
61. Rai SK, Dasgupta R, Das MK, Singh S, Devi R, Arora NK. Determinants of utilization of services under MMJSSA scheme in Jharkhand 'Client Perspective': a qualitative study in a low performing state of India. Indian J Public Health. 2012;55:254–9.
62. Randive B, Diwan V, De Costa A. India's conditional cash transfer Programme (the JSY) to promote institutional birth: is there an association between institutional birth proportion and maternal mortality? PLoS One. 2013;8:e67452–2.
63. Santhya KG, Jejeeboy SJ, Acharya R, Francis Zavier AJ. Effects of the Janani Suraksha Yojana on maternal and newborn care practices: women's experiences in Rajasthan. 2011. Population Council: New Delhi; 2011.
64. Santhya KG, Jejeeboy SJ, Francis Zavier AJ. Implementing the Janani Suraksha Yojana: perspectives and experiences of accredited social health activists in Rajasthan. 2011b. Population Council: New Delhi; 2011b.
65. Singh S, Chaturvedi R. Meeting the health needs of the poor: social audit in Uttar Pradesh. Reviewing Two Years of NRHM 2007. New Delhi: Centre for Health and Social Justice; 2007.
66. Sri BS, NS Khanna R. An investigation of maternal deaths following public protests in a tribal district of Madhya Pradesh, central India. Reproductive Health Matters. 2012;20:11–20.
67. Uttekar BP, Barge S, Deshpande Y, Uttekar V, Sharma J, Shahane S. Assessment of Janani Suraksha Yojana in Himanchal Pradesh. Vadodara, Gujarat: Centre for Operations Research & Training; 2007a.
68. Uttekar BP, Barge S, Khan W, Deshpande Y, Uttekar V, Sharma J, Chakrawar B, Shahane S. Assessment of ASHA and Janani Suraksha Yojana in Rajasthan. Vadodara, Gujarat: Centre for Operations Research & Training; 2007d.
69. Uttekar BP, Kumar N, Uttekar V, Sharma J, Shahane S: Assessment of Janani Suraksha Yojana in Assam. 2007e. Vadodara, Gujarat: Centre for Operations Research & Training; 2007e.
70. Uttekar BP, Kumar N, Uttekar V, Sharma J, Shahane S. Assessment of Janani avam Bal Suraksha Yojana in Bihar. Vadodara, Gujarat: Centre for Operations Research & Training; 2008b.
71. Uttekar BP, Uttekar V, Chakrawar B, Sharma J, Shahane S. Assessment of Janani Suraksha Yojana in West Bengal. Vadodara, Gujarat: Centre for Operations Research & Training; 2007b.
72. Uttekar BP, Uttekar V, Chakrawar BB, Sharma J, Shahane S. Assessment of ASHA and Janani Suraksha Yojana in Orissa. Vadodara, Gujarat: Centre for Operations Research & Training; 2007c.
73. Uttekar BP, Uttekar V, Chakrawar BB, Sharma J, Shahane S. Assessment of Janani Suraksha Yojana in Uttar Pradesh. Vadodara, Gujarat: Centre for Operations Research & Training; 2008a.
74. Vora KS: Implementation of Janani Suraksha Yojana and other maternal health policies in two Indian states: predictors of maternal health service utilization among poor rural women. 2012.
75. Powell-Jackson T, Hanson K. Financial incentives for maternal health: impact of a national programme in Nepal. J Health Econ. 2012;31:271–84.
76. Powell-Jackson T, Morrison J, Tiwari S, Neupane BD, Costello AM. The experiences of districts in implementing a national incentive programme to promote safe delivery in Nepal. BMC Health Serv Res. 2009;9:97.
77. Powell-Jackson T, Neupane BD, Tiwari S, Tumbahangphe K, Manandhar D, Costello AM. The impact of Nepal's national incentive programme to promote safe delivery in the district of Makwanpur. Adv Health Econ Health Serv Res. 2009;21:221–49.
78. Okoli U, Morris L, Oshin A, Pate MA, Aigbe C, Muhammad A. Conditional cash transfer schemes in Nigeria: potential gains for maternal and child health service uptake in a national pilot programme. BMC Pregnancy And Childbirth. 2014;14:408–8.
79. Ahmed S, Khan MM. A maternal health voucher scheme: what have we learned from the demand-side financing scheme in Bangladesh? Health Policy Plan. 2011;26:25–32.
80. Ahmed S, Khan MM. Is demand-side financing equity enhancing? Lessons from a maternal health voucher scheme in Bangladesh. Soc Sci Med. 2011;72:1704–10.
81. Hatt L, Nguyen H, Sloan N, Miner S, Magvanjav O, Sharma A, Chowdhury J, Chowdhury R, Paul D, Islam M, Wang H. Economic Evaluation of Demand-Side Financing (DSF) for Maternal Health in Bangladesh. In: *Review, Analysis and Assessment of Issues Related to Health Care Financing and Health Economics in Bangladesh* 2010. Bethesda, MD: Abt Associates; 2010.
82. Koehlmoos TLP, Ashraf A, Kabir H, Islam Z, Gazi R, Saha NC, Khyang J: Rapid Assessment of Demand-side Financing Experiences in Bangladesh. 2008. Dhaka: International Centre for Diarrhoeal Disease Research, Bangladesh (ICDDR,B); 2008.
83. Nguyen H, Hatt L, Islam M, Sloan N, Chowdhury J, Schmidt J-O, Hossain A, Wang H. Encouraging maternal health service utilization: an evaluation of the Bangladesh voucher program. Soc Sci Med. 2012;74:989–96.
84. Reproductive Health Vouchers Evaluation Team. The reproductive health vouchers program in Bangladesh. Summary of findings from baseline evaluation survey, Working draft. Population Council. 2011;2011
85. Rob U, Rahman M, Bellows B. Using vouchers to increase access to maternal healthcare in Bangladesh. Int Q Community Health Educ. 2009;30:293–309.
86. Ir P, Horemans D, Souk N, Van Damme W. Using targeted vouchers and health equity funds to improve access to skilled birth attendants for poor women: a case study in three rural health districts in Cambodia. BMC Pregnancy Childbirth. 2010;10
87. Van de Poel E, Flores G, Ir P, O'Donnell O, van Doorslaer E. Can vouchers deliver? An evaluation of subsidies for maternal health care in Cambodia. Bull World Health Organ. 2014;92:331–9.
88. Bhat R, Mavalankar DV, Singh PV, Singh N. Maternal healthcare financing: Gujarat's Chiranjeevi scheme and its beneficiaries. J Health Popul Nutr. 2009;27:249–58.
89. De Costa A, Vora KS, Ryan K, Sankara Raman P, Santacatterina M, Mavalankar D. The state-led large scale public private partnership 'Chiranjeevi Program' to increase access to institutional delivery among poor women in Gujarat, India: how has it done? What can we learn? PLoS One. 2014;9:e95704.
90. Ganguly P, Jehan K, de Costa A, Mavalankar D, Smith H. Considerations of private sector obstetricians on participation in the state led "Chiranjeevi Yojana" scheme to promote institutional delivery in Gujarat. India: a qualitative study *BMC Pregnancy Childbirth*. 2014;14:352.
91. Jega FM. Contracting out to improve maternal health: evaluating the quality of care under the Chiranjeevi Yojana in Gujarat, India. International Health Group: University of Liverpool; 2007.
92. Mohanan M, Bauhoff S, La Forgia G, Babiarz KS, Singh K, Miller G. Effect of Chiranjeevi Yojana on institutional deliveries and neonatal and maternal outcomes in Gujarat, India: a difference-in-differences analysis. Bull World Health Organ. 2014;92:187–94.
93. Abuya T, Njuki R, Warren CE, Okal J, Obare F, Kanya L, Askew I, Bellows B. A policy analysis of the implementation of a reproductive health vouchers program in Kenya. BMC Public Health. 2012;12:540.
94. Amendah DD, Mutua MK, Kyobutungi C, Buliva E, Bellows B. Reproductive health voucher program and facility based delivery in informal settlements in Nairobi: a longitudinal analysis. PLoS One. 2013;8:e80582–2.
95. Arur A, Gitonga N, O'Hanlon B, Kundu F, Senkaali M, Ssemujji R: Insights from innovations: lessons from designing and implementing family planning/reproductive health voucher programs in Kenya and Uganda. 2009: Abt Associates Inc.; 2009.
96. Bellows B, Kyobutungi C, Mutua MK, Warren C, Ezeh A. Increase in facility-based deliveries associated with a maternal health voucher programme in informal settlements in Nairobi. Health Policy Plan: Kenya; 2012.
97. Njuki R, Abuya T, Kimani J, Kanya L, Korongo A, Mukanya C, Bracke P, Bellows B, Warren CE. Does a voucher program improve reproductive health service delivery and access in Kenya? Health policies, systems and management. BMC Health Serv Res. 2015;15

98. Njuki R, Obare F, Warren C, Abuya T, Okal J, Mukuna W, Kanya L, Askew I, Bracke P, Bellows B. Community experiences and perceptions of reproductive health vouchers in Kenya. BMC Public Health. 2013;13:660.
99. Obare F, Warren C, Abuya T, Askew I, Bellows B. Assessing the population-level impact of vouchers on access to health facility delivery for women in Kenya. Soc Sci Med. 2014;102:183–9.
100. Obare F, Warren C, Njuki R, Abuya T, Sunday J, Askew I, Bellows B. Community-level impact of the reproductive health vouchers programme on service utilization in Kenya. Health Policy Plan. 2012;
101. Reproductive Health Vouchers Evaluation Team. The reproductive health vouchers program in Kenya. Summary of findings from program evaluation. Population Council. 2011:2011.
102. Watt C, Abuya T, Warren CE, Obare F, Kanya L, Bellows B. Can reproductive health voucher programs improve quality of postnatal care? A quasi-experimental evaluation of Kenya's safe motherhood voucher scheme. PLoS One. 2015;10:e0122828–8.
103. Agha S. Changes in the proportion of facility-based deliveries and related maternal health services among the poor in rural Jhang, Pakistan: results from a demand-side financing intervention. Int J Equity Health. 2011a;10
104. Agha S. Impact of a maternal health voucher scheme on institutional delivery among low income women in Pakistan. Reprod Health. 2011b;8
105. Okal J, Kanya L, Obare F, Njuki R, Abuya T, Bange T, Warren C, Askew I, Bellows B. An assessment of opportunities and challenges for public sector involvement in the maternal health voucher program in Uganda. Health Res Policy Syst. 2013;11:38.
106. Reproductive Health Vouchers Evaluation Team. The reproductive health vouchers program in Uganda. Summary of findings from program evaluation. Population Council. 2012:2012.
107. Alfonso YN, Bishai D, Bua J, Mutebi A, Mayora C, Ekirapa-Kiracho E. Cost-effectiveness analysis of a voucher scheme combined with obstetrical quality improvements: quasi experimental results from Uganda. Health Policy Plan. 2015;
108. Pariyo GW, Mayora C, Okui O, Ssengooba F, Peters DH, Serwadda D, Lucas H, Bloom G, Rahman MH, Ekirapa-Kiracho E. Exploring new health markets: experiences from informal providers of transport for maternal health services in eastern Uganda. BMC Int Health Hum Rights. 2011;11:S10.
109. Hanson K, Marchant T, Nathan R, Mponda H, Jones C, Bruce J, Mshinda H, Schellenberg JA. Household ownership and use of insecticide treated nets among target groups after implementation of a National Voucher Programme in the United Republic of Tanzania: plausibility study using three annual cross-sectional household surveys. BMJ. 2009;339:93–6.
110. Koenker HM, Yukich JO, Mkindi A, Mandike R, Brown N, Kilian A, Lengeler C. Analysing and recommending options for maintaining universal coverage with long-lasting insecticidal nets: the case of Tanzania in 2011. Malar J. 2013;12:150–0.
111. Mubyazi GM, Bloch P, Magnussen P, Olsen OE, Byskov J, Hansen KS, Bygbjerg IC. Women's experiences and views about costs of seeking malaria chemoprevention and other antenatal services: a qualitative study from two districts in rural Tanzania. Malaria J. 2010;9
112. Jain N, Srivastava NK, Khan AM, Dhar N, Adhish V, Menon S, Nandan D. Assessment of functioning of ASHA under NRHM in Uttar Pradesh. Health and Population: Perspectives and Issues. 2008;31:132–40.
113. Souza JP, Gülmezoglu AM, Vogel J, Carroli G, Lumbiganon P, Qureshi Z, Costa MJ, Fawole B, Mugerwa Y, Nafiou I, Neves I, Wolomby-Molondo J-J, Bang HT, Cheang K, Chuyun K, Jayaratne K, Jayathilaka CA, Mazhar SB, Mori R, Mustafa ML, Pathak LR, Perera D, Rathavy T, Recidoro Z, Roy M, Ruyan P, Shrestha N, Taneepanichsku S, Tien NV, Ganchimeg T, et al. Moving beyond essential interventions for reduction of maternal mortality (the WHO Multicountry Survey on Maternal and Newborn Health): a cross-sectional study. *The Lancet*. 2013;381:1747–55.

3

A review of measures of women's empowerment and related gender constructs in family planning and maternal health program evaluations in low- and middle-income countries

Mahua Mandal[1*], Arundati Muralidharan[2] and Sara Pappa[3]

Abstract

Background: Evidence suggests that gender-integrated interventions, which actively seek to identify and integrate activities that address the role of gender norms and dynamics, improve family planning (FP) and maternal health (MH). To understand the link between the gender components of interventions and FP and MH outcomes, it is critical to examine the gender measures used in evaluations.

Methods: We conducted a systematic review of evaluations of gender-integrated FP and MH interventions in low- and middle-income countries. We examine characteristics of the interventions and their evaluations, and summarize women's empowerment and related gender measures.

Results: Out of 16 evaluation articles, five reported the theoretical or conceptual model that guided the intervention. Twelve described how gender was quantitatively measured and identified 13 women's empowerment and related gender constructs. Gender scales or indexes were used in five evaluations, three of which noted that their scales had been validated. Less than one third of articles reported examining the effect of gender on FP or MH.

Conclusions: Evaluations of gender-integrated FP and MH interventions do not consistently describe how gender influences FP and MH outcomes or include validated gender measures within their studies. As a result, examining the pathways through which interventions empower women and the manner in which women's empowerment leads to changes in FP and MH outcomes remains a challenge. Valid measures of commonly reported women's empowerment and gender constructs, such as gender-equitable attitudes and women's decision-making power, must be adapted and used within evaluations to examine how empowerment and improvements in gender-related factors can produce positive FP and MH outcomes.

Keywords: Gender measures, Women's empowerment, Gender-integrated health interventions, Family planning, Maternal health, Low- and middle-income countries, Evaluations

* Correspondence: mmandal@email.unc.edu
[1]MEASURE Evaluation, Carolina Population Center, University of North Carolina at Chapel Hill, Chapel Hill, NC, USA
Full list of author information is available at the end of the article

Background

Gender-integrated health interventions actively seek to identify and integrate activities that address the role of gender norms and dynamics. They take into account the potential effect of gender on proposed program objectives and the impact of program results on gender relations. Gender-integrated health interventions include those that are gender transformative and gender accommodating. Gender transformative approaches actively strive to challenge and change gender inequalities while promoting health. These approaches encourage critical awareness of gender roles and norms, challenge the distribution of resources and allocation of responsibilities between men and women, address power relationships between men and women, and promote the position of women. For example, a national policy may require women to be accompanied by their husbands to family planning clinics in order to get contraception. A gender transformative intervention would work to change this policy so that women can access contraception without their husbands' permission or presence. Alternatively, gender accommodating interventions work around inequitable gender norms, roles, and relationships or adjust for these inequalities. While these approaches do not actively seek to change norms and inequalities, they strive to limit the harmful impact of interventions on gender relations and the harmful impact of gender norms and inequalities on health outcomes [1, 2]. Using the same example above, a gender accommodating intervention would increase knowledge of the existing policy among couples in a community and encourage husbands to accompany their wives to clinics so that women can access contraception.

An increasing number of gender-integrated health interventions have been implemented over the past decade to counter deeply rooted gender inequalities in order to improve family planning (FP) and maternal health (MH) outcomes [2, 3]. Concurrently, donors and national governments have focused on evaluating these interventions to determine their level of success and potential for scale-up. Evidence suggests that gender-integrated interventions improve FP and MH outcomes [3]. The Sustainable Development Goals (SGDs), building upon the Millennium Development Goals, provide impetus for continued action on gender equality by tackling inequalities and empowering women and girls. Goal 5 of the SDGs explicitly links gender equality to health and well-being through the key target (target 5.6) to ensure universal access to sexual and reproductive health and rights [4]. Given the greater programmatic attention and global political will to improve gender equality for health, especially women's health, it is necessary to examine how gender is measured, particularly in terms of women's empowerment, when evaluating gender-integrated health interventions. This in turn will help development researchers and practitioners identify and act on the pathways by which empowerment contributes to FP and MH outcomes.

Conceptualizations of women's empowerment often highlight one or more of a series of interconnected concepts of choice, options, control, and power — concepts that allude to "women's ability to make decisions and affect outcomes of importance to themselves and their families" [1]. Keller and Mbewe [5] offer a comprehensive definition of women's empowerment encompassing these concepts: "a process whereby women become able to organize themselves to increase their own self-reliance, to assert their independent right to make choices and to control resources which will assist in challenging and eliminating their own subordination". Other academics have focused on one central concept; for example, Gita Sen's [6] definition centers on altering the balance of power. In the era following the 1994 International Conference on Population and Development in Cairo, which articulated a people-centered approach to development, Kabeer's [7] description of empowerment as "the expansion in people's ability to make strategic life choices in a context where this ability was previously denied to them" has been widely accepted and used. Two salient characteristics of empowerment emerge as common across these definitions: that of empowerment as a process, and that of autonomy or choice.

There are several challenges to measuring women's empowerment. As a multidimensional latent construct, women can be empowered (or disempowered) within five broad dimensions: psychological, social (including familial), economic, legal, and political [8]. Recent work on measures has also attempted to capture empowerment within sexual relationships [9] and around contraceptive use, pregnancy, and childbearing [10], indicating the need to conceptualize a sixth dimension of health empowerment [8]. Recognizing various dimensions of empowerment is important, because empowerment in one dimension does not necessarily indicate empowerment in another [8]. Indicators of women's empowerment can also be organized according to the level or sphere of operation, at individual, household, and aggregate or population levels [4]. For instance, the individual level includes self-esteem and self-efficacy; the household level includes household decision-making and mobility; and at an aggregate level, Malhotra and colleagues identify indicators related to the labor market, education, and political and legal status. As with the six dimensions above, the process of empowerment may operate in some levels and not in others [1].

Women's empowerment is also contextually specific, in both place and time [8]. For example, restrictions on women's mobility, which is a measure of women's empowerment in Demographic and Health Surveys, is a relevant construct in South Asia but not in sub-Saharan Africa [11].

Finally, there is limited understanding of whether and how empowerment and related gender constructs are measured within the context of gender-integrated FP and MH interventions. While published reviews have explored the relationships between women's empowerment and fertility [10], gender-based power and reproductive health outcomes [12], and women's empowerment and maternal and child health [8], we found no reviews of health program evaluations that have examined the measurement of women's empowerment and related gender constructs and their relationship to FP and MH outcomes. This review builds on previous work by examining in depth women's empowerment and related gender measures within outcome and impact evaluations of gender-integrated FP and MH interventions.

Methods

This study draws from a broader, large-scale systematic review examining the influence of gender-integrated interventions on multiple health outcomes in low- and middle-income countries (LMICs) [3]. Using key search terms described elsewhere [3], we searched peer-reviewed and gray literature in electronic databases (e.g., PubMed, Population Information Online (POPLINE), Scopus) and sourced bibliographies (e.g., Bill & Melinda Gates Foundation), organizational websites, and relevant conference websites. The search yielded 2450 documents; 709 were excluded based on a title relevancy check.

To determine final relevancy for the remaining 1741 documents, we used the following inclusion criteria for review: (1) the intervention was gender-integrated, per the Interagency Gender Working Group's Gender Equality Continuum tool [13]; (2) the document was written in English; (3) the intervention was implemented in a LMIC, per the World Bank's definition; (4) methods and results of outcome or impact evaluations were discussed; (5) the intervention took place between January 1, 2008 to June 30, 2013; and (6) the evaluation measured FP or MH outcomes. For this review, we further excluded the gray literature, studies that included qualitative methods only, and evaluations that measured HIV or gender-based violence without also measuring FP or MH outcomes.

Original data abstraction methods are described elsewhere [3]. For this analysis, additional data were abstracted on the following: whether the article included in its theory of change or conceptual framework the role of gender in FP or MH outcomes; whether the evaluation measured a dimension of women's empowerment or other gender construct; the women's empowerment dimensions and related gender constructs measured; the level of operationalization of the construct (individual, couple, service delivery, community); the structure of the gender measures (single items, multi-item scale, multi-item index); whether the measures were validated in the current study or previous studies; and whether the gender measure mediated the relationship between the intervention and main FP or MH outcomes. We first describe the characteristics of the interventions and their evaluations. We then summarize the women's empowerment and related gender measures. Finally, we discuss measurement gaps in current evaluations of gender-integrated FP and MH interventions.

Results

Of the 196 documents from the broader systematic review, 180 documents were excluded because they did not fit the inclusion criteria for this review (Fig. 1). The resulting 16 articles describe evaluations of six transformative interventions [14–19] and ten accommodating interventions [20–29] (Table 1). The evaluations were

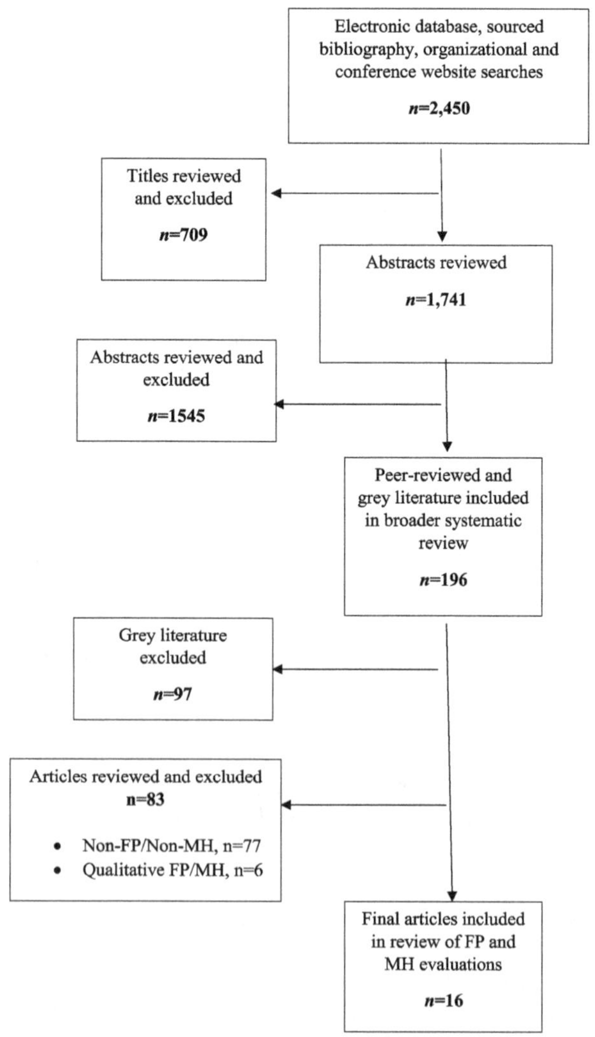

Fig. 1 Flow chart of literature search

Table 1 Women's empowerment constructs by level of operation and dimension of empowerment

	Women's empowerment dimension			
	Psychological	Social	Economic	Health
Level of operation				
Individual-level constructs				
Confidence/self-esteem	X			
Gender-equitable attitudes (of woman or partner) regarding sexual and reproductive health (SRH)				X
Gender-equitable attitudes (of woman or partner) regarding domestic matters		X		
Couple-level constructs				
Communication around SRH matters				X
SRH decision-making power				X
SRH control				X
Decision-making power regarding social life		X		
Support in pregnancy and health-seeking behaviors				X
Support in childcare and housework		X		
Household-level construct				
Domestic and financial decision-making power		X		
Service-delivery level constructs				
Provider-client interaction				X
Attitudes around women's health				X
Community and societal-level constructs				
Access to safe spaces		X		
Social networks		X		
Economic capabilities and assets			X	
Educational opportunities and participation			X	

conducted mostly by international non-government organizations and span 15 LMICs (Bangladesh, India, Nepal, Pakistan, China, Mexico, El Salvador, Iran, Ethiopia, Tanzania, Malawi, Nigeria, Senegal, Tanzania, and Turkey) (see Fig. 2). Most interventions were implemented in rural areas; four were in urban areas [16, 22, 26, 29] and two in both rural and urban areas [19, 21]. Interventions often focused on women and men, as individuals, to increase knowledge, change attitudes, and improve health-related behaviors. Five interventions focused on individuals [16, 19, 21, 22, 26], and one intervened with couples only [29]. Several interventions engaged influential members of the household [20] and service providers [27, 28] to improve the supportive environment for women and men. Almost half the interventions ($n = 7$) intervened on multiple levels [14, 15, 17, 18, 23–25, 30]. The majority of interventions aimed to improve FP and MH outcomes of married adults. Only two interventions focused

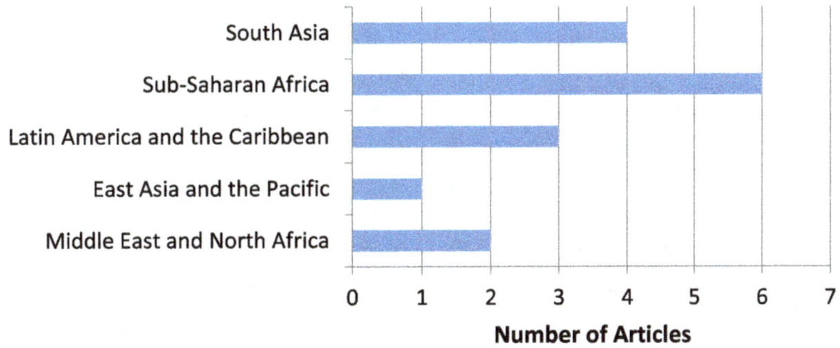

Fig. 2 Distribution of articles by region ($n = 16$)

on adolescents: one intervened with married couples to delay pregnancy and childbearing [14]; another attempted to empower unmarried girls to delay marriage [15].

Few articles (two transformative [18, 19] and three accommodating [20, 23, 29]) reported the theoretical or conceptual model that guided their interventions. Both accommodating interventions were guided by two or more published theories. Theories and conceptual models described include the framework for enabling agentic empowerment; information-motivation-behavioral skills; health-seeking model; tri-sectoral health system; household production of health; theory of reasoned action; health belief model; and three delays model. No article clearly articulated a customized theory of change describing how various components of the intervention worked together in a causal pathway to achieve the intended outcome.

Only one article described its intervention as primarily focused on increasing women's autonomy [21]. While most discussed gender-related constraints and power imbalances that affect access to and use of health services, and described their interventions as either attempting to transform or accommodate prevailing gender norms, they did not explicitly name their interventions as women's empowerment interventions. Despite this, 12 interventions described (either a priori or in the discussion) interventions focused on improving FP and MH through strategies that empower women directly (e.g., education, livelihoods training, social support) [14, 15, 21] or indirectly (e.g., training service providers on respectful interaction with female clients, promoting gender-equitable attitudes, and emphasizing gender equity in decision-making among men) [16, 17, 27]. Three of the 12 were male involvement interventions that included supporting or empowering women through greater male partner engagement in domestic matters such as childcare and household chores [26] or in health matters [25, 26, 29]. Because we included evaluations of all gender-integrated FP and MH interventions (i.e., they were not limited to women's empowerment and health), our review consisted of two additional male involvement interventions that targeted males as the main beneficiaries [18, 24]. These interventions did not describe strategies used to empower women or promote gender equality.

All evaluations collected primary data, and their study designs were considered of high or moderate rigor, per criteria used in the broader systematic review [3]. The majority were randomized control trials or quasi-experimental studies. One study sampled separate cross sections of individuals at baseline and endline in the intervention area only [17]; another compared baseline and endline measures of the same group of individuals in the intervention area only [24]. All but one evaluation [25] collected data at two or more time points.

Half the evaluations measured FP outcomes [14–18, 21, 22, 27], two measured MH outcomes [20, 24], and six measured both FP and MH outcomes [19, 23, 25, 26, 28, 29]. The majority of evaluations of transformative interventions ($n = 5$) examined FP outcomes [14–18]; one examined both FP and MH outcomes [19]. Half of the evaluations of accommodating interventions ($n = 5$) measured both FP and MH outcomes [23, 25, 26, 28, 29], one measured FP outcomes [27], and two measured MH outcomes [23, 25].

Despite describing the prevailing gender norms and dynamics that affect maternal health, two evaluations that used quantitative methods only did not report measurement of women's empowerment or gender indicators [14, 29]. In two evaluations that used mixed methods, gender constructs emerged from the qualitative methods; gender indicators were not quantitatively measured [20, 24].

Our review identified 13 constructs within four dimensions of women's empowerment: psychological, social, economic, and health; with most constructs falling within social and health empowerment. The majority of constructs operate at the individual and couple level. Only one household-level and two service-delivery-level constructs were identified. The remaining three constructs fall within the community and societal levels (Additional file 1). Individual-level measures of women's empowerment were used in evaluations of interventions focused on the individual level [19, 22, 26], service-delivery level [28], and at multiple levels [15, 17, 18, 25]. A couple-level empowerment measure was used in one evaluation of an intervention operating at multiple levels [23]; a service-delivery level measure was used in an evaluation of a service-delivery intervention [27]; and household measures were used in evaluation of two individual-focused interventions [16, 21]. Gender-equitable attitudes, and support in pregnancy and health-seeking behaviors were the only constructs that were measured by more than one article. Less than half ($n = 6$) of articles included a single empowerment or gender construct.

Additionally, male involvement interventions not explicitly designed to empower women measured the following indicators and constructs: men's knowledge of reproductive and maternal health; men's awareness of their wives' use of MH services; attitudes towards gender norms; couple communication around FP; frequency of male communication about FP with partners, extended family, or other men in the community; joint decision-making around FP and MH; and equitable gender norms.

Few studies measuring women's empowerment or related constructs used scales that were validated in that study (e.g., Cronbach's alpha) (Interpersonal Power, Relational Response to Condom Use, Comfort with Sexual Communication, Safer Sex Self-Efficacy) [16, 26] or in previous studies (Gender-Equitable Male scale and Supportive Behavior Questionnaire scale) [18]. One study reported using 13 scales but did not describe them in depth or report whether they were validated [19]. Two studies used indexes: Salutation, Assessment, Help, and Reassurance index [27] and Autonomy index [21]. The remaining studies used individual items or a series of items that were not combined into a composite or sum score. Four evaluations using validated scales or indexes were of FP interventions [16, 18, 21, 27], and one was of a combined FP and MH intervention [26].

Less than one third (n = 5) of studies reported examining the effect of gender on FP or MH outcomes. Four studies examined whether gender mediated the relationship between program participation (the main independent variable) and FP/MH outcomes [16, 18, 21, 27]. One study used separate statistical models to examine the effect of the intervention on the gender variable, and the gender variable on the FP outcome [21]. In two evaluations the gender variables were the same as or embedded within the dependent variable (e.g., men's awareness of their wives' use of antenatal care (ANC), attitudes around husbands participation in FP decisions) [22, 25]; thus, they were unable to examine the effect of women's empowerment or related gender constructs on FP and MH outcomes.

Discussion

Despite restricting articles to gender-integrated interventions evaluations, few studies clearly articulated a hypothesized theory of change or (set of) causal pathway(s) between the intervention components, women's empowerment and related gender constructs, and FP and MH outcomes. Theories of change assist program planners and implementers in conceptualizing and understanding how elements of a program are related to one another and to the final desired outcomes; and they assist evaluators in identifying and mapping the constructs and indicators that should be measured to pre-specified components of the intervention [31]. This is particularly important in evaluations of gender-integrated health interventions, since women's empowerment and related gender constructs are multidimensional, operate at multiple levels, and affect access to services, health behaviors, and health outcomes in complex ways.

While no study included a comprehensive set, in terms of level of operation, of women's empowerment measures, most studies captured, at least partially, its key characteristics: autonomy and empowerment as a process. Measures reflected women's autonomy (e.g., decision-making power, economic capabilities and assets) or determinants of women's autonomy (e.g., confidence/self-esteem). All evaluations except one measured changes over time, or the process of empowerment.

Surprisingly, none of the five evaluations of interventions in South Asia included women's mobility as a measure of empowerment, even though it is a commonly used indicator within research studies in the region [10]. This may be because the FP and MH interventions in the review's three South Asian countries did not attempt to address the lack of mobility as a barrier to FP or MH. Similarly, these evaluations did not include household-level measures of empowerment, even though parents and parents-in-law have substantial influence over a couple's family planning and childbearing practices, and reaching mothers- and fathers-in-laws was a strategy used in one intervention in India [14]. Such an exclusion results in incomplete mapping of the intervention components and strategies to appropriate indicators.

Some male involvement interventions designed to improve health through empowering their female partners also did not properly map indicators to program strategies. For example, the evaluation of an FP program emphasizing gender equality in decision-making among males measured two gender-related indicators: whether men communicated with their wives about FP, and men's attitudes around the role of men and women in FP decision-making. The first indicator measures merely the existence of couple communication and does not provide information regarding the quality of communication. Instances of communication may be characterized by coercion and male dominance rather than gender equality in decision-making. The second indicator more closely measures the desired concept, though it measures attitudes, not actual decision-making behaviors. Instead, the degree of joint decision-making (e.g., if the decisions are made mostly by the man, by the woman, or jointly; or who has the final say) is a more accurate measure of equality in decision-making.

Few articles described using validated measures of women's empowerment and related gender constructs, particularly evaluations of maternal health interventions; and several articles did not measure any gender construct. This finding is in contrast to the body of published studies of HIV and gender-based violence (GBV) program evaluations, which often use the Gender-Equitable Male scale [32–34] and Sexual Relationship Power Scale [35] to measure determinants or dimensions of women's empowerment. The lack of using validated measures in FP and MH interventions may be a result of FP and MH studies not adequately incorporating the latest knowledge from the SRH science base into evaluations of interventions.

Finally, we offer several considerations for the measurement of women's empowerment and related gender constructs for future evaluations of gender-integrated interventions in LMICs. First, in order to measure the most pertinent forms of empowerment in FP and MH interventions, i.e., those related to reproductive health, we recommend that evaluations identify existing reproductive empowerment and related scales that have been developed in more developed countries, such as the Reproductive Autonomy and Reproductive Coercion Scales [36, 37], and test and adapt them to various developing country contexts. Researchers should be cognizant of the applicability and validity of such scales across regions and cultures that vary in their conceptualization of women's empowerment.

Second, given the limited number of interventions focused on adolescents, our review identified few empowerment measures specific to this population. The meaning and process of empowerment, particularly reproductive empowerment, depend on where an individual is in his or her life course, whether he or she is married or in a partnership, and whether a female is pregnant or a mother. Additional empowerment measures should be developed specifically for adolescents who are married, unmarried, nulliparous, pregnant, and mothers to better understand the pathways between adolescents' empowerment and positive FP and MH outcomes.

Third, the majority of existing measures of women's empowerment are at the individual and couple levels. Given that women can be empowered or disempowered at the household, service-delivery, and community and society levels, there is a need to develop measures at these higher levels and to map the level of the measures used in evaluations to the level at which interventions operate. In particular, multiple levels of empowerment measures should be used in evaluations of interventions that are multilevel.

Fourth, we note that our review did not identify measures of policies or laws that encourage women's empowerment or protect women's rights. Given the recent body of work on measuring health and human rights [38–40], we recommend that evaluations of gender-integrated FP and MH interventions take advantage of the momentum to develop measures of policies and laws in order to examine their impact on FP and MH. For example, FP evaluations may consider developing indicators to measure the number, type, and scope of policies and laws that hinder women's rights to FP, including availability, accessibility, acceptability, and quality of contraceptives, and participation in decision-making [41].

Fifth, the FP and MH evaluation field should look to studies of male-focused gender transformative HIV and violence interventions [42, 43] to identify and adapt measures of male engagement and related gender constructs. Measures of normative change among males, including attitudes around gender roles and masculinity, may be particularly important in evaluations of FP and MH interventions that involve men with the explicit purpose of increasing gender equity and women's empowerment.

Next, to measure the added value of gender in a program, evaluations must examine the relationship between participating in the program and a gender construct; and the articulated gender construct and the desired health outcome. This can be done statistically by including gender variables as mediators in regressions models. Psychometric statistical methods, such as structural equation modeling, may be particularly well suited for evaluations of complex interventions that aim to examine the relationship between women's empowerment, other latent constructs, and FP and MH outcomes.

Finally, given the inter-relatedness of different dimensions of empowerment, evaluations may consider including multidimensional scales of empowerment (e.g., economic, social, and reproductive) within single studies. Including a broader construct with multiple women's empowerment dimensions within evaluations can help identify dimensions most malleable and predictive of positive FP and MH outcomes. Program planners and implementers can use the results to further support and improve relevant forms of empowerment in FP and MH interventions and policies.

Conclusions

Evaluations of gender-integrated FP and MH interventions do not consistently describe how gender influences FP and MH outcomes or include validated gender measures within their studies. As a result, examining the pathways through which interventions empower women and the manner in which women's empowerment leads to changes in FP and MH outcomes remains a challenge. Valid measures of commonly reported women's empowerment and gender constructs, such as gender-equitable attitudes and decision-making power, must be adapted and used within evaluations to examine how empowerment and improvements in gender-related factors can produce positive FP and MH outcomes.

Open peer review

Peer review reports for this article are available in Additional file 2.

Abbreviations

FP: Family planning; HIV: Human immunodeficiency virus; LMIC: Low- and middle-income countries; MH: Maternal and child health; SDG: Sustainable development goal; USAID: United States Agency for International Development

Funding

This article is part of a special issue on women's health and empowerment, led and sponsored by the University of California Global Health Institute, Center of Expertise on Women's Health, Gender, and Empowerment. The broader systematic review on which this study is based was conducted under MEASURE Evaluation Phase III and the Health Policy Project funded by the United States Agency for International Development.

About this supplement

This article has been published as part of BMC Pregnancy and Childbirth Volume 17 Supplement 2, 2017: Special issue on women's health, gender and empowerment. The full contents of the supplement are available online at https://bmcpregnancychildbirth.biomedcentral.com/articles/supplements/volume-17-supplement-2.

Authors' contributions

MM and AM conceptualized the study and wrote the manuscript. MM, AM, and SP analyzed and interpreted the data. All authors read and approved the final manuscript.

Consent for publication

Not applicable.

Competing interests

The authors declare that they have no competing interests.

Author details

[1]MEASURE Evaluation, Carolina Population Center, University of North Carolina at Chapel Hill, Chapel Hill, NC, USA. [2]WaterAid India, New Delhi, India. [3]Health Policy Plus (HP+), Palladium, Washington, DC, USA.

References

1. Malhotra A, Schuler SR, Boender C. World bank workshops on poverty and gender: new perspective. In: Measuring women's empowerment as a variable in international development. Washington, DC: World Bank; 2002.
2. Rottach E, Schuler S, Hardee K. A summary report of new evidence that gender perspectives improve reproductive health outcomes. Washington, DC: Population Reference Bureau; 2009.
3. Muralidharan A, Fehringer J, Pappa S, Rottach RE, Das M, Mandal M. Transforming gender norms, roles, and power dynamics for better health: evidence from a systematic review of gender-integrated health programs in low- and middle-income countries. Washington, DC: US Aid; 2015.
4. Sustainable Development Goals. 2017. https://sustainabledevelopment.un.org/sdg5. Accessed 5 Jun 2017.
5. Keller B, Mbewe DC. Policy and planning for the empowerment of Zambia women farmers. Rev Can Etud Dev. 1991;12(1):75–88.
6. Sen G. Women's empowerment and human rights: the challenge to policy. In: Graham-Smith F, editor. A report of the population summit of the World's scientific academies. London: Royal Society London; 1994.
7. Kabeer N. Discussing women's empowerment: theory and practice. In: Reflections on the measurement of women's empowerment, Volume Aida studies No. 3. Stockholm: L Novum Grafiska AB; 2001.
8. Pratley P. Associations between quantitative measures of women's empowerment and access to care and health status for mothers and their children: a systematic review of evidence from the developing world. Soc Sci Med. 2016;169:119–31.
9. Pulerwitz J, Gortmaker SL, DeJong W. Measuring sexual relationship power in HIV/STD research. Sex Roles. 2000;42(7-8):637–60.
10. Upadhyay UD, Gipson JD, Withers M, Lewis S, Ciaraldi EJ, Fraser A, Huchko MJ, Prata N. Women's empowerment and fertility: a review of the literature. Soc Sci Med. 2014;115:111–20.
11. Heckert J, Fabic MS. Improving data concerning women's empowerment in sub-Saharan Africa. Stud Fam Plann. 2013;44(3):319–44.
12. Blanc AK. The effect of power in sexual relationships on sexual and reproductive health: an examination of the evidence. Stud Family Plann. 2001;32(3):189–213.
13. Interagency Gender Working Group. Gender Equality Continuum. 2013. http://sbccimplementationkits.org/gender/wp-content/uploads/sites/7/2016/03/Activity-0.1_Understanding-and-Applying-the-Gender-Equality-Continuum.pdf. Accessed 2 Oct 2017.
14. Daniel EE, Masilamani R, Rahman M. The effect of community-based reproductive health communication interventions on contraceptive use among young married couples in Bihar, India. Int Fam Plan Perspect. 2008;34(4):189–97.
15. Erulkar AS, Muthengi E. Evaluation of berhane hewan: a program to delay child marriage in rural Ethiopia. Int Perspect Sex R H. 2009;35(1):6–14.
16. Exner TM, Mantell JE, Adeokun LA, Udoh IA, Ladipo OA, Delano GE, Faleye J, Akinpelu K. Mobilizing men as partners: the results of an intervention to increase dual protection among Nigerian men. Health Educ Res. 2009;24(5):846–54.
17. Lundgren RI, Gribble JN, Greene ME, Emrick GE, de Monroy M. Cultivating men's interest in family planning in rural El Salvador. Stud Fam Plann. 2005;36(3):173–88.
18. Shattuck D, Kerner B, Gilles K, Hartmann M, Ng'ombe T, Guest G. Encouraging contraceptive uptake by motivating men to communicate about family planning: the Malawi male motivator project. Am J Public Health. 2011;101(6):1089–95.
19. Venguer T, Pick S, Fishbein M. Health education and agency: a comprehensive program for young women in the Mixteca region of Mexico. Psychol Health Med. 2007;12(4):389–406.
20. Aubel J, Toure I, Diagne M. Senegalese grandmothers promote improved maternal and child nutrition practices: the guardians of tradition are not averse to change. Soc Sci Med. 2004;59(5):945–59.
21. Feldman BS, Zaslavsky AM, Ezzati M, Peterson KE, Mitchell M. Contraceptive use, birth spacing, and autonomy: an analysis of the oportunidades program in rural Mexico. Stud Fam Plann. 2009;40(1):51–62.
22. Mahamed F, Parhizkar S, Raygan SA. Impact of family planning health education on the knowledge and attitude among yasoujian women. Glob J Health Sci. 2012;4(2):110–8.
23. Midhet F, Becker S. Impact of community-based interventions on maternal and neonatal health indicators: results from a community randomized trial in rural Balochistan, Pakistan. Reprod Health. 2010;7:30.
24. Mushi D, Mpembeni R, Jahn A. Effectiveness of community based safe motherhood promoters in improving the utilization of obstetric care. The case of mtwara rural district in Tanzania. BMC Pregnancy Childbirth. 2010;10:14.
25. Nasreen HE, Leppard M, Al Mamun M, Billah M, Mistry SK, Rahman M, Nicholls P. Men's knowledge and awareness of maternal, neonatal and child health care in rural Bangladesh: a comparative cross sectional study. Reprod Health. 2012;9:18.
26. Sahip Y, Turan JM. Education for expectant fathers in workplaces in Turkey. J Biosoc Sci. 2007;39(6):843–60.
27. Sathar Z, Jain A, Ramarao S, ul Haque M, Kim J. Introducing client-centered reproductive health services in a Pakistani setting. Stud Fam Plann. 2005;36(3):221–34.
28. Tang S, Tian L, Cao WW, Zhang K, Detels R, Li VC. Improving reproductive health knowledge in rural China—a web-based strategy. J Health Commun. 2009;14(7):690–714.
29. Mullany BC, Lakhey B, Shrestha D, Hindin MJ, Becker S. Imapct of husbands' participation in antenatal health education servces on maternal health knowledge. J Nepal Med Assoc. 2009;48(173):28–34.
30. Midhet F, Becker S, Berendes HW. Contextual determinants of maternal mortality in rural Pakistan. Soc Sci Med. 1998;46(12):1587–98.

31. De Silva MJ, Breuer E, Lee L, Asher L, Chowdhary N, Lund C, Patel V. Theory of change: a theory-driven approach to enhance the medical research Council's framework for complex interventions. Trials. 2014;15:267.
32. Miller E, Tancredi DJ, McCauley HL, Decker MR, Virata MC, Anderson HA, Stetkevich N, Brown EW, Moideen F, Silverman JG. "Coaching boys into men": a cluster-randomized controlled trial of a dating violence prevention program. J Adolesc Health. 2012;51(5):431–8.
33. Pulerwitz J, Michaelis A, Verma R, Weiss E. Addressing gender dynamics and engaging men in HIV programs: lessons learned from horizons research. Public Health Rep. 2010;125(2):282–92.
34. Verma RK, Pulerwitz J, Mahendra V, Khandekar S, Barker G, Fulpagare P, Singh SK. Challenging and changing gender attitudes among young men in Mumbai, India. Reprod Health Matters. 2006;14(28):135–43.
35. Jewkes RK, Dunkle K, Nduna M, Shai N. Intimate partner violence, relationship power inequity, and incidence of HIV infection in young women in South Africa: a cohort study. Lancet. 2010;376(9734):41–8.
36. Miller E, Jordan B, Levenson R, Silverman JG. Reproductive coercion: connecting the dots between partner violence and unintended pregnancy. Contraception. 2010;81(6):457–9.
37. Upadhyay UD, Dworkin SL, Weitz TA, Foster DG. Development and validation of a reproductive autonomy scale. Stud Fam Plann. 2014;45(1):19–41.
38. Gruskin S, Ferguson L. Using indicators to determine the contribution of human rights to public health efforts. Bull World Health Organ. 2009;87:714–9.
39. Davis SL. Measuring the impact of the human rights on health in global health financing. Health Hum Rights. 2015;17(2):97–110.
40. Mullany LC, Richards AK, Lee CI, Suwanvanichkij V, Maung C, Mahn M, Beyrer C, Lee TJ. Population-based survey methods to quantify associations between human rights violations and health outcomes among internally displaced persons in eastern Burma. J Epidemiol Community Health. 2007; 61(10):908–14.
41. Hartmann M, Khosla R, Krishnan S, George A, Gruskin S, Amin A. How are gender equality and human rights interventions included in sexual and reproductive health programmes and policies: a systematic review of existing research foci and gaps. PLoS One. 2016;11(12):e0167542.
42. Dworkin SL, Fleming PJ, Colvin CJ. The promises and limitations of gender-transformative health programming with men: critical reflections from the field. Cult Health Sex. 2015;17 Suppl 2:S128–143.
43. Dworkin SL, Treves-Kagan S, Lippman SA. Gender-transformative interventions to reduce HIV risks and violence with heterosexually-active men: a review of the global evidence. AIDS Behav. 2013;17(9):2845–63.

4

Changing times? Gender roles and relationships in maternal, newborn and child health in Malawi

Lucinda Manda-Taylor[1*], Daniel Mwale[1], Tamara Phiri[1], Aisling Walsh[2], Anne Matthews[3], Ruairi Brugha[2], Victor Mwapasa[1] and Elaine Byrne[2]

Abstract

Background: For years, Malawi remained at the bottom of league tables on maternal, neonatal and child health. Although maternal mortality ratios have reduced and significant progress has been made in reducing neonatal morality, many challenges in achieving universal access to maternal, newborn and child health care still exist in Malawi. In Malawi, there is still minimal, though increasing, male involvement in ANC/PMTCT/MNCH services, but little understanding of why this is the case. The aim of this paper is to explore the role and involvement of men in MNCH services, as part of the broader understanding of those community system factors.

Methods: This paper draws on the qualitative data collected in two districts in Malawi to explore the role and involvement of men across the MNCH continuum of care, with a focus on understanding the community systems barriers and enablers to male involvement. A total of 85 IDIs and 20 FGDs were conducted from August 2014 to January 2015. Semi-structure interview guides were used to guide the discussion and a thematic analysis approach was used for data analysis.

Results: Policy changes and community and health care provider initiatives stimulated men to get involved in the health of their female partners and children. The informal bylaws, the health care provider strategies and NGO initiatives created an enabling environment to support ANC and delivery service utilisation in Malawi. However, traditional gender roles in the home and the male 'unfriendly' health facility environments still present challenges to male involvement.

Conclusion: Traditional notions of men as decision makers and socio-cultural views on maternal health present challenges to male involvement in MNCH programs. Health care provider initiatives need to be sensitive and mindful of gender roles and relations by, for example, creating gender inclusive programs and spaces that aim at reducing perceptions of barriers to male involvement in MNCH services so that programs and spaces that are aimed at involving men are designed to welcome men as full partners in the overall goals for improving maternal, neonatal and child health outcomes.

Keywords: Pregnancy, Maternal and child health, Male involvement, Antenatal care, Community systems, Health systems, Access, Barriers, Malawi

* Correspondence: mandal@medcol.mw
[1]University of Malawi, College of Medicine, Blantyre, Malawi
Full list of author information is available at the end of the article

Background

The United Nations Task Force on Child and Maternal Health recommends that the highest priority be given to strengthening the primary healthcare system, from community-based interventions to the first referral-level facility at which emergency obstetric care is available [1]. This recommendation is echoed in the 2007 Road Map for accelerating Maternal and Newborn Health in Malawi, which articulates the following two objectives: firstly, to increase availability, access, utilization of quality skilled obstetric care during pregnancy, childbirth and post natal care at all levels of the health care delivery system, and secondly, to strengthen the capacity of individuals, families, communities, civil society organizations and government to improve maternal health [2]. The emphasis on encouraging and supporting individuals, families, communities and civil society organizations to participate in maternal and newborn health comes from the recognition that maternal mortality and newborn survival can be reduced substantially through community or home-based initiatives [3–5].

Recent global trends in the delivery of maternal and child health services have been to move as many of those services as close to the community as possible [6]. Most obstetric complications occur unexpectedly around the time of delivery in women with no risk factors, which means that removing any potential obstacles that communities and individuals may experience in accessing health facilities is key [1]. Improved access not only depends on the availability of health services, but also on community factors that influence the decision-making of individuals. There is widespread recognition that involving men in maternal and child health services offers positive benefits [1]. Numerous studies have demonstrated that male involvement can have a positive impact on the utilization of maternal, newborn and child health (MNCH) services [7–11].

One area of published literature on male involvement in MNCH examines strategies on engaging men in HIV treatment and prevention strategies in the context of antenatal care (ANC) services. For example, there is evidence that in Maharashtra in India male partners can significantly impact women's uptake of HIV-related services and support adherence to antiretroviral drug regimens, especially in the context of ANC services [12]. Likewise, in Kenya, partner participation in HIV Counselling and Testing (HCT) and couples counselling not only increased partner attendance to 15%, but also increased Nevirapine and formula feeding uptake among HIV positive women attending antenatal clinics [13]. Furthermore, women who disclose their HIV status to their partners have a higher likelihood of accepting ARV prophylaxis, adhering to feeding choices and carrying out safer sex practices, unlike women who lack partner support [8, 14–17]. Several studies found that lack of male involvement can impact negatively on access and utilisation of services. For example, the majority of women in a number of studies refused HIV testing in Prevention of Mother to Child Transmission (PMTCT) settings because their partners had either not been present or had not given their permission to test [18–20]. While efforts to involve men have been addressed in the context of ANC/PMTCT this is only one component of addressing the health needs of women of reproductive age, newborns and children under-5 years of age.

Another area of published literature highlights the influence and implications male partners have more broadly in MNCH service utilisation. For example, Aarnio, Chipeta and Kulmala state that male partners in most cultures are the main decision makers in families; hence men affect women's health care seeking behaviour, such as the utilisation of ANC, family planning services, or the preferred institution for delivery [21]. A study in Ghana refers to the above as gatekeeping whereby compound heads and husbands who control the economic resources and household decisions impede women's prompt access to health care services [22]. Other studies in Uganda, Burkina Faso, Nigeria and Bangladesh echo the same dichotomous tension by highlighting the important role men play in their families and communities, which can support or compromise women's sense of autonomy and affect women's health seeking behaviour patterns [23].

Despite evidence that male partner support can increase women's uptake of maternal and child services, few men are reported as participating in MNCH programmes [15, 23]. Even when men want to be involved in maternity care, they are often discouraged from doing so because of societal and health system norms [24]. When men do get involved they can feel uncomfortable [24] particularly in confined or limited "spaces" at health facilities that have been traditionally reserved for women. There is therefore a contradiction between men's positive attitudes towards male involvement in MNCH and their actual low participation rates suggesting that external barriers play a large role in getting men involved [25]. It is important, therefore, to recognize the role of gender norms as determinants of male involvement and as a potential source of stress for men striving to adhere to multiple roles [21].

Gender constructions and male involvement in Malawi

The construction of masculinity in patriarchal societies often limits the ways in which men are "allowed" to engage in pregnancy, birth and child rearing [26]. In many patriarchal societies, men still have the final say on issues related to family planning, reproductive health, their wives' and daughters' labour market participation, and the use of family resources, including medical and educational expenditures [27]. Malawian society is largely male-dominated, even with regard to female reproductive health [28]. In Malawi, pregnancy and childbirth has traditionally been a woman's domain and maternal health care services have focused on women, with very little attention paid to male involvement [29]. In addition, in Malawi, as Kululanga et al. observe, women have been supported by other women during labour and birth [30]. Furthermore, the notion of male involvement during labour and birth is perceived as a foreign culture not commonly practiced in Malawi [31]. As such, programs and policies that seek to involve men in MNCH is a relatively new approach in Malawi [29]. However, because global trends recognise that men's involvement in maternal and child health is a key driving force in improving MNCH access and utilisation the Malawi government's policy document for accelerating the reduction of MNCH mortality and morbidity specifically articulates the need to empower communities, especially men, to contribute to timely referrals [2]. In addition, the Malawi National Sexual and Reproductive Health and Rights (SRHR) policy describes the need for male involvement in the development, promotion and delivery of SRHR in the context of maternal and neonatal health [32].

These policy documents have spurred the exploration and implementation of a number of strategies and programs to engage men in sexual and reproductive health programs in Malawi. For example, one study revealed the usefulness of an invitation card during pregnancy as a strategy to enhance male partner involvement in PMTCT services [33]. Another study, the Malawi Male Motivator Project, examined the role of peer educators as a strategy to engage men as partners in order to promote better sexual, reproductive and maternal health outcomes. Through the use of male peers in the community, the study reported men's increased understanding of and ability to discuss contraception and family planning [34]. In addition, a key program that encourages involving men in antenatal care to increase women's uptake of antenatal care services is the Safe Motherhood initiative. Under the Safe Motherhood project, women and men receive nutrition information and guidance at clinics [35]. Further, men receive advice on how to support their partners during pregnancy. Most importantly, the Safe Motherhood initiative in Malawi has empowered traditional leaders to make sure that all pregnant women deliver at a health facility [36]. This intervention is part of strategy number seven in the Road Map, which aims at empowering communities to ensure continuum of care between the household and health care facility [2].

The MNCH continuum of care is the operational context for health programming to ensure that there is continuity of care for women and children across the Reproductive Maternal Newborn and Child Health (RMNCH) services [37]. The first dimension of the continuum of care is the time from pre-pregnancy, through pregnancy, childbirth, and the early days and years of life [38]. The second dimension links the various levels of home, community and outreach, and health facilities [38]. The impact of the MNCH continuum of care programs depends on (1) high coverage of essential interventions throughout the continuum; (2) their quality; and (3) functional linkages between interventions and the health system [37].

The recently published Malawi Demographic and Health Survey (2015–2016) shows some improvements in key areas that point to the increasing uptake in maternal health services. For instance, the MDHS shows that most mothers (95%) received ANC services from a skilled health care provider [39]. Additionally, the proportion of women who received ANC in the first trimester has more than doubled from 9% in 1992 to 24% in 2015–2015 [39]. Moreover, institutional deliveries have increased from 55% in 1992 to 91% in 2015–2016 and over the same time period, home deliveries have decreased from 43% in 1992 to 7% in 2015–2016 [39].

In spite of the progress in Malawi, there are still some notable gaps. For example, the proportion of women (15–49) that received four or more ANC visits generally declined from 1992 (62%) to 2010 (46%) before rising modestly to 51% [39]. Furthermore, the 2015–2016 MDHS found that among women aged 15–49 giving birth in the 2 years before the survey, 42% had a postnatal check during the first 2 days after birth. Half of mothers (50%) did not receive postnatal check [39].

The above information provides an opportunity for reflection on male involvement in maternal, newborn and child health in Malawi. In this paper, male involvement refers to the actions and decisions men make at a community level to that either promote or hinder women's utilization of MNCH services.

Objectives

The research presented in this article was a component of a Community Systems Strengthening for Equitable Maternal, Newborn and Child Health (COSYST-MNCH) project in Malawi. The overall goal of the COSYST-MNCH project was to achieve a better understanding of community systems factors underpinning maternal, newborn and child health (MNCH) services in Malawi, focusing on the health dimensions of the first 1000 days of life. In Malawi, there is still minimal, though increasing, male involvement in ANC/PMTCT/MNCH services, but little understanding of why this is the case. The aim of this paper is to specifically explore the role and involvement of men in MNCH services, as part of the broader understanding of those community system factors.

Methods

A mixed method convergent research design within a transformative paradigm (that is seeking sustainable changes in behavior and systems to improve social development) was adopted for the COSYST-MNCH project [40]. The aim was to collect data, quantitative and qualitative, that would enable the identification and a better understanding of what community systems exist and how they function. This paper draws on the qualitative data collected in two districts (Mchinji and Nkhotakota) in Malawi to explore the role and involvement of men across the MNCH continuum of care, with a focus on understanding the community systems barriers and enablers to male involvement in the promotion of MNCH.

Setting

Two rural districts in Malawi were selected as case studies. A case study is a research strategy that involves an in-depth empirical investigation of a phenomenon within its real life context using a variety of data collection methods [41, 42]. The first phase of the research consisted of the selection of communities for the case studies. Two Traditional Authorities (T/As) in Mchinji (Mduwa and Mkanda) and Nkhotakota (Mwadzama and Malengachanzi) districts were selected. The main criteria for communities to be selected were that (i) the non-governmental organization (NGO) partner - Concern Worldwide had current (or recently completed) implemented projects/interventions; and (ii) that the NGO partner had established links with other stakeholders working in these districts. In addition, the District Health Officials (DHOs) in each of the two selected districts advised the researchers that the research participants would be able to provide valuable information and feedback on the enablers and barriers to MNCH service utilisation because of the distances that some of these villages have in terms of location to health centres and other health care services and facilities.

Health Surveillance Assistants (HSAs) in the two districts facilitated with identifying community members who were willing to participate in the research. This process required community sensitization and engagement in order to obtain project support, for identifying potential respondents in the community and to ensure good contextual understanding and knowledge of the communities and on-going activities. This was important for gaining entry into the communities.

The third stage involved conducting in-depth interviews (IDIs) and focus group discussions (FGDs) (refer to Additional files 1, 2, 3, 4 and 5), in each of the four selected Traditional Authorities. Data were collected from October 2014 to January 2015 by two Malawian research assistants (1 male and 1 female) who were trained on the protocol and data collection methods and conducted the interviews and focus group discussions. The research assistants were familiar with the local context, spoke the local language (Chichewa) and were not associated with the NGO operating in the traditional authorities. A female Malawian project coordinator provided local supervision.

A document review of existing literature on community systems and health systems, and a COSYST Community Systems Analytical Framework was drafted for analysing and describing community system enablers and barriers that explain the utilization of MNCH services. The framework, depicted in Fig. 1 below, informed the design of the interview guides. The broad ideas explored the formal and informal community systems enablers and constraining factors to MNCH service utilisation whereby a core set of questions focused on utilisation of specific MNCH services for example, ANC, delivery or PNC.

Prior to data collection, the questions were read for familiarization and to identify questions that were ambiguous or irrelevant; these were revised or removed. The tools were pretested/piloted in the two districts selected in order to check for clarity, relevance, comprehensiveness and flow of questions. Once again, questions that were identified as ambiguous or not relevant to answering the main study objectives were altered or omitted.

Interviews and FGD were held in private spaces. For instance, the FGDs were conducted in school halls or local churches and the IDIs were conducted in district health offices, private rooms in the health centres and at people's residences in the community. The FGDs comprised of a homogenous group of individuals in the following categories: women of child-bearing age who are using/not using MNCH services, and those affected by disease or vulnerabilities and household members such as husbands and grandmothers, mothers in law. Each FGD had 6–12 participants. The IDIs comprised of senior representatives of NGO and government departments units, District Assembly/Commission, and members of the District Health Management Team. We also interviewed village chiefs and religious leaders, traditional healers, nurses, HSAs, clinical officers and women who were utilizing MNCH services. A total of 85 IDIs and 20 FGDs were conducted. Tables 1 and 2 show the attributes of participants.

Participants were purposively sampled based on their socio-demographic characteristics including, age, occupation, parity, roles education and experiences. A diverse mix of educated (primary, secondary or tertiary) and uneducated (never been to school), singe, married, divorced and widowed men and women were interviewed whose occupations ranged from working as a manager for an NGO, in the hospital as a nurse, clinical officer or HSA to farming and owning small businesses in the community. The religious affiliations of the participants were Christian or Muslim. The community and religious

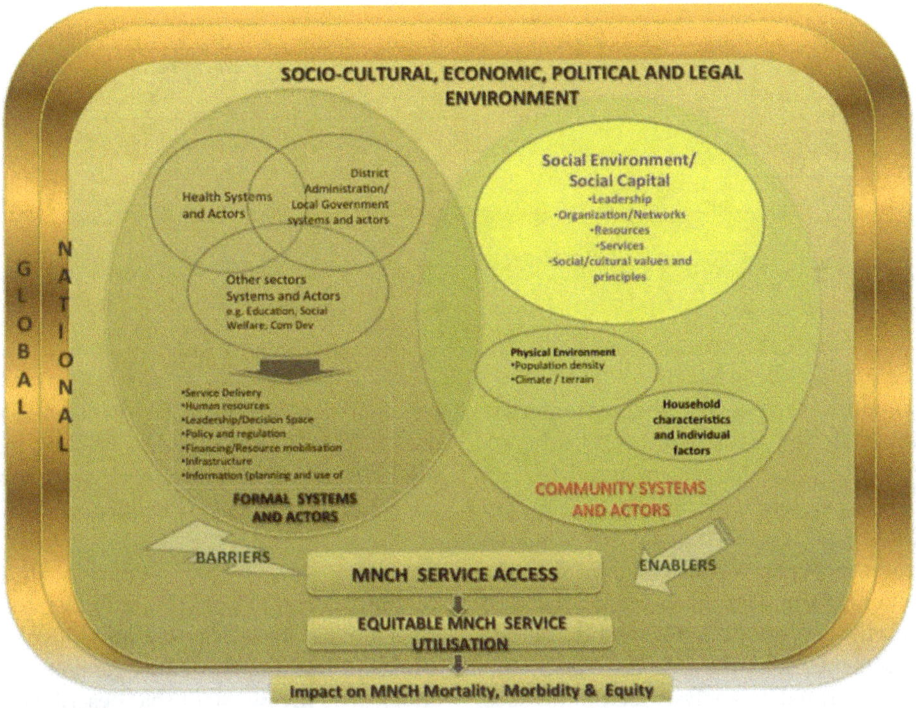

Fig. 1 COSYST-MNCH community systems analytical framework

leaders interviewed were all men. Traditional birth attendants (TBAs) were all women.

However, snowball sampling was also used to encourage interviewees to nominate other participants who met the eligibility criteria, but were hard-to-reach. In our study, snowball sampling was used to identify and interview TBAs and women of child-bearing age not using MNCH services as also asking interviewees to nominate other people they believed would have important contributions to make to the research. The IDIs and FGDs were conducted in Chichewa (the local language), audio-recorded (with permission) and later transcribed in Chichewa and then translated to English. Interviews continued until saturation was reached. The research assistants and the project coordinator checked the transcripts for completeness against the recorded interviews.

Data analysis

Data analysis was iterative, for instance, on-going throughout the data collection process. A point of saturation approach was also applied to the total sample of healthcare workers, local opinion leaders (traditional and religious), senior government and non-governmental officials, users and non-users of MNCH services and the relatives of mothers (husbands and grandmothers). Given that data analysis was iterative, saturation was

Table 1 In-depth interviews conducted

	MCHINJI							NKHOTAKOTA						
	Mduwa		Mkanda		Mchinji District Hospital		NUMBER	Malengachanzi		Mwadzama		Nkhotakota District Hospital		NUMBER
	M	F	M	F	M	F		M	F	M	F	M	F	
Traditional Leaders	6		2				8	3		6				9
Religious Leaders	5		2				7	4		3				7
Government Officials					4	1	5					3	2	5
Senior NGO officials					1	7	8				1	5	2	8
Health personnel	2	1		2			5	2		1	2			5
Health Surveillance Assistants	2		1				3	2	3	4				9
Traditional Birth Attendants		1		2			3		2		1			3
TOTAL	15	2	5	4	5	8	39	11	5	14	4	8	4	46

Table 2 Focus group discussions conducted

	MCHINJI					NKHOTAKOTA				
	Mduwa		Mkanda			Malengachanzi		Mwadzama		
	M	F	M	F	NUMBER	M	F	M	F	NUMBER
Caregiver-Husbands	1		1		2	2		1		3
Caregiver-Grandmothers + Mother in-law		2			2		1			1
MNCH users (pregnant women + women with under-5 children)		2		2	4		1		2	3
MNCH non-users (pregnant women + women with under-5 children)		1		1	2		1		2	3
TOTAL	1	5	1	3	10	2	3	1	4	10

achieved when no more patterns or themes emerged from the data. Once all the data had been gathered, translated and transcribed the Malawian and Irish researchers' coded data separately. The involvement of two separate coding teams experienced in qualitative research methods demonstrates the rigor, which was applied to the analysis and evaluation of the data. Each team presented key themes and sub-themes and a joint meeting agreed upon a final coding scheme for all the data collected.

Thematic analysis was the data analysis technique used to identify the main themes generated from the research. Thematic analysis was preferred because it best fit the search for evidence on the barriers and enablers to MNCH service utilization. Specific themes corresponding with the study objectives were immediately identified while additional themes emerged during the analytical process. Using NVivo 10, codes were developed from the responses and grouped into themes and sub-themes. The main themes were in the category of parent nodes and the sub-themes were in the category of child nodes. The main theme that is developed in this paper was that on male involvement. We used the structure of our interview guides, which we had based our literature review, to highlight what appeared to be system enablers and barriers to accessing MNCH services.

Ethical approval

The University of Malawi's College of Medicine Research and Ethics Committee (COMREC No granted ethical approval for the research. P.08/13/1443). In addition, permission to collect data in Mchinji and Nkhotakota was obtained from the Ministry of Health's Reproductive Health Unit. Written informed consent was obtained from individual participants. Literate participants provided a signature on the consent form, and illiterate participants provided a thumbprint. Interviews were conducted in a private space and participants were assured that their personal details would be omitted from transcripts to ensure confidentiality. Participants were also informed that any information generated by the research might be published, but that confidentiality would be maintained and no personal details would be divulged. Lastly, participants were informed that their involvement in the research was voluntary and that withdrawal was permitted at any time and without personal consequence.

Results

Within the context of community systems and actors, the main finding here was on male involvement in MNCH service utilization. Our study generated three main themes under male involvement that describe community systems and actors that enable or hinder women's utilization of MNCH services. In the context of this research, barriers are understood as any factors or reasons that impede or hinder women's utilization of MNCH services. Conversely, enablers are understood as factors or reasons that facilitate or support women's utilization of MNCH services. The themes identified to describe community system enablers and barriers of MNCH service utilisation in Mchinji and Nkhotakota were identified using the framework depicted in Fig. 1, above. Our three main specific themes included traditional gender roles at home; policy-changes to improve male involvement in MNCH, and; community/local initiatives to reinforce male involvement that operate within the socio-cultural milieu.

Gender roles at home

Barriers to MNCH utilisation were identified at household and facility levels. In spite of these obstacles, there was general agreement on the importance of male involvement in seeking healthcare and services for their families in particular in the decisions to attend antenatal care and to deliver at a healthcare facility.

> *"There is no appropriate treatment at home. In these years, most men encourage their wives to go to the hospital or maybe taking the children themselves" [NFGD5].*

> *"Men are the ones who encourage their wives to go for prenatal assistance and to go with a weak baby to the hospital" [MFGD3].*

Most of the men who were involved as participants in this study declared that they were involved in their family's health and well-being, particularly in reference to MNCH.

> *"When a woman is starting antenatal clinic they should all go together to receive counselling even if they have heard it before, but here they are advised again that you have to do this and that. Even if he parents are there, the man should take part as his family" [NFGD1].*

However, in terms of household level barriers, one of the issues that women reported was failure of their male partners in providing them with financial support for the purchase of the delivery items and transport costs for delivery. Women viewed this as a man's responsibility. As one participant remarked,

> *"Preparations of labour need cash so the husband is the one who is supposed to provide that cash" [N20].*

Without having the essential items required for the delivery, women were reluctant to deliver at the hospital as they would feel embarrassed and would fear being treated harshly by staff, or not receive treatment at all. Sometimes family members stepped in and purchased goods if husbands failed to do so. Sometimes the money was available, but used for other purposes, for example as reported by male participants, some men spent money on alcohol or on girlfriends and were therefore unable to cover the costs of their wives attending ANC and delivery at the hospital.

> *"We can say that we men cheat a lot - that is why we reject our women... We may have things to support our wives, but we give these things to girlfriends leaving our wives starving. If we stop cheating and give a little of what we have found to the wives, there will be less deaths" [MFGD3].*

Most participants voiced that women and men exercise an equal amount of power and authority within the family, but that each have different roles.

> *"All people are one family so the woman can also have power as a man as one family" [NFGD1].*

However, some women still needed permission from their husbands or other member of the family to attend clinic or hospital.

> *"There are others [other problems] that men cause maybe because of power and the way they speak in the home that maybe everything that happens he should be told first; so maybe a child is sick and they cannot go to the hospital unless they tell the man; so the man has to make the decision that you can go to the hospital" [N7].*

In terms of roles and responsibilities in the household it was expressed that women should look after the children in the daily care of the family, such as clothing, feeding and washing.

> *"When it comes to breastfeeding and cooking for the child it is the role of a woman. The role of the man is to just go out and search for food" [NFGD2].*

Men were expected to provide food or money for food, but also to encourage their wives to go to hospital when they or their children needed to, and arrange for this to happen. Men could encourage and persuade women to attend hospital and this was considered an important role for them to play. Men could also influence decisions over what food was given to children in his household; therefore, even though men might not have a direct responsibility in the preparing of food, he still needed to be informed on nutrition to make the right choices for his family.

The men who participated in the study were generally supportive of women attending hospitals:

> *"No individual can stop his wife from going to the hospital... Not nowadays... That cannot happen... since they know that this is dangerous"* [N27].

However, men were not generally comfortable to be in the delivery room with their spouses during delivery.

> *"This issue is very difficult for a man to go and watch how a woman is giving birth - as they have explained it can be difficult for a man to watch... Some of the women, because they are in pain during the time of labour, they say abusive language, and shout those words at a husband, so when coming back you can be concerned is that the way things are" [MFGD2].*

"Policy changes" to improve male involvement in MNCH

There is general support for the role of chiefs in MNCH. One participant in Nkhotakota suggested making it a law for men to attend ANC, whereas in an interview in Mduwa a participant noted that such a law exists and that it was the chiefs in Mchinji that passed this law in collaboration with the hospitals.

> *"It is really happening, men are going to the hospital with their wives because there is a rule in place, that those that fail to go to the hospital, for example, from Nkangala, they will be paying maybe K5000.00" [MFG 3].*

"They may pay also in terms of goats. So they really go to the hospital together because they are afraid of that payment" [MFGD3].

Community members generally accepted that these are 'good' laws and there is general support for a chief playing an active role in promoting MNCH attendance.

"And so far the punishment they put looks to be working here because these days we are seeing husbands escorting their wives to the hospital" [M24].

As one traditional leader informed us,

"But nowadays we [traditional leaders] have been taught by the HSAs that if a woman is pregnant we should follow her up, we allow one woman who has children to go and ask if she has started going to ANC, if she doesn't go, she will pay a goat we do not like that in the village" [N15].

However, some participants noted that ANC staff sent women away if their husbands did not accompany them. In Mchinji, when men are being unsupportive of their wives attending ANC the chief can intervene and write a letter to the health staff to state that the woman can still receive ANC. As one religious leader reported,

"They [health care workers] have come up with rules that every pregnant woman has to be accompanied by her husband during antenatal visits unless they present a letter from the chief justifying where the husband ran away; but every woman has to be accompanied by the husband" [M12].

Traditional leaders are providing letters of support for married, unmarried and divorced pregnant women in order for them to access MNCH services. Interviews with some religious leaders, husbands and female users of MNCH services revealed the following;

"Most men do not give their women to start pre-natal support when they are a month, two or three months. So when they go alone they are sent back because she is alone. When they go to pre-natal clinic at six months of pregnancy, they are told to bring a letter from the village headman that they may start prenatal support without their husband" [MFGD3].

"Even antenatal when she is a student and also she was impregnated outside the wedlock chiefs are providing letters for them so that they can be assisted at the hospital early" [MFDG1].

"There were some pregnant women in here, one of them was from Ntcheu but they left husbands behind. How would they go to the hospital, when it is required that the husband and the wife should go together? So, I had to write a letter of recommendation for her and she was welcomed" [M30].

For many of the men who participated in this study, feelings of discomfort and embarrassment were raised when discussing attending MNCH events. Some men reported feeling uncomfortable with participating in the health education component of the ANC visits because they felt shy and/or embarrassed about being asked to sing or dance with the women about reproductive health.

"It is embarrassing to have to sing in a choir about MNCH because it may be your first time and you are 50 years old say and young ones who maybe are 14 years. They are like teasing you because they know us (laughter)" [MFGD3].

"So men are like, so we should go there and clap hands as if we are dancing Chitelele while women are watching (laughter)?" [MFGD4].

One participant reported that men felt unwelcome by nurses and experienced long waiting times, but it was not clear whether these experiences were related to MNCH or to their own health needs.

Additionally, if they did attend, men reported that they felt uncomfortable sitting with women, interacting with young nurses and discussing things like sanitary pads with doctors. In some cases, men still did not feel that maternal and child health is their responsibility. As one participant observed:

"We are not yet there, most men are not involved in issues of maternal child health, despite the information, but there is something that needs to be done to change the attitude of the male figures in the houses. It's an issue of attitudes... Maybe they think that the issue of maternal health, the issue of bearing children, and the issue of child health are the issues of a woman. The message has been there for years, but we are not yet there" [N20].

Furthermore, one woman noted that sometimes men do not believe that attending the under-five clinic is a priority in the home. Some men feel that once a baby is born, husbands try to convince mothers that there is no need to attend a clinic if the baby is well by saying:

"My wife I do not want my baby to go to under-five clinics let us do other things at home. So, what would

you do as a wife because the baby belongs to the two of you it is not illegitimate because if it is illegitimate child you can do your own things. So if the husband says the money that he has is for drinking there is no money for soap it's enough that we have a baby and he/she will grow" [FFGD].

The fear of a going for a HIV test in case the result was positive (testing is done of both parents when ANC commences) was also raised as a barrier for men in attending ANC.

"Not all of us will go along with the blood testing as we are afraid that my friends will isolate me (if found to be HIV)" [MFGD3].

Despite this unease, it was noted in one of the FGDs that even though they are mocked for going to ANC men feel they are doing the right thing.

"We do accompany our women going to the ANC and there is no problem because people conclude that is how you show love to your family. Though people talk that you are charmed you only accept the talk and respond to them by saying that she is my wife whom I chose. I don't stop escorting them at ANC because it is our choice" [MFGD2].

Community and health care provider initiatives for male involvement

Men in our study reported to be involved in initiatives, which foster communication about family planning. As one religious leader from Mkanda in Mchinji district noted,

"... We have a group called Mai Mwana in our area and we meet them on the 22nd. 22nd is a day that we all meet like an umbrella meeting... all groups like CBOs, Mai Mwana, and from agriculture. In that meeting everybody is asked to give information they have to the people.... Mai Mwana teaches us on family planning to avoid over-population in our area" [RL1].

A male participant provided an example of the collaboration between health service providers and community leaders, which was supported by funding from the UNICEF known as the "male championship model."

"Previously...we had male championship. There was a competition to see which part of the Traditional Authority (TA) is doing very fine on these issues. So, there was a completion on which areas is doing well on male championship, that is men who are also trying to disseminate information about family planning in all the TAs in Mchinji... And after that there was dissemination in Dowa, it was like a big event because there was an invitation of Ministry of Health's personnel that presided over that function" [M5].

Another man told us of the "male motivator" program which was supported by the Mai Mwana programme (translated from Chichewa to mean Mother and Child in English), in Mchinji, which trained about 10 men in each village to go and talk to other men on the importance of being involved in MNCH.

In Nkhotakota, a non-governmental official (NGO) reported that at community level they had established male only groups to encourage men to support women accessing MNCH services,

"...at community level what we have done is that we have established also what we call: one man can. There are only male groups. They are mainly involved in male involvement influencing the information; the decision of men to make sure that there is support from men to makes rue that they support the women accessing these services" [N4].

Another health care provider in the same district reported that collaborations between the community and health care providers have increased the involvement of men in MNCH issues.

"The community involvement is high because people meet frequently. Village chiefs call for meetings with the people and nowadays you will find that the number of malnourished children has decreased. MNCH issues are discussed and, for instance, women are encouraged to take part in health issues, and men should also take part by taking their wives to the hospital. Moreover, if a child is sick they are advised to take him/her to the hospital. Nowadays men understand if the mother is not there they take the child to the hospital" [N6].

The role of faith-based organizations, like churches, was mentioned as crucial to getting men involved in MNCH services. However, despite all these community and health care provider initiated activities, one government official from Nkhotakota district hospital observed that male involvement in MNCH issues is still a challenge.

"...I do monthly assessment of how many men are attending those health talks.... We were surprised that over the past year from September 2013 to September 2014 we only had 4.6% of men attending these health talks" [N19].

Discussion

This study adds to the existing literature on male involvement in MNCH in Malawi by reflecting on the community system factors that encourage or impede men from supporting women's utilisation of MNCH services. The involvement of men in the health of women and newborns around the time of childbirth – including but not limited to support for women during and after pregnancy, seeking skilled care for birth and complications, newborn care, nutrition and breastfeeding, family planning after childbirth and maternal health – has the potential to directly address gender influences on maternal and newborn health outcomes [43].

Changing perceptions of traditional gender roles and power in decision-making?

The findings from our study echo findings from other qualitative studies on the perceived barriers and enablers to MNCH service utilisation. The main barriers to male involvement in MNCH identified in this study were at the household level, whereby husbands continue to retain control of the finances and decision-making in the home. In addition, men reported on the stigma men face when participating in activities thought of as "women's business" [44]. Men reported to be shy to go to ANC as they were asked to sing or dance with the women and the fear of an HIV test being positive also emerged from the narratives of men. While most participants in our study expressed general agreement that men should accompany women to ANC, it is clear that in Malawi, dichotomous tensions exist between men being viewed as the providers and decision makers in their families and men being supportive of and engaging in women's health seeking practices. It remains apparent that culturally defined gender roles and power relationships continue to serve as an obstacle to male involvement in MNCH.

However, our study also reveals positive strategies to involve "men as partners" and "men as positive agents of change" even if traditional constructions of masculinity and power remain unchallenged. In particular, getting men involved into peer groups, encouraging men to accompany their wives to ANC and participate in educative components of ANC services deliberately help target gender relations in order to challenge patriarchal structures that reinforce pre-existing roles and norms surrounding masculinity. Our findings reveal the community and health care provider efforts to transform gender relations, norms and structures in order to improve MNCH outcomes in Mchinji and Nkhotakota. We also note that some of the strategies employed can produce the opposite effect, if not carefully initiated. What is promising about these strategies is the intention to change the behaviour of men in the community.

"Policy-changes" and community-based initiatives to engage men

Community leaders play a significant role in influencing health service use among rural communities in sub-Saharan Africa. Our findings reveal community leaders in our study (all who were men), played an active role in the promotion of knowledge on the MNCH services provided and the role of men in supporting women in utilising these services. As mentioned earlier, in Malawi, the Safe Motherhood program has empowered traditional leaders to make sure that all pregnant women deliver at a health facility. In Malawi, the engagement of chiefs has provided an opportunity for involving men in MNCH, and the narratives of the men we interviewed revealed that they were likely to follow the advice when a respected member of the community delivers it. As Kululanga et al., observe, "Involvement of chiefs and village headmen/women in public health interventions demonstrate the importance of the issue and therefore motivate greater participation of other community members" [45]. In addition, the authority and respect that traditional leaders command offer a vehicle "through which social and cultural changes can be realized" [45, 46]. Moreover, chiefs, in Malawi, have instituted bylaws that penalize men if they do not accompany women to ANC ("go to scale") and are present at the delivery. Tanzania, Zimbabwe and Malawi have reported on the perceived effectiveness of the implementation of bylaws initiated by community leaders on engaging community members for better MNCH outcomes [47]. Despite the deployment of punitive tactics such as the imposition of fines, chiefs provide the leadership that may be necessary to create an environment that encourages the use of MNCH services. To this extent, traditional leaders have collaborated with the formal health care system to promote the involvement of men in MNCH service utilization. In short, traditional leaders are community level enablers and can strengthen community systems to support the utilisation of MNCH services; however, we note that this practice should be undertaken in a supportive (rather than coercive) manner so as to avoid counter-productive health seeking behavioural practices.

Another strategy to engage men involved the health care providers in collaboration with community leaders. The "male championship" and Mai Mwana programmes in Mchinji were mentioned by participants as important initiatives for involving men to improve the health of mothers and infants. Both programmes are anchored on the use of peer educators. The use of peer educators (male motivators) was perceived as an effective community-based strategy to include and involve men by targeting men with messages focused on the benefits of utilizing MNCH services. From the narrative accounts provided by participants in Mchinji, it became clear that such activities helped challenge traditional gender norms. Our findings are similar to observations made by Kadomoto et al., in the Philippines whereby it was reported that teaching men about maternal and child health improved men's involvement in the services, but also enabled the same men to become educators of other men in the community [46]. In essence, peer-educators are useful for influencing men and encouraging greater participation in MNCH services.

Health facility initiatives to engage men

The use of incentives to encourage male involvement is employed as a strategy to reward positive behaviour to improve MNCH. The use of incentives is what was reported in our study from participants in Mchinji district. In fact, a similar finding was revealed in a study done by Kululanga et al., in Mwanza district, where participants at Mwanza district hospital described the same type of competition organized by UNICEF in 2008 [29]. In addition, incentives also come in the form of receiving priority care at health centres and hospitals. Our study also confirmed that women who are accompanied with their husbands to ANC clinic are assisted and attended to first. A current practice at hospitals and health centres in Malawi is to incentivise women who come with their husbands by providing the couple with priority services. Even promotional messages are displayed to encourage and reward partners that attend ANC together. In an urban hospital in Malawi, for example, a caption under a picture in the ANC facility reads as follows: "Go to the hospital during the first three months together with your husband" [48] A husband accompanying his pregnant spouse rewards the couple with priority service and this type of treatment is not unique to Malawi. In Kenya, for example, health staff promoted the involvement of husbands in ANC through giving preferential treatment and a free shawl for their child if the husband attended ANC with his wife [48]. However, as Kululanga et al. warn, the use of incentives for couples attending ANC together can result in stigmatisation and unfair treatment of women who are unsupported and/or must choose to attend without a male partner [46]. Ultimately though, despite this concern, we acknowledge the potential role that incentives can play in encouraging behaviour change in men.

Study limitations

Our study participants were mainly from the two districts we selected as case studies and our findings reflect the opinions of the individuals we interviewed in these two districts. In order to further contribute to a holistic understanding on the community system barriers and enablers to MNCH service utilization it may have been useful to interview key informants such as policy makers, NGO officials, technocrats and donor partners as their opinions may have further enriched our findings.

Conclusion

Traditional notions of men as decision makers and socio-cultural views on maternal health continue to present challenges to male involvement in MNCH programs. The main obstacles to male involvement do not only centre on the traditional constructions on masculinity and power. Overall, what is critical to catalysing social change are approaches that view men as partners or view men as agents of positive change. The informal bylaws of traditional leaders, health facility initiatives and the health care provider strategies provide a range of opportunities to engage and involve men in supporting women's use of MNCH services. However, the use of coercive or punitive measures as well as competitions to drive men to participate in what for them can be a threatening space, is not the best approach to creating deep and meaningful behaviour change. At a programmatic and content level, community-led initiatives need to use entertainment for example, drama and plays, that are culturally acceptable to both men and women, during community meetings to address gender-related barriers and facilitators of MNCH service utilisation. Health care provider initiatives need to be sensitive and mindful of gender roles and relations by, for example, creating gender inclusive programs and spaces that aim at reducing perceptions of barriers to male involvement in MNCH services so that programs and spaces that are aimed at involving men are designed to welcome men as full partners in the overall goals for improving maternal, neonatal and child health outcomes.

Additional files

Additional file 1: Appendix 1. In-depth interview guide.
Additional file 2: Appendix 2. In-depth interview guide.
Additional file 3: Appendix 3. In-depth interview guide.
Additional file 4: Appendix 4. In-depth interview guide.
Additional file 5: Appendix 5. Focus Group Discussion guide.

Abbreviations

ANC: Antenatal care; COMREC: College of Medicine Research and Ethics Committee; COSYST-MNCH: Community systems strengthening for equitable maternal, newborn and child health; FGDs: Focus group discussions; HSAs: Health surveillance assistants; IDIs: In-depth interviews; MNCH: Maternal, newborn and child health; NGOs: Non-governmental organizations; PMTCT: Prevention of mother-to-child transmission; T/A: Traditional authority; TBAs: Traditional birth attendants

Acknowledgements

The authors wish to thank Mr. Lyle Taylor for the professional language editing services.

Funding

Community Systems Strengthening for Equitable Maternal, Newborn and Child Health (COSYST-MNCH) project was funded by Irish Aid/Higher Education Authority (of Ireland) 2012–2015 (Grant Number: COSYST_MNCH 1513: Irish Aid.), as part of the Programme of Strategic Cooperation between

Irish Aid and Higher Education and Research Institutes The project was a partnership of experienced development workers, researchers and practitioners in the Royal College of Surgeons in Ireland (RCSI – lead); College of Medicine (CoM), University of Malawi; Concern Worldwide (CWW), Ireland and Malawi, and; Dublin City University (DCU), Ireland. The funders of the project had no role in the design of the study' in the collection, analyses, or interpretation of data; in the writing of the manuscript, and in the decision to publish the results.

Authors' contributions

RB, VM, EB, AM, AW, conceived and designed the study; LMT, DM, TP, collected the data, transcribed and performed preliminary data coding and analysis. EB, AM, and AW performed separating coding on the data and all teams – Malawian and Irish – agreed upon the final codes; LMT initially conceived the manuscript and wrote the first draft of the article. All authors were involved in reviewing and providing comments and revisions the paper. All authors read and approved the final manuscript.

Ethics approval and consent to participate

The University of Malawi's College of Medicine Research and Ethics Committee (COMREC No granted ethical approval for the research. P.08/13/1443). In addition, permission to collect data in Mchinji and Nkhotakota was obtained from the Ministry of Health's Reproductive Health Unit. Written informed consent was obtained from individual participants. Interviews were conducted in a private space and participants were assured that their personal details would be omitted from transcripts to ensure confidentiality. Participants were also informed that any information generated by the research might be published, but that confidentiality would be maintained and no personal details would be divulged. Lastly, participants were informed that their involvement in the research was voluntary and that withdrawal was permitted at any time and without personal consequence.

Consent for publication

Not applicable.

Competing interests

The authors declare that they have no competing interests.

Author details

[1]University of Malawi, College of Medicine, Blantyre, Malawi. [2]Royal College of Surgeons in Ireland, Dublin, Ireland. [3]Dublin City University, Dublin, Ireland.

References

1. UN Millennium Project. Who's Got the Power? Transforming Health Systems for Women and Children. Summary version of the report of the Task Force on Child Health and Maternal Health. New York, USA; 2005. https://www.k4health.org/sites/default/files/whos%20got%20the%20power%20TF4Childandmaternalhealth.pdf. Accessed 22 Nov 2016.
2. Ministry of Health [Malawi]. Road Map for accelerating the reduction of Maternal and Neonatal Morbidity and Mortality in Malawi. Lilongwe: MOH; 2007.
3. Manandhar DS, Osrin D, Shrestha BP, Mesko N, Morrison J, Tumbahangphe KM, Tamang S, Thapa S, Shrestha D, Thapa B, Shrestha JR, Wade A, Borghi J, Standing H, Manandhar M, Costello AM. Effect of a participatory intervention with women's groups on birth outcomes in Nepal: cluster-randomised controlled trial. Lancet. 2004;364(9438):970–9.
4. Bang AT, Bang RA, Baitule SB, Reddy MH, Deshmukh MD. Effect of home-based neonatal care and management of sepsis on neonatal mortality: field trial in rural India. Lancet. 1999;354:1955–61.
5. Martines J, Paul VK, Butta ZA, Koblinsky M, Soucat A, Walker N, Bahl R, Fogstad H, Costello A. Neonatal survival: a call for action. Lancet. 2005;365(9465):1189–97.
6. Cleason M, Waldman RJ. The evolution of child health programmes in developing countries: from targeting diseases to targeting people. B World Health Organ. 2000;78:1234–45.
7. UNICEF. Improving male involvement to support elimination of mother-to-child-transmission of HIV in Uganda: A case study. 2016. file:///C:/Users/user/Downloads/Uganda%20Case%20Study%203_15%20HR_0.pdf. Accessed 27 Feb 2016.
8. Aluisio A, Richardson BA, Bosire R, John-Stewart G, Mbori-Ngacha D, Farquhar C. Male antenatal attendance and HIV testing are associated with decreased infant HIV infection and increased HIV-free survival. J Acquir Immune Defic Syndr. 2011;56(1):76–82. doi:10.1097/QAI.0b013e3181fdb4c4.
9. Brusamento S, Ghanotakis E, Tudor Car L, van Velthoven MH, Majeed A, Car J. Male involvement for increasing the effectiveness of prevention of mother-to-child HIV transmission (PMTCT) programmes. Cochrane Database Syst Rev 2012, doi:10.1002/14651858.CD009468.pub2.
10. Reece MHA. Assessing male spousal engagement with prevention of mother-to-child transmission (PMTCT) programs in western Kenya. AIDS Care. 2010;22(6):743–50.
11. Dudgeon MR, Inhorn MC. Men's influences on women's reproductive health: medical anthropological perspectives. Soc Sci Med. 2004;59(7):1379–95.
12. Peltzer K, Jones D, Weiss M, Shikwane E. Promoting male involvement to improve PMTCT uptake and reduce antenatal HIV infection: a cluster randomized controlled trial protocol. BMC Public Health. 2011;11:778. doi:10.1186/1471-2458-11-778.
13. Panditrao M, Darak S, Kulkarni V, Kulkarni S, Parchure R. Sociodemographic factors associated with loss to follow-up of HIV-infected women attending a private sector PMTCT program in Maharashtra, India. AIDS Care. 2011;23(5):593–600.
14. Jones SA, Sherman GG, Varga CA. Exploring socio-economic conditions and poor follow-up rates of HIV-exposed infants in Johannesburg, South Africa. AIDS Care. 2005;17(4):466–70.
15. Msuya SE, Mbizvo EM, Hussain A, Uriyo J, Sam NE, Stray-Pedersen B. Low male partner participation in antenatal HIV counselling and testing in northern Tanzania: implications for preventive programs. AIDS Care. 2008;20(6):700–9.
16. Mepham S, Zondi Z, Mbuyazi A, Mkhwanazi N, Newell ML. Challenges in PMTCT antiretroviral adherence in northern KwaZulu-Natal, South Africa. AIDS Care. 2011;6:741–7.
17. Peltzer K, Sikwane E, Majaja M. Factors associated with short-course antiretroviral prophylaxis (dual therapy) adherence for PMTCT in Nkangala district, South Africa. Acta Paediatr. 2011;100(9):1253–7.
18. Homsy J, Kalamya JN, Obonyo J, Ojwang J, Mugumya R, Opio C, Mermin J. Routine intrapartum HIV counseling and testing for prevention of mother-to-child transmission of HIV in a rural Ugandan hospital. J Acquir Immune Defic Syndr. 2006;42(2):145–54.
19. Dahla V, Mellhammar L, Banjunirwe F, Bjorkman P. Acceptance of HIV testing among women attending antenatal care in south-western Uganda: risk factors and reasons for test refusal. AIDS Care. 2008;20(6):726–52.
20. Aarnio P, Chipeta E, Kulmala T. Men's perception of delivery care in rural Malawi: exploring community level barriers to improving maternal health. Health Care Women Int. 2013;34(6):419–39.
21. Story WT, Barrington C, Fordham C, Sodzi-Tettey S, Barker PM, Singh K. Male Involvement and accommodation during obstetric emergencies in rural Ghana: a qualitative analysis. Int Perspect Sex Reprod Health. 2016;42(4):211–9.
22. Ngom P, Debpuur C, Akweongo P, Adongo P, Binka FN. Gate-keeping and women's health seeking behaviour in Navrongo, Northern Ghana. Afr J Reprod Health. 2003;7(1):17–26.
23. Kurewa EN, Kandawasvika GQ, Mhlanga F, Munjoma M, Mapingure MP, Chandiwana P, Chirenje MZ, Rusakaniko S, Stray-Pedersen B. Realities and Challenges of a Five Year Follow Up of Mother and Child Pairs on a PMTCT Program in Zimbabwe. Open AIDS J. 2010;5:51–8.
24. Mullick S, Kunene B, Wanjiru M. Agenda Special Focus. In: Involving men in maternity care: health service delivery issues; 2005. http://citeseerx.ist.psu.edu/viewdoc/download?doi=10.1.1.192.5507&rep=rep1&type=pdf. Accessed 20 Mar 2017.
25. Dumbaugh M, Tawian-Agyemang C, Manu A, ten Ashbroek GHA, Kirkwood B, Hill Z. Perceptions of, attitudes towards and barriers to male involvement in

newborn care in rural Ghana, West Africa: a qualitative analysis. BMC Pregnancy Childbirth. 2014;14:269.

26. Farre L. The role of men in the economic and social development of women: Implications for gender equality. World Bank Res Obs. 2013;28(1):22–51.
27. Palamuleni ME, Adebowale AS. Women empowerment and the current use of long-acting and permanent contraceptive: Evidence from 2010 Malawi Demographic and Health Survey. Malawi Med J. 2014;26(3):63–70.
28. Kululanga LI, Sundby J, Chirwa E, Malata A, Maluwa A. Barriers to husbands' involvement in maternal health care in a rural setting in Malawi: a qualitative study. J Res Nurs Midwifery. 2012;1:1–10.
29. Kululanga LI, Sundby J, Malata A, Chirwa E. Striving to promote male involvement in maternal health care in rural and urban settings in Malawi – a qualitative study. BMC Reprod Health. 2011;8:36. Accessed 25 June 2017
30. Kululanga LI, Malata A, Chirwa E, Sundby J. Malawian fathers; views and experiences of attending the birth of their children: a qualitative study. BMC Pregnancy Childbirth. 2012;12:141. doi:10.1186/147-2393-12-141. Accessed 20 June 2017.
31. Ministry of Health. Sexual and Reproductive Health Policy. Lilongwe: MOH; 2015. http://malawi.unfpa.org/en/publications/sexual-and-reproductive-health-policy. Accessed 22 Sept 2017.
32. Nyondo AL, Choko AT, Chimwaza A, Muula AS. Invitation cards during pregancy enhance male partner involvement in prevention of mother to child transmission of Human Immunodeficiency Virus (HIV) in Blantyre, Malawi: a randomized controlled open label trial. PLoS One. 2015;10(3):e0119273.
33. Shattuck D, Kerner B, Gilles K, Hartman M, Ng'ombe T, Guest G. Encouraging contraceptive uptake by motivating men to communicate about family planning: The Malawi Male Motivation Project. Am J Public Health. 2011;101(6):1089–95.
34. Hendriks SL, Mkandawire E, Mkandawire-Valhmu L. Why men tackle mother and child health: lessons from Malawi. Conversation. 2016; https://theconversation.com/when-men-tackle-mother-and-child-health-lessons-from-malawi-69501. Accessed 9 June 2017.
35. UNFPA: Giving birth should not be a matter of life and death. Dec, 2012 https://www.unfpa.org/sites/default/files/resource-pdf/EN-SRH%20fact%20sheet-LifeandDeath.pdf. Accessed 22 Feb 2017.
36. Maternal, Newborn and Child Health Framework. International Federation of Red Cross and Red Crescent Societies. http://www.ifrc.org/PageFiles/93927/1232600-MNCH%20Framework%20report_LR%20(2).pdf. Accessed 22 June 2017.
37. PMCH Fact Sheet: RMNCH Continuum of Care. Reproductive, maternal, newborn and child health. 2011. http://www.who.int/pmnch/about/continuum_of_care/en/ Accessed 22 June 2017.
38. National Statistics Office (NSO) [Malawi] and ICF. Malawi Demographic and Health Survey 2015–16. Zomba, Malawi and Rockville, Maryland, USA. NSO and ICF; 2017. https://dhsprogram.com/pubs/pdf/FR319/FR319.pdf. Accessed 22 June 2017.
39. Creswell JW, Piano Clark VL. Designing and Conducting Mixed Methods Research. 2nd ed. London: SAGE Publications; 2011.
40. Gilson L: Health policy and Systems Research: A Methodology Reader. AHPSR and WHO. 2012. http://www.who.int/alliance-hpsr/alliancehpsr_reader.pdf. Accessed 20 Feb 2017.
41. Yin RK. Enhancing the Quality of Case Studies in Health Services Research. Health Serv Res. 1999;34(5-part 2):1209–24.
42. Comrie-Thomson L, Tokhi M, Ampt F, Portela A, Chersich M, Khanna R, Luchters S. Challengeing gender inequity through male involvement in maternal and newborn health: critical assessment of an emerging evidence base. Clut Health Sex. 2015;17(sup2):177–89.
43. Mullany BC. Barriers and attitudes towards promoting husbands in maternal health in Katmandu, Nepal. Soc Sci Med. 2006;62(11):2789–809.
44. Wambui T, Alehagen S. Perceptions of family planning among low-income men in Western Kenya. Int Nurs Rev. 2009;56:340–5.
45. Kululanga LI, Sundby J, Malata A, Chirwa E. Male involvement in maternity health care in Malawi. Afr J Reprod Health. 2012;16(1):145–57.
46. Kadomoto N, Iwasa H, Takashi M, Dulnuan MM, Kai I. Ifugao males, learning and teaching for the improvement of maternal and child health status in the Philippines: an evaluation of a program. BMC Public Health. 2011;11(280):1–10.
47. Manda-Taylor L, Dealy D-A, Roberts J. Factors associated with delayed antenal care attendance in Malawi: Results from a qualitative study. Med J Zambia. 2017;44(1):17–25.
48. Pell C, Menaca A, Were F, Afrah NA, Chatio S, Manda-Taylor L, Hamel MJ, Hodgson A, Tagbor H, Kalilani L, Ouma P, Pool R. Factors affecting Antental Care Attendance: Results from qualitative studies in Ghana, Kenya and Malawi. PLoS ONE. 2013;8(1):e53747. Accessed 7 July 2017.

5

The specific and combined role of domestic violence and mental health disorders during pregnancy on new-born health

Alexandre Archanjo Ferraro[1*], Luis Augusto Rohde[2,3], Guilherme Vanoni Polanczyk[2], Adriana Argeu[2], Euripides Constantino Miguel[2], Sandra Josefina Ferraz Ellero Grisi[1] and Bacy Fleitlich-Bilyk[2]

Abstract

Background: Addressing impaired foetal growth is recognized as a public health priority. Certain risk factors for this condition, such as poor nutritional status at birth, have been found to be highly correlated with poverty. However, the role of psychosocial factors, specifically the mother's mental health and exposure to violence during pregnancy, have yet to be further explored. Our objective was to determine if there is a measurable association between combined psychosocial factors, specifically domestic violence and mental disorders, and birth outcomes, specifically birth nutritional status and preterm delivery.

Methods: We followed 775 women from an underserved, urban area, beginning their 28th week of gestation. Diagnostic interviews were performed to determine if any of the mothers had any of the following disorders: mood disorder, anxiety, obsessive–compulsive disorder (OCD), substance dependence, psychotic disorder, or anti-social personality disorder. Physical, psychological, and sexual domestic violence were also assessed.

Results: Domestic violence and mental disorders were highly correlated in our sample. About 27.15% of the women in our study experienced domestic violence, and about 38.24% of them were diagnosed with mental disorders. The main association we found between combined psychosocial factors and neonate outcomes was between anxiety (IRR = 1.83; 95%CI = 1.06–3.17)/physical violence (IRR = 1.95; 95%CI = 1.11–3.42) and the rate of small-for-gestational age (SGA) in new-borns. More specifically, the combination of anxiety (beta = −0.48; 95%CI = −0.85/−0.10) and sexual violence (beta = −1.58; 95%CI = −2.61/−0.54) was also associated with birth length. Maternal risk behaviours such as smoking, drinking, inadequate prenatal care, and inadequate weight gain could not sufficiently explain these associations, suggesting that these psychosocial factors may be influencing underlying biological mechanisms.

Conclusion: Domestic violence against women and mental disorders amongst pregnant women are extremely prevalent in under-resourced, urban areas and ultimately, have detrimental effects on birth outcomes. It is imperative that actions be taken to prevent violence and improve mental health during pregnancy.

Keywords: Domestic violence, Mental health disorders, Birth weight, Birth length

* Correspondence: ferraro@usp.br
[1]Department of Pediatrics, School of Medicine, Universidade de Sao Paulo, Av Dr Eneas Carvalho Aguiar, 647, Sao Paulo 05403-900, Brazil
Full list of author information is available at the end of the article

Background

Around eighteen million babies worldwide are born with low birth weight (LBW) every year – constituting 14% of all yearly births. Addressing impaired foetal growth and development, such as LBW, is recognized as a key public health priority because there are clear links between LBW and adverse outcomes later in life. For example, children born with LBW have higher chances of developing diabetes, hypertension, stroke, obesity, and mental health disorders as adults [1, 2]. Birth size largely reflects the quality of the intrauterine environment, which in turn, reflects the mother's environment during the child's early development [3]. For example, birth weight is highly influenced by the mother's nutritional status, which in turn, is highly influenced by family income, maternal education, health-seeking attitudes of the family, feeding practices, and 'risky' environments [4]. Although a strong consensus exists in support of the relationship between nutrition and birth outcome, the role of psychosocial factors has yet to be further explored. In the last decade, both maternal experience of violence and mental health, mainly depression, have been linked with threats to the health of a child [5–8] and further research should be conducted to deepen our understanding of their underlying mechanisms.

A meta-analysis of 14 published studies from developed countries found a small but significant effect of violence during pregnancy on low birth weight (OR = 1.4; 95% CI 1.1–1.8) [9]. However, few studies of this sort have been carried out in developing countries. In a review of all research concerning the relationship between psychosocial factors and pregnancy outcomes, Paarlberg et al. [10] concluded that "studies on the association between maternal stressor exposure and birth weight have yielded mixed results" and thus, a firm conclusion could not be drawn. However, these psychosocial factors have generally been studied separately, and have remained limited in the number of mental disorders covered. This is an important research question because, if a connection between maternal psychological stress/mental disorders and specific developmental neonate outcomes is established, then preventative actions in clinical practice and public health efforts can be taken to ameliorate their effects.

The aim of this work is to measure the association between domestic violence and different mental disorders during pregnancy and neonate outcomes in a middle-income country. Our hypothesis is that these psychosocial stressors are linked to negative birth outcomes; that their combined presence will result in increased negative birth outcomes; and that the pathway in which they act is by influencing maternal risky behaviours during pregnancy.

Methods

Study design

The Butantan birth cohort is a population-based birth cohort following mothers from their 28th week of gestation to the present. The present analysis used data from the T0 (28th gestational week) and T1 (2nd month after birth) phases.

Population and sample

All pregnant women who were attending pre-natal care in 5 primary care facilities in the region of Butantan – a health district in the western region of the city of Sao Paulo, Brazil – from July 2010 to December 2012, were eligible to enrol in the study. Although this area receives good pre-natal care coverage in the form of monthly home visits through the Family Health Strategy [11], the region is considered an area of great social vulnerability. The region is far from the city centre, is densely populated, and consists of mostly poor families along with a few, newly formed lower-middle income class families. Violence, such as constant encounters between drug dealers and police, co-exists with nurseries, schools, and churches.

Although theoretically, all eligible mothers could have participated in our study, we only included the first 5 eligible subjects assessed per week from each primary health facility. The criterion for eligibility included residence in the area described. Twins and children who were born with any disease associated with impaired development were excluded from analysis.

The planned sample size of the study was 900 women. This size would produce a statistical power of 90% in identifying an association between depression and LBW – assuming a 20% frequency of depression, a 9% incidence of low birth weight, and a relative risk of 1.80.

Variables

The outcome variables included birth weight (BW), birth length (BL); being born small for gestational age (SGA); and preterm birth (PTB). BW (g) and BL (cm) were outcomes treated as continuous variables. This information was measured according to routine hospital protocol and collected from the clinical reports taken on the birth. SGA was determined according to the Williams reference curve [12]. Gestational age was evaluated using ultra sound: 51.79% of the sample had the ultra sound performed by their 12th week of gestation, while the rest of the mothers did not have an ultra sound until after this period. In this later case, gestational age was based on the mother's reported last menstrual period or through the Capurro Somatic Method [13], which was assessed by a paediatrician at birth. The Capurro Somatic Method was used in cases where the gestational age determined by the ultrasound differed by more than

2 weeks from the gestational age determined by the last reported menstrual period. All women delivered in maternity hospitals.

Trained psychologists began data collection in the beginning of the third trimester – around the 28th week – during routine pre-natal care visits. Domestic violence against women was measured according to the WHO Domestic Violence Questionnaire [14]. Questions 704 to 706 in the Questionnaire assess for 7 types of physical abuse, 4 types of psychological abuse, and 3 types of sexual abuse perpetrated by the husband/partner in the last 12 months. Given that the mothers were in their 6th month of gestation when assessed, violence may have occurred immediately before or during gestation (or, in some cases, during both these periods). Mental health disorders were measured according to the Mini International Neuropsychiatric Interview (MINI) – a short and structured diagnostic interview used to reveal current disorders [15]. Both instruments had been previously adapted to the Brazilian population before being used in this study [16, 17]. Physical, psychological, and sexual violence were analyzed separately and then pooled in one variable named "violence". Recurrent episodes of domestic violence reported within the last 12 months were considered positive. Mental disorders were pooled in the following groups: *"mood disorder"* – current hypomanic episode (ICD-10 F31.8), current manic episode (ICD-10 F30.x), current dysthymic disorder (ICD-10 F34.1), current major depression (ICD-10 F32.x); *"anxiety"* – current panic disorder without agoraphobia (ICD-10 F40.01), current panic disorder with agoraphobia (ICD-10 F40.0), social phobia (ICD-10 F40.1), post-traumatic stress disorder (ICD-10 F43.1), general anxiety disorder (ICD-10 F41.1); *"OCD-obsessive compulsive disorder"* – (ICD-10 F42.8); *"substance dependence"* – alcohol and illicit drugs dependence (ICD-10 F10.2× and F11.0 - F19.1), *"anti social personality disorder"* – (ICD-10 F60.2), and *"psychotic disorder"* – (ICD-10 F32.3 and F33.3).

Professionals were trained according to the WHO guidelines presented in "Putting Women First: ethical and safety recommendations for research on domestic violence against women" [18]. The training also focused on how to cope with the challenges of such field-work. Women who were diagnosed with a mental disorder were advised to refer to their general practitioners. Those who were identified as victims of domestic violence were advised to look for the closest Center for Victims of Domestic Violence. Field researchers only directly referred cases to local health facilities (doctor, nurse or social worker) in high risk cases, in which it had been concluded that the woman was unable to follow the previous advice.

Other independent variables were family socioeconomic status (according to the Brazilian Association of Population Studies – ABEP [19], where "A" is the wealthiest and "E" the poorest), years of maternal schooling (stratified into three categories: 0–7 years, 8–10 years, and 11 or more years of completed education – where federal mandatory schooling is 8 years), occupation of the father of the offspring (based on the International Classification of Occupation [20] and classified as *"non-manual"* or *"qualified, semi-qualified"* and *"unskilled manual"*), maternal age (adolescent or non-adolescent mother), maternal migration (being born in Sao Paulo or not), birth order (categorized as primipara or not), reported drinking and smoking habits during gestation (yes or no), unwanted pregnancy (negative feelings towards pregnancy, having considered an abortion – yes or no), sex of the offspring (male or female), number of prenatal care visits (classified as adequate or inadequate for the gestational age), and gestational weight gain - a proxy of maternal nutritional habits (classified as adequate or inadequate for the gestational age, taking into account the pre-gestational body mass index - BMI). These last two variables were classified according to the standards provided by the Brazilian Ministry of Health.

Data bases and analysis

Data was collected on paper and later transferred to an Excel database (version 6.01). Double entry and verification of data were incorporated in this process to minimize data input errors. Statistical analysis was done using STATA software (version 10.0). Dichotomous variables had their proportion calculated in %, with a respective 95% confidence interval. Continuous variables had their mean and standard deviation calculated and were checked for outliers (defined as below "1st quartile-1.5 × interquartile interval" and above "3rd quartile + 1.5 × interquartile interval").

We began our analysis by calculating the loss-to-follow-up rate using the chi-square method to test for any selection bias (Additional file 1: Table S1). Then, the description of the studied sample was determined according to exposure of the psychosocial variables: violence or mental disorders. Next, we tested for associations between each exposure (not specified in their categories, but as pooled information) and the outcomes through bivariate Poisson regression (for binary outcome variables, which produced incidence rate ratios - IRR) and linear regression (for continuous outcome variables, which produced beta scores). Violence and mental disorders were analysed both separately and together, and finally presented in graphs. Models using non-pooled violence and mental disorders were then built. Confounders for which models were adjusted were chosen based on the assumption that they must be antecedent of exposure *and* outcome [21]. Since the violence measurement only encompassed the last 12 months, the independent variables that fulfilled this assumption were maternal schooling, maternal migration, family socioeconomic status, and being an adolescent mother. Finally, we tested whether the associations could be explained by the presence of maternal risk behaviours, namely smoking, drinking, inadequate prenatal care, and inadequate weight gain. Stressful events could increase the likelihood of these behaviours, which in turn could affect foetal development. If the association disappears when these variables are included in the models it means that these variables completely explain the link between mental disorders/domestic violence and neonate outcomes, since they would be in the pathway between exposure and outcome.

Ultimately, the null hypothesis was rejected when the probability of occurring type I error was smaller than 5%.

Ethics

All mothers who were invited to take part in the study were presented with a term of agreement by a professional trained in clarifying the terms in cases where the mother exhibited difficulty in reading or understanding. Mothers read and signed an informed consent after it was determined that they understood the scope of the project, and data from hospital charts were used only after the mothers' consent. The local ethics in research committee (CAPPesq) approved this research protocol (research protocol number 0054/09).

Results

Nine hundred women were assessed during pregnancy and 775 of them were followed up to the T1 phase (puerperium). Seven mothers had twins and one mother had a child with Down syndrome, none of which were included in the present analysis. The other mothers lost in the study (n = 117, or 13.1%) resulted from their migration out of the sample neighbourhood and loss of contact after repeated telephone calls and home visits. The subjects that were followed-up did not differ from the original enrolled sample in regards to the occupation of the father of the child, family socioeconomic status, maternal schooling, having an unwanted pregnancy, reported smoking and drinking during gestation (Additional file 1: Table 1), and being an adolescent, migrant, or primipara mother. Six children also died between the 28th week of gestation and the first week of life.

Most families in our sample belonged to the socioeconomic class C (low middle-income class), and were headed by "manual, non-skilled professionals." Table 1 shows that pregnant women with mental disorders and victims of domestic violence were more likely to have a partner with a less qualified job, were more likely to come from a lower income class, and were more likely to not be primipara. They also had higher incidences of unwanted pregnancy, and they reported smoking and drinking more than the national average. Furthermore,

Table 1 Description of the sample of pregnant women from the Butantan birth cohort according to their exposure to mental disorder or to domestic violence in the last 12 months

Variable	Category	w/ Mental Disorder (n = 296) % (95%CI)	no Mental Disorder (n = 478) % (95%CI)	w/ Abuse (n = 205) % (95%CI)	no Abuse (n = 550) % (95%CI)
Paternal occupation	Non-manual	11.90 (0.08–0.16)	20.92 (17.18–24.65)**	12.11 (7.42–16.79)	19.77 (16.34–23.20)*
	Qualified manual	18.22 (13.57–22.86)	18.30 (14.75–21.85)	17.37 (11.93–22.80)	18.62 (15.26–21.97)
	Nonqualified manual	69.89 (64.37–75.41)	60.78 (56.30–65.27)	70.53 (63.98–77.07)	61.61 (57.42–65.80)
Family Economic Class	A + B	13.85 (9.89–17.81)	20.29 (16.67–23.91)**	18.54 (13.17–23.90)	17.82 (14.61–21.03)*
	C	63.85 (58.35–69.35)	66.32 (62.07–70.57)	58.54 (51.74–65.34)	67.45 (63.53–71.38)
	D + E	22.30 (17.53–27.07)	13.39 (10.33–16.45)	22.93 (17.12–28.73)	14.73 (11.76–17.70)
Maternal Schooling	< 8 year	21.62 (16.90–26.34)	17.19 (13.79–20.59)	17.56 (12.31–22.81)	19.31 (16.00–22.62)
	8–10 years	40.20 (34.58–45.82)	37.53 (33.17–41.89)	43.42 (36.57–50.26)	36.25 (32.21–40.28)
	11 or + years	38.18 (32.61–43.74)	45.28 (40.80–49.77)	39.02 (32.29–45.76)	44.44 (40.27–48.61)
Adolescent Childbearing	–	21.28 (16.59–25.97)	21.97 (18.24–25.69)	25.85 (19.81–31.90)	20.90 (17.50–24.32)
Maternal Migration	–	40.13 (34.50–45.77)	46.53 (42.02–51.03)	34.80 (28.21–41.40)	47.17 (42.97–51.36)**
Primipara	–	40.20 (34.58–45.82)	51.15 (46.65–55.66)**	40.00 (33.24–46.76)	50.46 (46.26–54.65)*
Unwanted pregnancy	–	29.15 (23.94–34.37)	13.24 (10.18–16.29)**	29.76 (23.44–36.07)	15.15 (12.14–18.16)**
Smoking in pregnancy	–	23.31 (18.47–28.16)	11.55 (8.67–14.44)**	24.39 (18.46–30.32)	12.96 (10.14–15.78)**
Drinking in pregnancy		10.47 (6.96–13.98)	8.60 (6.07–11.12)	15.12 (10.18–20.07)	7.10 (4.95–9.26)*
Prenatal care	Inadequate n. of visits	36.82 (31.30–42.35)	30.54 (26.40–34.69)	37.07 (30.41–43.74)	31.09 (27.21–34.97)
Gestational weight gain	Inadequate for pre gest BMI	40.50 (33.64–47.36)	45.68 (40.50–50.86)	39.44 (31.30–47.57)	45.05 (40.18–49.92)

One missing data for mental disorder and 20 missing data for domestic violence; inadequate number of visits took into account the gestational age; inadequate gestational weight gain took into account the pre-gestational body mass index (IMC); * $p < 0.05$; ** $p < 0.01$

women who suffered abuse in the study were more likely to have been born in the sample area than they were to have been a migrant to the community.

Violence, in one form or another, was reportedly experienced by 27.15% of the women, while 38.24% exhibited some form of mental disorder. More specifically, psychological, physical, and sexual violence were reported by 24.77%, 13.46% and 2.23% of the women, respectively. Mental disorders were prevalent in the mothers as follow: 29.97% for mood disorders; 16.26% for anxiety disorder; 4.52% for Obsessive Compulsive Disorder (OCD); 4.13% for substance dependence; 3.61% for psychotic disorder and 2.19% for anti-social personality disorder.

Among the 775 neonates, 47.95% were born male, 9.29% were born small for gestational age (SGA), 5.81% were born low birth weight (LBW) and 7.11% were born premature. Hypoxia was present in 7.47% of the newborns. Averages for weight and length (sd) were 3221 (492) and 48.49 (2.04), respectively.

Domestic violence against women was highly linked to mental disorders during gestation. Among women who reported having experienced violence in the last 12 months, 62.9% ($p < 0.001$) them were diagnosed with a mental disorder, while only 28.7% of women who did not report experiencing violence were diagnosed. Figure 1 shows the unadjusted effect size of the association of pooled mental disorders and pooled violence with birth outcomes. Birth weight was statistically associated with domestic violence (DV) (*beta* = −138.08; 95% CI -260.45 / -15.71) and presented a stronger association with mental disorders (MD) plus DV (*beta* = −163.01; 95% CI -287.51 / -38.51). Birth length had no association. Being exposed to both MD and DV increased the likelihood of being SGA (IRR = 2.25; 95% CI 1.12–4.54). Moreover, DV alone increased the risk of preterm birth (2.17; 95% CI 1.04–4.54).

Tables 2 and 3 show the unadjusted and adjusted analysis of the association between all types of violence and mental disorders on birth outcomes. SGA was associated with physical violence, anxiety, and OCD – these first two factors are shown in the unadjusted and adjusted analysis, while the latter is shown only in the unadjusted analysis. Anti-social personality disorder doubled the risk for preterm birth. This finding takes into account that there were only 4 women that presented these exposures and outcomes together, and therefore, serves as an estimate with large confidence intervals. Birth weight was associated with physical and sexual violence in both unadjusted and adjusted analyses, and anxiety disorder presented a tendency towards significance (p = 0.067 in the adjusted model). Finally, length was associated with sexual violence and anxiety disorder in both the unadjusted and adjusted analyses.

These findings did not change considerably when maternal risk behaviours were included in the models (Tables 2 and 3). This suggests that the pathway, which explains the association, does not pass exclusively through these behaviours. Ultimately, we could not confirm the hypothesis that the pathway through which mental disorders and violence have an effect

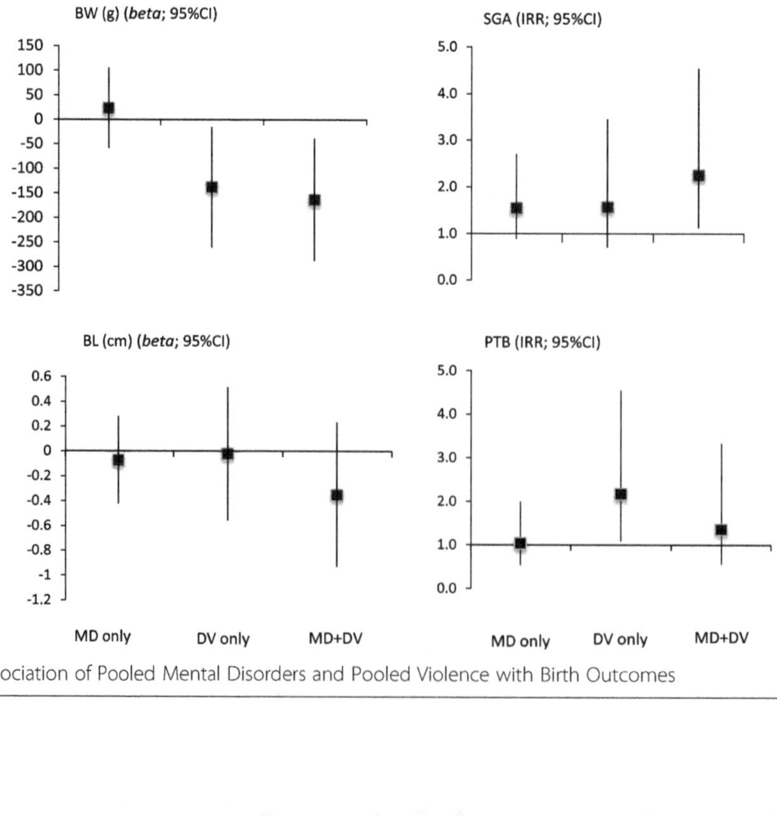

Fig. 1 Effect Size of the Association of Pooled Mental Disorders and Pooled Violence with Birth Outcomes

Table 2 Bi and multivariate regression analysis between current mental disorders in pregnancy and birth outcomes in the Butantan birth cohort

Birth Outcome	Unadjusted Models	p	Adjusted Models[a]	p	p*
SGA	IRR (95%CI)		IRR (95%CI)		
Mood dis	1.52 (0.95–2.45)	0.084	1.40 (0.85–2.29)	0.182	
Anxiety dis	1.72 (1.01–2.93)	0.047	1.83 (1.06–3.17)	0.030	0.023
OCD	2.28 (1.04–4.97)	0.039	2.00 (0.90–4.43)	0.087	
Substance dep	1.37 (0.50–3.74)	0.545	1.23 (0.44–3.40)	0.691	
Psychotic dis	0.38 (0.05–2.70)	0.331	0.36 (0.05–2.61)	0.311	
AS Personality dis	1.94 (0.61–6.16)	0.262	1.65 (0.51–5.38)	0.407	
PTB					
Mood dis	0.96 (0.53–1.72)	0.881	1.06 (0.58–1.92)	0.854	
Anxiety dis	0.76 (0.35–1.69)	0.506	0.81 (0.36–1.82)	0.616	
OCD	0.85 (0.21–3.48)	0.818	0.92 (0.22–3.82)	0.914	
Substance dep	0.88 (0.21–3.59)	0.853	0.93 (0.23–3.84)	0.922	
Psychotic dis	0.49 (0.07–3.57)	0.484	0.55 (0.08–4.03)	0.557	
AS Personality dis	3.50 (1.26–9.68)	0.016	4.62 (1.60–13.35)	0.005	0.003
Weight (g)	beta (95%CI)		beta (95%CI)		
Mood dis	−28.97 (−105.73/47.80)	0.459	−20.46 (−98.38/57.47)	0.606	
Anxiety dis	−80.29 (−175.53/14.95)	0.098	−89.89 (−186.01/6.24)	0.067	
OCD	32.15 (−137.36/201.66)	0.710	51.70 (−118.13/221.52)	0.550	
Substance dep	−82.97 (−259.81/93.87)	0.357	−66.77 (−243.26/109.73)	0.458	
Psychotic dis	92.32 (−96.21/280.85)	0.337	98.73 (−90.60/288.07)	0.306	
AS Personality dis	−184.90 (−424.87/55.08)	0.131	−163.68 (−405.18/77.81)	0.184	
Length (cm)					
Mood dis	−0.04 (−0.34/0.26)	0.795	−0.03 (−0.34/0.28)	0.851	
Anxiety dis	−0.41 (−0.78/−0.04)	0.030	−0.48 (−0.85/−0.10)	0.013	0.017
OCD	−0.20 (−0.89/0.49)	0.566	−0.21 (−0.91/0.48)	0.549	
Substance dep	−0.34 (−1.04/0.36)	0.341	−0.32 (−1.02/0.386)	0.379	
Psychotic dis	0.26 (−0.47/0.99)	0.479	0.24 (−0.49/0.97)	0.518	
AS Personality dis	−0.66 (−1.57/0.24)	0.150	−0.70 (−1.61/0.21)	0.132	

IRR incidence rate ratio from Poisson regression analysis; "beta" from linear regression analysis, *95% CI* (95% confidence interval), *SGA* small for gestational age, *PTB* preterm birth, *dis* disorder, *dep* dependence, *OCD* obsessive compulsive disorder, *AS* anti-social

*Same adjustments plus for maternal risk behaviours: smoking during gestation, drinking during gestation, inadequate number of prenatal care visits for the gestational age and inadequate weight gain for the gestational age considering the pre-gestational BMI

[a]Adjusted for socio-demographic variables: maternal schooling, economic class, adolescent childbearing, maternal migration

on the offspring is by influencing maternal risk behaviours during pregnancy.

Discussion

Violence is a major public health issue in developing countries, where 90% of these events occur [22]. In Latin America, this has been found to be primarily an urban phenomenon, with the highest concentrations of violence occurring in the peripheries of major cities [23, 24]. The global estimate for repeated intimate partner violence among ever-partnered women is 30.0% (95% CI 27.8–32.2) [25]. A recent meta-analysis found that violence towards women during pregnancy remains at an average of 14.4% (IQR 13.2–25.7) [26]. In developed countries, physical violence against the female partner has been estimated to occur in up to 20% of pregnancies [27]. Meanwhile, in Latin America, a Mexican [28] study reported rates of 33.5%, while a Brazilian study reported a rate of 33.8% [29]. Moreover, maternal mental disorders are also highly prevalent. A systematic review [30] of studies of depression during pregnancy, which included 21 studies (only one from a developing country) reported a prevalence of 7.4%, 12.8% and 12% for the first, second, and third trimesters, respectively. Heron et al. [31] revealed anxiety disorder in 7.3% of mothers in a British population during their third

Table 3 Bi and multivariate regression analysis between different types of domestic violence during the last year and birth outcomes in the Butantan birth cohort

Birth Outcome	Unadjusted Models	p	Adjusted Models[a]	p	p*
SGA	IRR (95%CI)		IRR (95%CI)		
Physical violence	2.06 (1.19–3.56)	0.009	1.95 (1.11–3.42)	0.021	0.168
Psychological violence	1.03 (0.60–1.76)	0.910	0.94 (0.54–1.62)	0.816	
Sexual violence	1.96 (0.62–6.25)	0.252	2.13 (0.66–6.82)	0.205	
PTB					
Physical violence	1.27 (0.62–2.60)	0.512	1.30 (0.63–2.70)	0.478	
Psychological violence	1.51 (0.86–2.66)	0.153	1.51 (0.85–2.67)	0.159	
Sexual violence	1.65 (0.40–6.79)	0.485	1.94 (0.47–8.02)	0.362	
Weight (g)	beta (95%CI)		beta (95%CI)		
Physical violence	−166.61 (−269.74/−63.49)	0.002	−148.52 (−252.95/−44.09)	0.005	0.016
Psychological violence	−72.00 (−153.55/9.55)	0.083	−62.25 (−144.05/19.55)	0.136	
Sexual violence	−232.26 (−471.79/7.27)	0.057	−244.78 (−483.72–5.84)	0.045	0.082
Length (cm)					
Physical violence	−0.40 (−.82/0.02)	0.061	−0.34 (−0.76/0.09)	0.122	
Psychological violence	−0.10 (−0.43/0.23)	0.540	−0.06 (−0.39/0.27)	0.715	
Sexual violence	1.53 (−2.56/−0.49)	0.004	−1.58 (−2.61/−0.54)	0.003	0.008

IRR incidence rate ratio from Poisson regression analysis; "beta" from linear regression analysis, *95% CI* (95% confidence interval), *SGA* small for gestational age, *PTB* preterm birth, *dis* disorder, *dep* dependence, *OCD* obsessive compulsive disorder, *AS* anti-social

*Same adjustments plus for maternal risk behaviours: smoking during gestation, drinking during gestation, inadequate number of prenatal care visits for the gestational age and inadequate weight gain for the gestational age considering the pre-gestational BMI

[a]Adjusted for socio-demographic variables: maternal schooling, economic class, adolescent childbearing, maternal migration

trimester. However, limited data exists from developing countries [32, 33].

This study adds to the literature on violence and mental health during pregnancy by providing a follow-up research study in an underserved, urban population in a middle-income country – a context still vastly underrepresented in studies – and by assessing a larger range of mental health problems than has been done in the past. Detailed assessments measuring psychological stress and evaluating mental disorders were performed using diagnostic interviews and screening scales; high incidences of domestic violence and mental disorders were recorded.

This relation between violence and poor mental health is not new. In a meta-analysis, Golding [34] found that the weighted Odds Ratios of the association between different mental disorders and violence varied from 3.5 to 5.6; the most common disorders among those who suffered violence were depression and post-traumatic stress disorders. A cross-sectional study in Brazil [35] found that adolescents who were victims of violence during pregnancy were 4.3 times more likely to also suffer from common mental disorders (95% CI 1.7–10.9). More recently, the WHO reported a pooled OR = 1.97 (95% CI 1.56–2.48) in a review of 6 studies about the association between depression and violence [25]. Recent trends in urbanization and westernization have been thought to contribute to the rise in violence and mental health problems, as a result of changes in family structure, deterioration of traditional social networks, new environments challenging traditional values and beliefs, and other emerging categories of vulnerability [36]. Moreover, adverse life events, such as violence, are known risk factors for poor mental health [37], thus supporting our finding that the magnitude of negative effects would be even higher when both factors were present.

Although the association we found between violence and mental disorders and neonate outcomes had been confirmed in some parts of the literature, many studies yielded mixed results. However, there is evidence that suggests that this association may only be apparent in communities of lower socioeconomic status. Anderson et al. [6] did not find an association when conducting a study among Swedish women, and neither did Chung et al. [7] among women in Hong Kong. Hoffman et al. [38], on the other hand, found a positive association, but only among women from an under-resourced African-American community in the United States. Rahman et al. [8] also found an independent association between maternal antenatal depression and low birth weight among 632 mothers in rural Pakistan, and Patel & Prince [39] found it in a study of 270 pregnant women in Goa. In Nicaragua [40], Mexico [28], China [41], India [42] and a previous study in Brazil [43] reported negative outcomes as well.

Nonetheless, our findings suggest that a positive association persists even after controlling for socio-economic and demographic confounders (socioeconomic status, maternal schooling, maternal migration and being an adolescent mother). We found that in this under-resourced, urban area, domestic violence and mental health in pregnant women are highly prevalent and intimately correlated. From this study, we can extrapolate that violence (physical and sexual) and anxiety disorder have a negative effect on birth variables, i.e., birth weight, birth length, and the likelihood of being a SGA new-born. We also found that anti-social personality disorder increased the risk for PTB. However, although we also found an association between anti-social personality disorder and PTB, these results are not conclusive due to the few cases we had in our sample. Ultimately, it must be noted that these findings could not be merely explained by neglected prenatal care, lower gestational weight gain, smoking, or drinking – as previously thought. It must be noted that although we did not find any effects from depression, this may be due to the high rates of co-morbidity in this sample – among mood disorders 37.9% of women also exhibited anxiety, in comparison to just 7.1% in the group with no mood disorder.

The mechanisms through which violence and mental disorders affect birth outcomes are not clear. Violence might have a direct impact on foetal growth through trauma, by indirectly causing low weight gain and/or increasing smoking and drinking during pregnancy. It is known, however, that female victims of sexual violence are more likely to have sexually transmitted diseases and urinary tract infections, both of which cause impaired foetal growth [44]. Similarly, poor mental health may affect the infant outcome by leading to poor self-care, such as poor appetite or lesser access to antenatal services. However, our findings seem to contradict this and suggest that pathways beyond maternal behaviours may contribute more to the outcomes.

Biological pathways may explain our findings. For example, the mechanisms underlying both of these exposures and physiological alterations may involve epigenetically-mediated changes in gene expression. Extensive animal studies have demonstrated that the association between maternal psychosocial stress and low birth weight is mediated by changes in the hypothalamic-pituitary-adrenal (HPA) axis. There is also increasing evidence in humans that the HPA axis is in overdrive in pregnant women subjected to psychosocial stress [45]. In these cases, cortisol crosses the placenta, which has been demonstrated to inhibit intrauterine growth when present in high levels [46, 47]. In addition, measures of psychosocial stress, even in utero, are correlated with oxidative stress, inflammation, and telomere length. Therefore, risk factors may act through common biological pathways yielding a common phenotype: low birth weight [48]. A recent work summarized possible mechanisms that could explain the biological pathway behind growth impairment in the offspring of women exposed to psychosocial stress [49].

Higher rates of impaired foetal growth in developing countries might be explained by a higher prevalence of risk factors for violence during pregnancy, such as, poor education, adolescent pregnancy, unplanned pregnancy, low social support, relationships encouraging alcohol and drugs usage, and easy access to weapons. Moreover, in some of these countries, social and cultural norms around masculinity may endorse gendered power relationships and violence [50]. It must be noted that there may also be potential cultural biases in the various instruments used to measure violence that may skew the results.

It is important to establish if there is a common biological mechanism mediating the association between violence and impaired foetal growth, and mental disorder and impaired foetal growth. If the gestational cortisol axis were the final common pathway in the association between psychosocial stress during pregnancy and negative birth outcomes, the cortisol stress system could be a potential target for therapeutic intervention in vulnerable women. Furthermore, it is also important to establish whether the subjective experience of stress (i.e., mental disorder) in association with violence will result in relatively greater overdrive of the cortisol stress axis than either risk factor alone: i.e., whether the effects of violence and depression are additive on HPA axis measures. If there existed a cumulative effect of these risk factors, it would help in the future to identify high-risk groups.

Our study should be understood in the context of its limitations. We had a 13.1% loss of mothers in our follow up. Even if there was no statistical difference in the descriptive variables among the followed up and lost women, those who have higher rates of migration could have also had greater health risks. It must also be noted that our measurement of violence encompassed the last 7 months of gestation and a pre-conception period, making a total of 12 months. During this period, we conducted routine data collections for our outcome variables. If any measurement bias were introduced during this period, it would not be a differential bias, since exposed and non-exposed groups were submitted to similar neonatal procedures.

Conclusion

In conclusion, domestic violence against women and mental disorders amongst pregnant women have detrimental effects on birth outcomes and unfortunately, are extremely prevalent in under-resourced, urban areas. It is imperative that actions be taken to prevent violence and improve mental health during pregnancy, especially in disadvantaged populations that may be more at risk.

Abbreviations
ABEP: Brazilian association of population studies; BL: Birth length; BMI: Body mass index; BW: Birth weight; DV: Domestic violence; HPA: Hypothalamic-pituitary-adrenal; ICD: International classification of diseases; IRR: Incidence rate ratio; LBW: Low birth weight; MD: Mental health disorder; OCD: Obsessive–compulsive disorder; OR: Odds ratio; PTB: Preterm birth; SGA: Small for gestational age; WHO: World Health Organization

Acknowledgements
We would like to acknowledge all mothers and children who decided to take part in this study. We also would like to acknowledge our field workers and central staff.

Funding
CNPQ - National Council for Scientific and Technological Development; FAPESP – Foundation for the Support of Research of the State of Sao Paulo, Brazil.

Authors' contributions
AAF – study design, data analysis and drafting the manuscript.
LAR – study design, interpretation of the data and manuscript critically revision. GVP - research admnistration, interpretation of the data and manuscript critically revision. AA - data collection, data management and drafting the manuscript. ECM - study design, fund raising and manuscript critically revision. SJFEG - study design, fund raising and manuscript critically revision. BFB - research admnistration, data collection and drafting the manuscript. All authors read and approved the final manuscript.

Competing interests
The authors declare that they have no competing interests

Author details
[1]Department of Pediatrics, School of Medicine, Universidade de Sao Paulo, Av Dr Eneas Carvalho Aguiar, 647, Sao Paulo 05403-900, Brazil. [2]Department of Psychiatry, School of Medicine, Universidade de Sao Paulo, Sao Paulo, Brazil. [3]Department of Psychiatry and Legal Medicine, School of Medicine, Universidade Federal do Rio Grande do Sul, Porto Alegre, Brazil.

References
1. Gluckman PD, Hanson MA, Bateson P, Beedle AS, Law CM, Bhutta ZA, Anokhin KV, Bougneres P, Chandak GR, Dasgupta P, et al. Towards a new developmental synthesis: adaptive developmental plasticity and human disease. Lancet. 2009;373(9675):1654–7.
2. Fall CH. Fetal programming and the risk of noncommunicable disease. Indian J Pediatr. 2013;80(Suppl 1):S13–20. doi:10.1007/s12098-012-0834-5.
3. Gluckman PD, Hanson MA. Living with the past: evolution, development, and patterns of disease. Science. 2004;305(5691):1733–6.
4. Ferrari AA, Solymos GM, Castillo RM, Sigulem DM. Risk factors for protein-energy malnutrition in pre-school shantytown children in São Paulo, Brazil. Sao Paulo Med J. 1998;116(2):1654–60.
5. Patel V, Rahman A, Jacob KS, Hughes M. Effect of maternal mental health on infant growth in low income countries: new evidence from South Asia. BMJ. 2004;328:820–3.
6. Andersson L, Sundstrom-Poromaa I, Wulff M, Astrom M, Bixo M. Neonatal outcome following maternal antenatal depression and anxiety: a population-based study. Am J Epidemiol. 2004;159(9):872–81.
7. Chung TK, Lau TK, Yip AS, Chiu HF, Lee DT. Antepartum depressive symptomatology is associated with adverse obstetric and neonatal outcomes. Psychosom Med. 2001;63(5):830–4.
8. Rahman A, Iqbal Z, Bunn J, Lovel H, Harrington R. Impact of maternal depression on infant nutritional status and illness: a cohort study. Arch Gen Psychiatry. 2004;61(9):946–52.
9. Murphy CC, Schei B, Myhr TL, Du MJ. Abuse: a risk factor for low birth weight? A systematic review and meta-analysis. CMAJ. 2001;164(11):1567–72.
10. Paarlberg KM, Vingerhoets AJ, Passchier J, Dekker GA, Van Geijn HP. Psychosocial factors and pregnancy outcome: a review with emphasis on methodological issues. J Psychosom Res. 1995;39(5):563–95.
11. Victora CG, Barreto ML, do Carmo Leal M, Monteiro CA, Schmidt MI, Paim J, Bastos FI, Almeida C, Bahia L, Travassos C, Reichenheim M, Barros FC, Lancet Brazil Series Working Group. Health conditions and health-policy innovations in Brazil: the way forward. Lancet. 2011;377(9782):2042–53.
12. Williams RL, Creasy RK, Cunningham GC, Hawes WE, Norris FD, Tashiro M. Fetal growth and perinatal viability in California. Obstet Gynecol. 1982;59(5):624–32.
13. Capurro H, Konichezky S, Fonseca D, Caldeyro-Barcia R. A simplified method for diagnosis of gestational age in the newborn infant. J Pediatr. 1978;93:120–2.
14. Garcia-Moreno C, Jansen HA, Ellsberg M, Heise L, Watts CH et al. Prevalence of intimate partner violence: findings from the WHO multi-country study on women's health and domestic violence. Lancet. 2006;368(9543):1260–9.
15. Sheehan DV, Lecrubier Y, Sheehan KH, Amorim P, Janavs J, Weiller E, Hergueta T, Baker R, Dunbar GC. The Mini-International Neuropsychiatric Interview (M.I.N.I.): the development and validation of a structured diagnostic psychiatric interview for DSM-IV and ICD-10. J Clin Psychiatry. 1998;59(Suppl 20):22–33. quiz 34-57
16. Schraiber LB, Latorre Mdo R, França I Jr, Segri NJ, D'Oliveira AF. Validity of the WHO VAW study instrument for estimating gender-based violence against women. Rev Saude Publica. 2010;44(4):658–66.
17. Amorim, P. Mini International Neuropsychiatric Interview (MINI): validação de entrevista breve para diagnóstico de transtornos mentais. Rev Bras Psiquiatr 2000, vol.22, n.3, pp. 106-115.
18. World Health Organization – WHO, 2001. URL: http://www.who.int/gender/violence/womenfirtseng.pdf. Accessed 14 May 2014.
19. ABEP. Criterio de Classificaçao Econômica Brasil. Associacao Brasileira de Estudos Populacionais. Sao Paulo: ABEP; 2007.
20. Olsen J, Frische G. Social differences in reproductive health. A study on birth weight, stillbirths and congenital malformations in Denmark. Scand J Soc Med. 1993;21(2):90–7.
21. Textor J, Hardt J, Knüppel S. DAGitty: a graphical tool for analyzing causal diagrams. Epidemiology. 2011;5(22):745.
22. Krug EG, editor. World report on violence and health. Geneva: World Health Organization; 2002.
23. Cardia N. Urban violence in Sao Paulo. Washington D.C.: Woodrow Wilson International Centre for Scholars (Comparative Urban Studies Occasional Paper Series, 33), 2000.
24. Sanjuan AN. [Youth and violence in Caracas – Paradox of a process of citizenship loss]. [Portuguese]. In: Pinheiro PS, editor. Sao Paulo without fear – a diagnose of urban violence. Rio de Janeiro: Garamond; 1998. p. 254.
25. World Health Organisation. Global and regional estimates of violence against women: prevalence and health effects of intimate partner violence and non-partner sexual violence. Geneva: WHO; 2013. p. 52.
26. Howard LM, Oram S, Galley H, Trevillion K, Feder G. Domestic violence and perinatal mental disorders: a systematic review and meta-analysis. PLoS Med. 2013;10(5):e1001452. doi:10.1371/journal.pmed.1001452.
27. Gazmararian JA, Lazorick S, Spitz AM, Ballard TJ, Saltzman LE, Marks JS. Prevalence of violence against pregnant women. [erratum appears in JAMA 1997 Apr 9;277(14):1125]. JAMA. 1996;275(24):1915–20.
28. Valdez-Santiago R, Sanin-Aguirre LH. Domestic violence during pregnancy and its relationship with birth weight. Salud Publica de Mexico. 1996;38(5):352–62.
29. Moraes CL, Reichenheim ME. Domestic violence during pregnancy in Rio de Janeiro, Brazil. Int J Gyn Obst. 2002;79:269–77.
30. Bennett HA, Einarson A, Taddio A, Koren G, Einarson TR. Prevalence of depression during pregnancy: systematic review. [erratum appears in Obstet Gynecol. 2004 Jun;103(6):1344]. Obstet Gynecol. 2004;103(4):698–709.
31. Heron J, O'Connor TG, Evans J, Golding J, Glover V, The ALSPAC Study

Team. The course of anxiety and depression through pregnancy and the postpartum in a community sample. J Affect Disord. 2004;80(1):65–73.
32. Fatoye FO, Adeyemi AB, Oladimeji BY. Emotional distress and its correlates among Nigerian women in late pregnancy. JObstetrics Gynaecol. 2004;24(5):504–9.
33. Lovisi GM, López JR, Coutinho ES, Patel V. Poverty, violence and depression during pregnancy: a survey of mothers attending a public hospital in Brazil. Psychol Med. 2005;35(10):1485–92.
34. Golding JM. Intimate partner violence as a risk factor for mental disorders: a meta-analysis. J Fam Violence. 1999;14(2):99–132.
35. Ferri CP, Mitsuhiro SS, Barros MC, Chalem E, Guinsburg R, Patel, et al. The impact of maternal experience of violence and common mental disorders on neonatal outcomes: a survey of adolescent mothers in Sao Paulo, Brazil. BMC Public Health. 2007;7(147):209.
36. Harpham T. Urbanization and mental health in developing countries: a research role for social scientists, public health professionals and social psychiatrists. Soc Sci Med. 1994;39(2):233–345.
37. Browm EW, Harris TO. Social origins of depression. London: Tavistock; 1978.
38. Hoffman S, Hatch MC. Depressive symptomatology during pregnancy: evidence for an association with decreased fetal growth in pregnancies of lower social class women. Health Psychol. 2000;19(6):535–43.
39. Patel V, Prince M. Maternal psychological morbidity and low birth weight in India. Br J Psychiatry. 2006;188:284–5.
40. Valladares ME. Low birth weight newborns and domestic violence: case-control study. Leon, Nicaragua, Universidad Nacional Autonoma de Nicaragua, 1996. Source ID: PIP/143376.
41. Leung WC, Wong YY, Leung TW, Ho PC. Pregnancy outcome following domestic violence in a Chinese community. Int J Gynaecol Obstet. 2001; 72(1):79–80.
42. Jejeebhoy SJ. Associations between wife-beating and fetal and infant death: impressions from a survey in rural India. Stud Fam Plan. 1998;29(3):300–8.
43. Menezes TC, Amorin MMR, Santos LC, Faundes A. [Domestic physical violence and pregnancy: results of a survey in the postpartum period] [Portuguese]. RBGO. 2003;25(5):309–16.
44. Campbell JC. Health consequences of intimate partner violence. Lancet. 2002;359(9314):1331–6.
45. O'Keane V, Scott J. From 'obstetric complications' to a maternal-foetal origin hypothesis of mood disorder. Br J Psychiatry. 2005;186:367–8.
46. Gitau R, Cameron A, Fisk N, Glover V. Fetal exposure to maternal cortisol. Lancet. 1998;352:707–8.
47. French NP, Hagan R, Evans SF, Godfrey M, Newnham JP. Repeated antenatal corticosteroids: size at birth and subsequent development. Am J Obstet Gynecol. 1999;180(1.1):114–21.
48. Newsome CA, Shiell AW, Fall CHD, Phillips DIW, Shier R, Law CM. Is birth weight related to later glucose and insulin metabolism? — a systematic review. Diabet Med. 2003;20:339–48.
49. Entringer S, Buss C, Wadhwa PD. Prenatal stress and developmental programming of human health and disease risk concepts and integration of empirical findings. Curr Opin Endocrinol Diabetes Obes. 2010;17(6):507–16.
50. Naved RT, Huque H, et al. Men's attitudes and practices regarding gender and violence against women in Bangladesh. Preliminary findings. Dhaka: ICDDR, B; 2011.

6

Male involvement in maternal health: perspectives of opinion leaders

Raymond A. Aborigo[1,2*], Daniel D. Reidpath[1], Abraham R. Oduro[2] and Pascale Allotey[1]

Abstract

Background: Twenty years after acknowledging the importance of joint responsibilities and male participation in maternal health programs, most health care systems in low income countries continue to face challenges in involving men. We explored the reasons for men's resistance to the adoption of a more proactive role in pregnancy care and their enduring influence in the decision making process during emergencies.

Methods: Ten focus group discussions were held with opinion leaders (chiefs, elders, assemblymen, leaders of women groups) and 16 in-depth interviews were conducted with healthcare workers (District Directors of Health, Medical Assistants in-charge of health centres, and district Public Health Nurses and Midwives). The interviews and discussions were audio recorded, transcribed into English and imported into NVivo 10 for content analysis.

Results: As heads of the family, men control resources, consult soothsayers to determine the health seeking or treatment for pregnant women, and serve as the final authority on where and when pregnant women should seek medical care. Beyond that, they have no expectation of any further role during antenatal care and therefore find it unnecessary to attend clinics with their partners. There were conflicting views about whether men needed to provide any extra support to their pregnant partners within the home. Health workers generally agreed that men provided little or no support to their partners. Although health workers had facilitated the formation of father support groups, there was little evidence of any impact on antenatal support.

Conclusions: In patriarchal settings, the role of men can be complex and social and cultural traditions may conflict with public health recommendations. Initiatives to promote male involvement should focus on young men and use chiefs and opinion leaders as advocates to re-orient men towards more proactive involvement in ensuring the health of their partners.

Keywords: Ghana, Maternal health, Safe motherhood, Male involvement, Role of men, Maternal morbidity, Near miss

Background

A number of international instruments have acknowledged the critical role of men in increasing access to and utilisation of maternal health services [1, 2]. As decision makers, men are central to preparations for birth and the actions needed in case of an emergency [3]. In patriarchal communities such as those in most African settings, the influence of men is even more profound. Men in these settings control household resources and often make critical decisions that affect maternal health including the choice of health services [4, 5].

Globally, the involvement of men in maternal health programs has been associated with positive reproductive health outcomes, such as increase in the use of contraceptives [6, 7], improved maternal health outcomes [8] and increased uptake of interventions to prevent HIV transmission [9–12]. Despite these benefits, few men participate in maternal health services [9, 13].

A number of studies in Africa have explored male involvement in maternal health programs. In Kenya, although men were aware of the benefits of their involvement in maternal health, perception of pregnancy support as a female role, negative health worker attitudes, and unfriendly antenatal care services limited male involvement [4, 14]. In Malawi, a study found that using peers to encourage male involvement was effective and sustainable

* Correspondence:rayborigo@yahoo.com; raymond.aborigo@navrongo-hrc.org
[1]Global Public Health and SEACO, JC School of Medicine and Health Sciences, Monash University, Subang Jaya, Malaysia
[2]Navrongo Health Research Centre, Post office Box 114, Navrongo, Ghana

[15]. In Uganda, a study that investigated perceived benefits of male attendance of antenatal care (ANC) found that knowledge of three or more antenatal care services, obtaining health information from facility health workers, and a spouse having skilled attendance at last childbirth were all predictive of increased male attendance at ANC [16].

In Ghana, involving men in maternal health programs has focused on reproductive health campaigns that emphasise the value of responsible sexual behaviour, small family size, and mutual respect for women [17]. Most studies that have examined these initiatives have focused on their impact on family planning uptake [6, 18–20] with limited attention to the critical role of men in caring for their pregnant partners, support during child birth and seeking care when complications occur. Although some studies in Ghana report that majority of women have negative opinions and attitudes towards male involvement [21], it nonetheless negates the many health benefits that are associated with male involvement.

A large study which was undertaken by one of the lead authors as part of his PhD research investigated severe maternal morbidities in the community [22, 23]. The findings highlighted men's reluctance in participating in antenatal care and their significant influence in the choice of place of delivery and health seeking in the event of complications. We fed these results back to opinion leaders in order to gain a better understanding of men's resistance to the adoption of a more proactive role in pregnancy care and their enduring influence in the decision making process during health seeking.

Methods

Study setting

The study was carried out in the East and West Kassena-Nankana Districts in the Upper East Region; the poorest region of Ghana. The Kassena-Nankana District (KND) has a population of about 150,000 with a population growth rate of less than 1% [24, 25]. There are two major ethnic groups – the Kassena and the Nankani. The two ethnic groups largely share a homogeneous socio-cultural system although there are some minor differences in cultural practices and festivals. Polytheism is common with animism co-occurring with various denominations of Christianity and Islam. Illiteracy is high 55% within the KND especially among women [26].

The district is largely patriarchal and male dominance is ensured through marriage customs such as the patrilineal inheritance and polygamy. Individuals live in relatively isolated compounds made up of physically linked household units headed by males with absolute authority over members. This gives men control over the use of family resources and decisions about health seeking [27].

Villages which are made up of several scattered compounds are headed by traditional chiefs. Political governance is through a district assembly with elected representatives from sections within the villages. Ten paramount chiefs and several divisional and sub-chiefs with their elders, zealously guard the cultural traditions of the people.

As gate keepers, chiefs play a critical role in implementing health programs within their villages. Maternal health programs therefore require the support of the traditional hierarchy in order to facilitate men's understanding of women's health and support the empowerment of women to make decisions regarding their health.

In terms of health care, public health facilities have been strategically located throughout the district to improve geographical access to services. The community has access to 33 community health compounds with resident community health nurses, six health centres, two public and four private clinics [28, 29]. The only hospital in the district is located in the urban centre and serves as a referral facility for all cases in need of emergency obstetric care. Financing of health services in the district is largely through a district mutual health insurance scheme and all maternal healthcare services are provided free within accredited health facilities.

This research was part of a bigger study which used data from a demographic surveillance system run by the Navrongo Health Research Centre to identify severe maternal morbidities within the community. The surveillance system which covers the study district, collects routine data on marriages, pregnancies, births, deaths and migrations every 120 days [25]. The surveillance platform also has an address system that facilitates the tracing of research participants in the community. The study was therefore sited within the surveillance system in order to facilitate the tracing of severe maternal morbidities.

Study design

A qualitative research approach was used to gain an understanding of men's perception of their role in maternal health. Opinion leaders who were mostly male and health professionals who have direct contact with community members shared their views through focus group discussions and in depth interviews respectively. The bigger study was carried out as a PhD project [22, 23, 30]. The main study obtained local explanations for severe maternal morbidities from interviews with traditional healers and traditional birth attendants and used that explanation to screen over 900 women who recently gave birth in order to identify those who suffered severe maternal complications based on the local definition. Women who suffered severe maternal complications responded to an audit tool with an open narrative section that enabled to collection of qualitative data. The results from the audit which had a community focus were shared with opinion leaders within the research setting and the reactions of the community leaders regarding the role of men in maternal health are shared in this paper. Specifically, the opinion leaders offered their views on the role of men in delaying access to an appropriate place of care, lack of support for their partners during pregnancy, delays in initiating antenatal care and challenges with complying with drug regimes and nutritional requirements.

Sampling procedure

Communities were purposively selected based on their relative isolation from the district hospital. This was to explore the influence of geographical access to the referral centre for emergency obstetric care. In all, 10 communities beyond a 15 km radius of the district hospital were selected. Selection of opinion leaders (chiefs, elders, assembly members, leaders of women groups) was done through the village chiefs. The study team requested each chief to invite between 10 and 12 opinion leaders to discuss issues related to maternal health.

The Ghana Health Service is implementing a primary health care policy which makes community participation led by the Chiefs, an integral part of the implementation strategy. Beyond that, the Navrongo Health Research Centre (NHRC) has been carrying out research in the study district for over 25 years and as part of the requirements for initiating any research project, researchers have to conduct community entry activities which involves meetings with chiefs and their elders to discuss the research project and to seek permission to implement the study in their communities. Also, each of the chiefs has been involved in research at some point during the period of NHRC'S existence but this is rare. Apart from the current study, the only other study that directly involved opinion leaders as respondents was one that involved the lead author. That study determined the appropriateness of community engagement strategies as used by the research Centre [31].

In-depth Interviews (IDIs) were held with health professionals whose work demands regular interaction with opinion leaders or the provision of direct maternal health services to community members. Four members of the district health management team (public health nurses and District directors of health) and four staff of the health centres. These categories of professionals were considered key stakeholders in maternal health in the various villages. We also interviewed eight community health officer-midwives. Community health officer-midwives are nurses who have been trained to proficiency in midwifery skills and placed in health compounds within the community to offer basic obstetric care to women.

Data collection

The student researcher who has over 14 years experience in conducting qualitative research, assisted in conducting the 16 in-depth interviews with the health workers. The researcher also moderated ten Focus Group Discussions (FGDs) with the opinion leaders. The discussions with opinion leaders were conducted in the local languages - Kasem or Nankani - while the interviews with the health workers were in English (Additional file 1). Each focus group discussion lasted about 2 hours and the in-depth interviews, 1 hour. All the interviews and discussions were audio recorded and labeled with unique identifiers. For ethical reasons, quotes from the in-depth interviews are attributed generically to "health workers". The study guides were pre-tested to ensure that they elicited the right information to meet the research objectives. Data collection lasted from March to November 2012.

The discussions focused on gender specific concerns that were raised in the larger study. Male support for women over the duration of pregnancy and the opinions of males on broader gender dynamics during pregnancy were explored. Specifically, men's enduring role in making decisions related to place for delivery or health care when complications occur were discussed.

Based on the sampling approach, only 10 communities qualified to participate in the study. Considering that we had an average of 10 people participate in each focus group discussion, it meant about 120 individuals participated in the focus groups. This was in addition to the 16 IDIs with the health workers.

Although there is currently no consensus on how saturation is reached for one to stop interviewing, we think the number of interviews we conducted were enough for us to achieve saturation. Creswel suggests 20 to 30 interviews [32] while Morse suggests 30 to 50 [33] but they both failed to explain why these number of interviews and not any other. In studies with a high level of homogeneity like the current study, a sample of six interviews is deemed sufficient to enable the development of meaningful themes and useful interpretations [34].

Data processing and analysis

All the focus group discussions were transcribed into English. In transcribing the discussions, culture specific terminologies were retained and transcribed verbatim in the local languages. Transcripts and field notes were imported into QSR NVivo 10.0 software [35] for thematic analysis. Initial coding was based directly on the research questions. Themes were derived inductively by reading every sentence in all transcripts, identifying answers to repeated questions and naming them, and segmenting the data into similar groupings to form preliminary categories of information about male involvement in maternal health. Segments of texts in the respondents' own words and expressions relating to the themes were extracted and labeled. Subsequent coding was based on emergent themes. Patterns, similarities and differences in these codes and themes were examined. This was to ensure that negative and deviant views were considered in the research report.

Observations and field notes were coded together with the main transcripts and used to provide further contextual information.

Results

The study offered an opportunity to opinion leaders to participate in research. Generally, involvement of opinion leaders in research has been limited to granting permission for research to take place in their communities. Rarely are they engaged in research as participants. As a male dominated group who were mostly married, the opinion leaders found the themes intriguing and discussed them exhaustively. Motivation to participate in the study was driven by their constant neglect from discussing critical issues that affect the health of their spouses.

Delays in the decision making process

Health seeking decisions, particularly relating to pregnancy and childbirth, are traditionally made primarily on consultation with a soothsayer for a preliminary diagnosis and advice about the plan of action. Communication with the soothsayer is the responsibility of the head of the compound who are mostly men. The role of the soothsayer is critical because according to the traditional belief system, there are circumstances under which pregnant women could not present to health facilities. The consequences of choosing the wrong place for care could spell misfortune for the family. A woman in need of emergency obstetric care may therefore have to wait for the consultation of sooth-sayers to be completed before care can be sought. A women's group leader who participated in the focus groups confirmed that:

> *"We are only women. If a woman who has just delivered falls sick, it is the responsibility of the man to go out and consult a soothsayer to know why it is so. Women cannot know why the newly delivered woman is sick. The men also find out whether the visit (to the health facility) would affect her survival". FGD-OL-MA.*

Women who exercise some level of autonomy are considered disrespectful. Women cannot unilaterally initiate care seeking without causing offense. Women who act independently disrupt the social hierarchy and challenge the power structure. This was a common theme and for some community members, not even a life-threatening event such as a severe maternal morbidity provides sufficient justification for a woman to override the deep-rooted social norm. Women who encounter misfortune after independently seeking care risk being labeled as witches. The excerpt below conveys some of the views held by men.

> *"Infact, traditionally, a woman cannot go to the hospital without the knowledge of the compound head. If the husband is not at home, they will ask her to wait for him to come. It may take him a whole day or two to return; is it true or not? Meanwhile the woman is suffering and they are waiting for someone to come. It is a problem; if she goes without informing anyone and the pregnancy miscarries, they will say she is a witch and she will not be allowed into the house. That is what also leads to the delay". FGD-OL-NA.*

Women's lack of urgency in the decision making process is compounded by their economic dependence on their husbands. Although maternal health care services are free within public health facilities in Ghana, indirect costs associated with utilisation of these facilities such as expenditure on transportation and food, generally require that the woman has cash when seeking care. In the absence of the man, such resources may not be available and the woman has to wait for the husband.

> *"She has to inform her husband because he has to give her some money to go to the hospital. Even if she has health insurance and will not pay for the treatment, she will drink water over there and she may even go in a vehicle". FGD-OL-GA.*

The participants admitted that some of the women make more money than their husbands. They reported that some women are wage earners or work in the informal sector as traders or farmers and therefore do not need any financial support to seek care. However, regardless of the woman's personal access to financial resources, she risks offending her husband if she initiates care seeking without first obtaining the consent of her husband. As a women's group leader put it, *once you have decided to attach yourself to (marry) him, you have no right to have your own thoughts". FGD-OL-YU (Women Group Leader).* Once a decision is made by the head of the family, women can neither contest nor disobey because they risk incurring the wrath of their husbands.

Men's role in the decision making process includes the place of delivery. Preference for home delivery was common among the opinion leaders who argued that prior to the arrival of modern health care, women were already experiencing safe deliveries at home.

"Our parents did not go to the hospital and yet we are living. Look, my wife has delivered nine children without going to the hospital". FGD-OL-PI.

Despite the prevailing cultural norms, there was some evidence of changing views of women's autonomy, particularly from those who had had the experience of travel outside the district. Most of the young men who expressed acceptance of women's right to independently access care were literate and had been exposed to alternative cultures of the tribal groups in the southern part of the country. The Ashanti tribe, for instance, is matrilineal with power vested in women to make critical decisions for the community including nominating the next chief. The young men reported that it was within the woman's right to initiate care seeking or choose a place for delivery in the absence of the husband or compound head, especially for maternal emergencies. They however added that it is imperative for the woman to inform the husband about her decision as soon as possible.

"She can go without informing you; if you leave home for your farm and she falls sick, she can go to the hospital. You cannot quarrel with her when she comes back home; who knows what will happen if she delays. She can go." FGD-OL-PI.

Lack of support from men during pregnancy

The health workers were of the view that as stakeholders in maternal health, men can support their pregnant partners and participate in maternal health interventions. They defined support to include better education of their partners to take control of their health by reminding them of clinic days and assisting them comply with drug regimens, financing and facilitating their health facility visits and ensuring the use of health facilities for delivery and health care. The reluctance of men to perform these roles was communicated strongly by the health workers and the cultural context was viewed as the main limiting factor.

"That is the problem here, they don't even ask their wives to know what happened at the clinic and that is why some of the women collect the drugs and keep them in the house and don't take them. If the men were interested, they can ask that what drugs did you receive? How are you going to be take them? They will tell them and they will support them to take the drugs but they just don't care". IDI-HEALTH WORKER.

The men claimed that they often assist their partners with household chores such as fetching water or firewood because they recognise the risk involved if pregnant women engage in strenuous physical activity. Support was also in the form of increased affection and care, transportation in case of illness, provision of good food, money for clinic expenses, consulting sooth-sayers and pouring of libation. The men reported that it was necessary for them to continuously monitor the health of their partners by pouring libation and consistently consult sooth-sayers throughout the period of the pregnancy. This traditional role was deemed necessary to prevent illnesses caused by evil spirits, witches and charms or show appreciation to the ancestors for recovery from illnesses.

"If your wife is pregnant, your enemies can interfere with the pregnancy, witches can also interfere with the pregnancy and kill the woman. So the man won't sit down; he will go round (consult sooth-sayers) to see to it that his wife gives birth safely." FGD-OL-PI.

Men's support during antenatal care

The health workers reported that there was a new health policy to encourage men to accompany their partners for antenatal care. According to the health workers, the initiative was because tests for HIV for instance, require that the couple be tested to reduce the risk to the foetus. Men who attend antenatal care also have access to critical information on the reproductive health of their partners, information on obstetric danger signs and information on birth preparedness. Also, as heads of the household, men in antenatal care could increase adherence to guidance provided at the clinic.

Most of the male opinion leaders were unaware of the initiative to encourage them to attend antenatal care. For those who were aware of the initiative, a few supported it. They argued that since it took two of them to make the pregnancy, both of them have responsibility for the health of the woman and the outcome of the pregnancy. They also recognised that some women feel reluctant to go for antenatal care after the first visit and men can ensure that they adhere to the schedules. Besides, "*Your wife is your friend; if you have time to go with her, it does not spoil anything; it is good" (FGD-OL-PU).* Some shared stories to highlight the relevance of the policy.

"Let me tell you a true story; a woman went for weighing and she was told the type of foods to eat. When she got home and told her husband, the man asked her to go back to the hospital for those foods (laughter by respondents.) If the man had gone with his wife to the clinic, he would have also heard the type of foods his wife should eat. It would have been more helpful". FGD-OL-MA.

Some men were of the view that normally, they would not accompany their partners for antenatal care but a health policy could encourage such attendance. They said compliance was more likely if the policy had the support of the chiefs, because *if your chief tells you to dance, you cannot say your hips are hurting. FGD-OL-KO.*

Men's perceptions about antenatal care

The question of whether men in the community accompanied their partners to the ANC surprised some participants because generally, men in the KND do not accompany their partners for antenatal care. One community member reported that *"there is no man in [community A] who does that (accompanies the wife for antenatal care); not even a single one" (FGD-OL-PI).*

Socially, the idea of attending antenatal care with one's wife was strange to most community members. Statements such as *"we are not used to that (FGD-OL-PI)", "I have never seen that"(FGD-OL-SI)* and *"they say women should go for weighing and not men" (FGD-OL-KU)",* were common. Health workers were of the view that men often assume that issues in the clinic are for women and therefore their presence there is irrelevant.

> *"They think it is the woman's issue and they don't see their importance in coming". IDI-Health worker.*

In both Kasem and Nankani, the words used for antenatal care are *maŋem* and *makrɜ* which translate as "weighing" in English. Men wondered what their role was at the antenatal clinic when the purpose was to "weigh" pregnant women. Also, men prioritised other roles over supporting their partners in this way. The responsibility of men to work and provide for the family takes precedence over public health recommendations such as accompanying their partners to the clinic. Concerns about what the family will eat and who will attend to other children if both husband and wife are absent were raised by participants.

> *"The reason why we cannot do that is we are always engaged in one activity or the other. When we wake up, we sweat before we get something to eat. So while the woman is attending the antenatal clinic, the man will remain at home and work so that when she returns there will be something for both of us to eat. That is why we have no time to go with them". FGD-OL-AA.*

Men's concerns about attending antenatal care

Underlying men's reluctance to attend antenatal care is a cultural perception that the overt expression of one's affection and concern for his wife is inappropriate. Some participants said the practice of publicly expressing affection is shameful and can only be a borrowed culture from other tribal groups such as the Akans in southern Ghana or the "Whiteman".

> *"We are not used to it; we are not "Gambue" (Akan tribe in southern Ghana) Gambue like holding their wives and putting their arms around their necks. Here, if you even touch your wife while you are walking with her, people will see you in a different manner". FGD-OL-AA.*

> *"It is not our tradition; our forefathers did not do that. If you do that, they will say you are a useless man. They will mock and insult you". FGD-OL-KU.*

Men who accompanied their wife's to the clinic were called "kana-kadona" (women's rivals) or "bakana" which means "man-woman"; suggesting that the man exhibits female tendencies. Most of the men were of the view that accompanying their partners to the clinic is embarrassing and cannot be promoted within their communities.

Factors that influence men's attendance of antenatal care

Women with complications were more likely to have their husbands attend antenatal care with them. This was due to two reasons; first, because the woman cannot walk due to the illness and therefore has to be transported and second, because they want to have first-hand information on her recovery. Women who have to travel long distances to access antenatal care were also more likely to be accompanied by their male partners as indicated by one male participant.

> *"My house is far from the clinic so when she was pregnant and paddled a bicycle to the clinic and back, she lost the pregnancy. So when she became pregnant again, I had to pick her on the bicycle to and from the clinic. I heard everything she was told at the clinic". FGD-OL-MA.*

Attendance of antenatal clinic was also reported to be influenced by trust among couples. The men said they would attend antenatal care if they suspected that the woman was not interested in keeping the pregnancy. This was mainly to prevent any attempt to terminate a pregnancy.

The men also reported that clinic infrastructure was not built to accommodate them. Men at antenatal care have restricted access to treatment and examination rooms, thus, they often remain under trees and do not feel part of the antenatal care process.

Increasing male involvement

The need to increase male involvement in maternal health was recognised by most participants. Initiatives that were pursued by health workers included a conscious effort to consistently engage men in reproductive health discussions during routine home visits and at community meetings or durbars. According to the health workers, community meetings were preferred as men were usually absent during home visits. Durbars were reportedly effective in reaching a critical mass of males and attendance was best on market days but men often got drunk before arriving at the durbar ground. Other suggested strategies included drama and radio programs to reach out to men.

Current incentives to increase male involvement in antenatal care included giving women who attended antenatal care with their husbands' preferential treatment throughout the antenatal care process. Men who attended antenatal care were also publicly acknowledged and commended. Health workers also facilitate the formation of father support groups within the communities to promote the sharing of knowledge and to encourage peer support for young fathers. Surprisingly, none of the opinion leaders mentioned the work of the groups in the discussions. This raises concerns about either the effectiveness of the intervention or the appropriateness of the approach to the formation of the groups.

> *"It is because they have realised these problems like men not (being) interested in accompanying their wives to the facilities, and their refusal to ensure that women should be provided good nutritional foods and clothing during pregnancy to ensure safe delivery, Ghana Health Services said that any time they have a community durbar or workshop, we should go and educate the people on the importance of these things. Why the men need to give all the necessary support to their wives during pregnancy and even after. Also, in our home visits we have been doing all these and yet they don't want to change. We will also not stop; time will come when they will change and pay attention to their wives." IDI-Health Worker.*

The health workers acknowledged that changing behaviour is a challenge, especially in societies where individuals can suffer social derision and stigma after embracing change. Consequently, it was suggested that the approach be gradual and tactful in order not to offend communities with strong opposing cultural values.

> *"My suggestions would be that, areas where male involvement in the activities are low, we should do more community sensitisation through drama or radio, organise durbars and we should take this thing slowly because we are changing human behaviour. These are people who are 40 to 50 years old who have been living with the women and thinking that once a woman is pregnant it is hers; till the child comes out, I have nothing to do and all of a sudden you want them to start accompanying their wives to antenatal care, when the wife has laboured they should come for postnatal care and family planning. They have not been doing it for a long time so my suggestion is that we should involve them slowly." IDI-Health Worker.*

Participants suggested the use of chiefs to mobilise and disseminate information on male involvement. The effectiveness of this approach lies in the traditional role of the chief as the community gate-keeper and the custodian of traditional norms and practices. Traditional norms which conflict maternal health interventions are best altered using chiefs and elders as advocates. Traditional chiefs have the power to sanction community members who go against the status quo in the community and this was often mentioned in the data. For instance, a health worker reported that some chiefs have instituted by-laws which compel men to ensure that their partners attend antenatal care or face potential fines.

> *"Just to add, if they want to implement such a law, they need to come down to our chief and he can also organise his elders together with a fixed date and time just like we were told to do so here today. We will agree and do but if you meet me on the way and put such an issue to me, I wouldn't even listen to you. I will only be saying yes, yes to you but I wouldn't agree afterwards and if the chief should ask me that did you meet people on your way, I will reply no, I never met anyone on my way (laughs)." FGD-OL-MA.*

> *"In my former station, the chief told the men that if they don't allow their wives to attend ANC, they will pay a fine and all the men agreed and allowed their wives to attend ANC and it was fine. We even formed male groups and we talked about family planning, child health and pregnancy issues and it was helping us". IDI-Health Worker.*

Most of the opinion leaders said they were too old to learn new initiatives in maternal health. They were however of the view that young men could benefit from targeted health campaigns so that as they transition into adulthood, they would view support for their partners during pregnancy as a way of life. They emphasised the need to properly articulate the kind of support that women need from men during pregnancy and how that support should be offered.

Discussion

The study revealed both cultural and social constraints to female empowerment in the KND. Men view female autonomy as disrespectful and an affront to their authority and this includes any unilateral initiative to seek care for maternal complications. Women risk rejection by their husbands and negative societal labels if they fail to respect the hierarchy in the decision-making process. This is particularly so if misfortune occurs after acting independently. Fortunately, men are transitioning from restricting female autonomy to allowing women to independently initiate care seeking for maternal emergencies. Although riddled with caveats including making such decisions only when the male partner is absent, the change nevertheless is positive and calls for the adoption of innovative strategies such as the use of chiefs and other opinion leaders to positively engage men. In addition, thoughtful restructuring of maternal health programs to increasingly engage men could increase male involvement. Previous initiatives such as female education and women economic empowerment which have proved successful in other settings [36, 37] are necessary but not sufficient in accelerating the needed change in men to improve maternal health.

Men in the KND demonstrated adequate knowledge of the type of support they ought to give to their partners during pregnancy and claimed to offer it. However, both health worker reports and findings from the severe maternal morbidity audit showed that men offer little support to their pregnant partners. This disconnect suggests that men are not necessarily translating their desire to support their partners into actual behaviours. In patriarchal settings, there are strict gender roles which are often adhered to, yet some men reported a desire to rise above role stereotypes to support their partners during pregnancy. Programs that aim to improve the role of men in maternal health especially in supporting their partners to take control of their lives, could capitalise on this desire to accelerate male involvement. This must however be pursued with caution in order not to further disenfranchise women.

Men in the KND reported many barriers to accompanying their partners to the ANC. ANC services in Ghana are dominated by females - providers and clients - with hardly any content or infrastructural adaptation to make services attractive or useful to men. Traditionally, males have viewed ANC as a female dominated environment and thus inappropriate for them. Men in the KND risk social derision and stigma if seen accompanying their partners to the ANC. Studies in other African countries report similar findings [4, 15, 38]. In societies such as the KND where spousal communication is limited [6] and where public display of one's affection for the wife is traditionally prohibited, the health system would require the support of chiefs and other opinion leaders to break through cultural barriers. With the support of the opinion leaders, program planners can re-align male involvement programs to fit the socio-cultural context. This can be done through behaviour change programs that focus on using chiefs as champions in re-orienting adult males and young men towards more proactive involvement in ensuring the health of their partners during pregnancy and the puerperium.

Unlike men in rural western Kenya [4], men in the KND lack knowledge on the importance of accompanying their partners to the ANC. The few who do so are usually left under trees and do not actively participate in ANC activities because antenatal infrastructure and services are not designed to accommodate them. Meanwhile, men have other competing social obligations that are necessary for the sustenance of the family. Consequently, men find attendance of ANC unnecessary and a waste of time. If ANC programs are to make progress with male involvement, then programs will have to be restructured to accommodate men to ensure that time spent at the ANC is worth the while. Incentives geared towards encouraging male involvement would have to go beyond applauding men and giving their partners preferential treatment to include participation in ANC activities such as listening to the foetal heart beat, counseling on obstetric danger signs, HIV testing, and access to information on their partners' medications and ANC schedule.

A review of the risk approach to ANC in the 1980s in Ghana revealed that progress in maternal health was not significant after several years of implementation and therefore the couple centered approach was adopted [17]. Sadly however, 30 years after adopting the approach, the system is still grappling with strategies to engage men. The impact of father support groups which have been demonstrated in other settings to be effective [15], are yet to be realised within the health system in Ghana. An opportunity however exists within the Community-Based Health Planning Services [39] to adopt a family-centered approach which would not only ensure that a wider number of men have access to information provided during ANC but that all significant others at the family level have access to such information. When community health nurses conduct routine compound visits, all significant others should participate in discussions related pregnancy. This would showcase maternal health as a shared responsibility and not that of women alone.

Strengths of the study

This study is unique because it arose out of critical concerns raised by women who suffered a life-threatening maternal condition and felt little support from their husbands. Also, the focus on opinion leaders who are the drivers of change at the community level, especially where cultural norms need to be addressed, ensured that findings would be useful in understanding and modifying cultural behaviours that negatively affect maternal health at the community level.

Another strength is that data collection and analysis was completed primarily by a local male researcher with an in-depth understanding of local customs and fluency in the local languages. This was likely to reduce the perceived barriers between interviewer and respondent and likely allowed for deeper exploration of the issues that may have been missed had the primary researcher not been so knowledgeable about the local context.

Weaknesses of the study

One potential weakness of this study is that we relied upon self-reported behaviour on the part of men, without including direct observations. It is possible that men may have reported behaviours that they believe would reflect well upon them, rather than the actual behaviours. However, given the variety of responses – including those who report supporting their partners and those who openly reported disdain for participation in ANC – we do not believe such social desirability biases unduly affected our data.

Conclusions

In patriarchal societies, men play an important role as facilitators of their wives' access to timely and appropriate care. An understanding of the dynamics of male influence is therefore crucial in negotiating compromises to improve the health of women. As custodians of traditions, opinion leaders can play a critical role in shaping gender roles and traditions to promote maternal health. This complex role is particularly relevant where cultural traditions conflict with public health recommendations.

Although significant progress has been made in the realisation of women's rights and gender equality globally, pockets of gender discrimination remain mainly due to cultural norms and these areas are likely to continue to skew indicators of safe motherhood and other gender related measures. Without working with chiefs and other pinion leaders to design innovative strategies for engaging men in maternal health interventions and to give more autonomy to women to take decisions related to their health, reducing maternal mortality and disabilities due to pregnancy would continue to progress at a slow pace.

Abbreviations

ANC: Antenatal Care; FGDs: Focus Group Discussions; IDIs: In-depth Interviews; KND: Kassena-Nankana District; NHRC: Navrongo Health Research Centre; NHRCIRB: Navrongo Health Research Centre Institutional Review Board

Acknowledgements

The authors would like to acknowledge the support of the Navrongo Health Research Centre for providing the platform for the study. Mr. Gideon Logonia provided critical support in data collection and the Global Public Health team of Monash University, Malaysia and staff of the Navrongo Health Research Centre gave invaluable, constructive feedback. Finally, our profound gratitude goes to the women, chief, elders and opinion leaders of the Kassena-Nankana districts.

Funding

This study was funded by Global Public Health, Monash University, Malaysia and the INDEPTH Network educational support initiative.

Authors' contributions

RAA conceived of the study, participated in its design, coordination, acquisition of data and drafted the manuscript. PA and DR participated in the design of the study, analysis and interpretation of the data and reviewed the manuscript critically for important intellectual content. AO assisted in the interpretation and reviewed the manuscript critically for intellectual content. All authors gave final approval to the version of the manuscript to be published.

Competing interests

The authors declare that they have no competing interests.

References

1. United Nations. Report of the Fourth World Conference on Women. Beijing, 4–15 September 1995 [Internet]. United Nations, New York; 1996. Report No.: A/CONF:177/20/Rev.1. Available: http://www.un.org/womenwatch/daw/beijing/pdf/Beijing%20full%20report%20E.pdf
2. UNFPA. ICPD and Human Rights: 20 years of advancing reproductive rights through UN treaty bodies and legal reform [Internet]. Jun 2013 [cited 20 Oct 2013]. Available: http://www.unfpa.org/webdav/site/global/shared/documents/publications/2013/icpd_and_human_rights_20_years.pdf
3. Maternal and Neonatal Health Program. Birth Prepardness and Complication Readiness: A Matrix of Shared Responsibility [Internet]. 2004 [cited 22 Oct 2013]. Available: http://pdf.usaid.gov/pdf_docs/PBAAC805.pdf
4. Kwambai TK, Dellicour S, Desai M, Ameh CA, Person B, Achieng F, et al. Perspectives of men on antenatal and delivery care service utilisation in rural western Kenya: a qualitative study. BMC Pregnancy Childbirth. 2013;13: 134. doi:10.1186/1471-2393-13-134.
5. Ngom P, Debpuur C, Akweongo P, Adongo P, Binka FN. Gate-keeping and Women's health seeking behaviour in Navrongo, northern Ghana. Afr J Reprod Health Rev Afr Santé Reprod. 2003;7:17–26. doi:10.2307/3583341.
6. Bawah AA. Spousal communication and family planning behavior in Navrongo: a longitudinal assessment. Stud Fam Plan. 2002;33:185–94. doi:10.1111/j.1728-4465.2002.00185.x.
7. Terefe A, Larson CP. Modern contraception use in Ethiopia: does involving husbands make a difference? Am J Public Health. 1993;83:1567–71. Available: http://www.ncbi.nlm.nih.gov/pmc/articles/PMC1694882/
8. Yargawa J, Leonardi-Bee J. Male involvement and maternal health outcomes: systematic review and meta-analysis. J Epidemiol Community Health. 2015; jech-2014-204784. doi:10.1136/jech-2014-204784
9. Farquhar C, Kiarie JN, Richardson BA, Kabura MN, John FN, Nduati RW, et al. Antenatal Couple Counseling Increases Uptake of Interventions to Prevent HIV-1 Transmission. J Acquir Immune Defic Syndr 1999. 2004; 37: 1620–1626. Available: http://www.ncbi.nlm.nih.gov/pmc/articles/PMC3384734/
10. Theuring S, Nchimbi P, Jordan-Harder B, Harms G. Partner involvement in perinatal care and PMTCT services in Mbeya region, Tanzania: the providers' perspective. AIDS Care. 2010;22:1562–8. doi:10.1080/09540121003758572.
11. Celentano DD, Nelson KE, Lyles CM, Beyrer C, Eiumtrakul S, Go VF, et al. Decreasing incidence of HIV and sexually transmitted diseases in young Thai men: evidence for success of the HIV/AIDS control and prevention program. AIDS Lond Engl. 1998;12:F29–36.
12. Homsy J, Kalamya JN, Obonyo J, Ojwang J, Mugumya R, Opio C, et al. Routine intrapartum HIV counseling and testing for prevention of mother-to-child transmission of HIV in a rural Ugandan hospital. J Acquir Immune Defic Syndr 1999. 2006;42: 149–154. doi:10.1097/01.qai.0000225032.52766.c2

13. Natoli L, Holmes W, Chanlivong N, Chan G, Toole MJ. Promoting safer sexual practices among expectant fathers in the Lao People's Democratic Republic. Glob Public Health. 2012;7:299–311. doi:10.1080/17441692.2011.641987.
14. Ganle JK, Dery I. "What men don"t know can hurt women's health': a qualitative study of the barriers to and opportunities for men's involvement in maternal healthcare in Ghana. Reprod Health. 2015;12:93. doi:10.1186/s12978-015-0083-y.
15. Kululanga LI, Sundby J, Malata A, Chirwa E. Striving to promote male involvement in maternal health care in rural and urban settings in Malawi - a qualitative study. Reprod Health. 2011;8:36. doi:10.1186/1742-4755-8-36.
16. Tweheyo R, Konde-Lule J, Tumwesigye NM, Sekandi JN. Male partner attendance of skilled antenatal care in peri-urban Gulu district. Northern Uganda BMC Pregnancy Childbirth. 2010;10:53. doi:10.1186/1471-2393-10-53.
17. Odoi-Agyarko H. Profile of reproductive health situation in Ghana. Ghana: WHO; 2003.
18. Adongo PB, Tapsoba P, Phillips JF, Tabong PT-N, Stone A, Kuffour E, et al. The role of community-based health planning and services strategy in involving males in the provision of family planning services: a qualitative study in southern Ghana. Reprod Health. 2013;10:36. doi:10.1186/1742-4755-10-36.
19. Bawah AA, Akweongo P, Simmons R, Phillips JF. Women's fears and men's anxieties: the impact of family planning on gender relations in northern Ghana. Stud Fam Plan. 1999;30:54–66. Available: http://onlinelibrary.wiley.com/doi/10.1111/j.1728-4465.1999.00054.x/abstract
20. Hindin MJ, Kincaid DL, Kumah OM, Morgan W, Kim YM, Ofori JK. Gender differences in media exposure and action during a family planning campaign in Ghana. Health Commun. 1994;6:117–35. doi:10.1207/s15327027hc0602_3.
21. Ganle JK, Dery I, Manu AA, Obeng B. "If I go with him, I can't talk with other women': Understanding women's resistance to, and acceptance of, men's involvement in maternal and child healthcare in northern Ghana". Soc Sci Med 1982. 2016;166: 195–204. doi:10.1016/j.socscimed.2016.08.030
22. Aborigo RA. Contextualizing maternal mortality and morbidity through maternal health audits. Monash University, Malaysia: PhD thesis in preparation; 2014b.
23. Aborigo RA, Allotey P, Reidpath D. Contextualizing maternal morbidity through community case reviews. J Womens Health Care. 2013;2 doi:10.4172/2167-0420.1000e112.
24. Ngom P, Debpuur C, Akweongo P, Adongo P, Binka FN. Gate-keeping and women's health seeking behaviour in Navrongo, northern Ghana. Afr J Reprod Health. 2003;7:17–26.
25. Oduro AR, Wak G, Azongo D, Debpuur C, Wontuo P, Kondayire F, et al. Profile of the Navrongo health and demographic surveillance system. Int J Epidemiol. 2012;41:968–76. doi:10.1093/ije/dys111.
26. Nyarko P, Wontuo P, Alex Nazzar, Philips JF, Ngom P, Binka F. Navrongo Demographic Surveillance System (NDSS) Ghana. INDEPTH Network, Accra; 2002.
27. Adongo PB, Phillips JF, Kajihara B, Fayorsey C, Debpuur C, Binka FN. Cultural factors constraining the introduction of family planning among the Kassena-Nankana of northern Ghana. Soc Sci Med. 1997;45:1789–804. doi:10.1016/S0277-9536(97)00110-X.
28. DHMT-E. Kassena-Nankana District East District Annual report. Dist Health Manag Team Ghana Health Serv. 2011;
29. DHMT-W. Kassena-Nankana District West District Annual report. Dist Health Manag Team Ghana Health Serv. 2011;
30. Aborigo RA, Allotey P, Reidpath DD. The traditional healer in obstetric care: a persistent wasted opportunity in maternal health. Soc Sci Med. 2015;133: 59–66. doi:10.1016/j.socscimed.2015.03.046.
31. Tindana PO, Rozmovits L, Boulanger RF, Bandewar SVS, Aborigo RA, Hodgson AVO, et al. Aligning community engagement with traditional authority structures in global health research: a case study from northern Ghana. Am J Public Health. 2011;101:1857–67. doi:10.2105/AJPH.2011.300203.
32. Creswell JW. Qualitative Inquiry & Research Design: choosing among five approaches [internet]. 2nd ed. thousand oaks. London. New Delhi: SAGE Publications; 2007. Available: https://charlesbickenheuserdotcom.files.wordpress.com/2015/03/creswell_2007_qualitative_inquiry_and_research_design__choosing_among_five_approaches__2nd_edition.pdf
33. Morse J. The significance of saturation. Qual Health Res. 1995;5:147–9. Available: http://qhr.sagepub.com/content/5/2/147.short?rss=1&ssource=mfc
34. Guest G, Bunce A, Johnson L. How many interviews are enough?: an experiment with data saturation and variability. Field Methods. 2006;18:59–82. Available: http://fmx.sagepub.com/content/18/1/59.full.pdf
35. QSR International Pty Ltd. NVivo 10 research software for analysis and insight [Internet]. 2014 [cited 24 Aug 2014]. Available: http://www.qsrinternational.com/products_nvivo.aspx
36. Do M, Kurimoto N. Women's empowerment and choice of contraceptive methods in selected African countries. Int Perspect Sex Reprod Health. 2012; 38: 23+. Available: http://go.galegroup.com/ps/i.do?id=GALE%7CA295326724&v=2.1&u=monash&it=r&p=EAIM&sw=w&asid=28cce1d0e023184aae05a11c5ffe4cfe
37. Crissman HP, Adanu RM, Harlow SD. Women's sexual empowerment and contraceptive use in Ghana. Stud Fam Plan. 2012;43:201–12. doi:10.1111/j.1728-4465.2012.00318.x.
38. Onyango MA, Owoko S, Oguttu M. Factors that influence male involvement in sexual and reproductive health in western Kenya: a qualitative study. Afr J Reprod Health. 2010;14:32–42.
39. Nyonator FK. The Ghana community-based health planning and services initiative for scaling up service delivery innovation. Health Policy Plan. 2005;20:25–34. doi:10.1093/heapol/czi003.

7

Factors influencing access of pregnant women and their infants to their local healthcare system

Shabir A. Madhi[1,2,3*], Luis M. Rivera[4], Xavier Sáez-Llorens[5,6], Clara Menéndez[7,8], Nazira Carrim-Ganey[9], Mark F. Cotton[10], Darren Katzman[11], Mariëtha M. Luttig[11], Rosalba Candelario[12], Sherryl Baker[12] and Mahua Roychoudhury[12]

Abstract

Background: The successful implementation of maternal vaccination relies on results of clinical trials, considering the prenatal and postnatal attendance at selected healthcare institutions. This study evaluated factors influencing maternal/infant access to healthcare facilities to identify potential barriers to participation in future clinical trials on maternal vaccination.

Methods: In this prospective, multi-centre, observational study, pregnant women ($N = 3243$) were enrolled at ten sites across Panama, the Dominican Republic, South Africa, and Mozambique between 2012 and 2014. They completed questionnaires at enrolment, delivery, and infant follow-up (90 days post-partum) visits, including questions on transportation, phone accessibility, alternative childcare, gestational age at enrolment, delivery location, and health status of their infant. Logistic regression was used to identify factors significantly associated with return to study site for delivery or infant follow-up visits.

Results: Among 3229 enrolled women with delivery information, 63.6% (range across sites: 25.3–91.5%) returned to study site for delivery. Older women and those at later gestational age at enrolment were more likely to deliver at the study site. While heterogeneities were observed at site level, shorter travel time at delivery and increased transportation costs at enrolment were associated with increased likelihood of women returning to study site for delivery. Among 3145 women with live-born infants, 3077 (95.3%) provided 90-day follow-up information; of these, 68.9% (range across sites: 25.6–98.9%) returned to study site for follow-up visits. Women with other children and with lower transportation costs at delivery were more likely to return to study site for follow-up visits. Among 666 infants reported sick, 94.3% were taken to a healthcare facility, with only 41.9% (range across sites: 4.9–77.3%) to the study site.
(Continued on next page)

* Correspondence: madhis@rmpru.co.za
[1]Medical Research Council: Respiratory and Meningeal Pathogens Research Unit, University of the Witwatersrand, Johannesburg, South Africa
[2]Department of Science and Technology/National Research Foundation: Vaccine Preventable Diseases, University of the Witwatersrand, Johannesburg, South Africa
Full list of author information is available at the end of the article

(Continued from previous page)

Conclusion: Although high retention was observed from enrolment through 90 days after delivery, post-partum surveillance should be broadened beyond the study sites and additional follow-up visits should be planned within the neonatal period. The factors influencing maternal/infant access to healthcare facilities and the issues identified in this study should be taken into consideration in planning future clinical studies on maternal immunisation in low- and middle-income countries.

Keywords: Developing countries, Group B *Streptococcus*, Healthcare system, Immunisation, Infants, Pregnant women

Background

Between 1990 and 2015, the global under-five annual mortality rate has declined by 53%, from 91 to 43 deaths per 1000 live births [1]. Moreover, an acceleration in the improvement of child survival has been observed during this period, with annual rates of reduction in mortality increasing from 1.8% in 1990–2000 to 3.9% in 2000–2015 [1]. The decline in mortality has been slower in neonates than in post-neonatal under-five children (47% versus 58% globally), with neonatal mortality rates that fell from 36 to 19 deaths per 1000 live births between 1990 and 2015. Almost 45% of the 5.9 million deaths reported worldwide among children younger than 5 years in 2015 occurred in neonates, and the neonatal period remains the most vulnerable time for a child's survival [1–4]. The vast majority of newborn deaths and almost all maternal deaths (99%) take place in developing countries [3, 5]. As lack of access to quality healthcare at critical time points prior to, during, and after delivery may influence mortality rates [4, 5], identifying barriers to healthcare utilisation could reduce infant and maternal deaths.

Immunisation of pregnant women can protect neonates from diseases which may present within the first days of life: tetanus vaccination is recommended by the World Health Organisation [6], some countries have introduced routine seasonal influenza vaccination [7], and others recommend primary or booster vaccination against pertussis [8, 9]. Maternal vaccination against other diseases, such as Group B *Streptococcus* (GBS), which can kill infants in the first hours of life, is currently under investigation [10, 11]. GBS is a major cause of neonatal sepsis and meningitis, and is classified as early-onset disease when presenting between 0 to 6 days of age and late-onset disease when presenting between 7 to 89 days of age [12]. In previous clinical trials, a single dose of an investigational GBS vaccine was administered to women at 24–35 weeks of gestation, but the optimal vaccination schedule has not been determined [10, 11].

The successful implementation of maternal vaccination will rely on results of clinical trials, taking into account the prenatal and postnatal attendance at the selected healthcare institutions serving as study sites. This study identified factors influencing whether pregnant women would enrol in clinical trials and return to study site for delivery, infant follow-up visits, or medical assistance in case of infant disease. The aim was to identify potential barriers to participation in future large-scale efficacy trials of investigational GBS vaccines administered during pregnancy.

Methods

This prospective, multi-centre, observational study was conducted between November 2012 and January 2015 in potential sites for a phase 3 maternal immunisation clinical efficacy study in which pregnant women from countries with reported high incidence of GBS disease in infants could be enrolled. Although 13 sites originally qualified for participation, three sites, one each in Malawi, South Africa and Panama, did not recruit any participants. The study was therefore conducted at ten sites: three in Panama, two in the Dominican Republic, four in South Africa, and one in Mozambique (Table 1). The study sites were urban, except the semirural site in Mozambique.

The study was conducted in accordance with the principles of Good Clinical Practice and the Declaration of Helsinki. The study protocol and related documents were approved by the institutional review boards or ethics committees in each study country: Comite de Docencia e Investigación, Hospital Santo Tomás, Panama; Consejo Nacional de Bioetica en Salud, the Dominican Republic; University of the Witwatersrand Human Research Ethics Committee (Medical), South Africa; Health Research Ethics Committee Research Development and Support Division, Stellenbosh University, South Africa; and National Bioethics Health Committee, Mozambique. Written informed consent was obtained from all women, or their parent/legal representative if minors, prior to enrolment in the study. Informed assent was also obtained from women who were classified as minors. The study was registered at www.clinicaltrials.gov (NCT01734434).

Women who sought antenatal care at the study site were eligible for participation if they were at ≥24 weeks (Panama, the Dominican Republic, and site SA_1 in South Africa) or 28–34 weeks (sites SA_2, SA_3, and SA_4 in South Africa and the site from Mozambique) of gestation at enrolment, and if they provided written

Table 1 Demographics and baseline characteristics of women included in the full analysis set

	Panama			Dominican Republic		South Africa				Mozambique
	PA_1	PA_2	PA_3	DR_1	DR_2	SA_1	SA_2	SA_3	SA_4	MO_1
	N = 263	*N* = 63	*N* = 174	*N* = 276	*N* = 224	*N* = 500	*N* = 499	*N* = 500	*N* = 490	*N* = 251
Age (years)										
Mean ± SD	24.3 ± 5.2	28.8 ± 6.0	25.0 ± 5.6	24.1 ± 5.1	25.0 ± 5.4	29.0 ± 6.4	25.8 ± 5.9	27.4 ± 5.9	26.0 ± 5.4	25.0 ± 6.3
< 18, n (%)	0 (0)	0 (0)	1 (0.6)	1 (0.4)	2 (0.9)	1 (0.2)	0 (0)	1 (0.2)	0 (0)	0 (0)
18–22, n (%)	113 (43.0)	10 (15.9)	71 (40.8)	132 (47.8)	92 (41.1)	92 (18.4)	182 (36.5)	125 (25.0)	150 (30.6)	111 (44.2)
23–27, n (%)	94 (35.7)	20 (31.7)	50 (28.7)	74 (26.8)	67 (29.9)	134 (26.8)	147 (29.5)	147 (29.4)	164 (33.5)	55 (21.9)
28–32, n (%)	32 (12.2)	13 (20.6)	32 (18.4)	43 (15.6)	40 (17.9)	124 (24.8)	93 (18.6)	126 (25.2)	112 (22.9)	47 (18.7)
33–37, n (%)	19 (7.2)	16 (25.4)	15 (8.6)	25 (9.1)	15 (6.7)	97 (19.4)	50 (10.0)	66 (13.2)	47 (9.6)	28 (11.2)
≥ 38, n (%)	5 (1.9)	4 (6.3)	5 (2.9)	1 (0.4)	8 (3.6)	52 (10.4)	27 (5.4)	35 (7.0)	17 (3.5)	10 (4.0)
Gestational age (weeks)										
Mean ± SD	28.7 ± 3.7	32.7 ± 4.0	29.6 ± 4.4	33.5 ± 4.8	31.1 ± 4.4	32.7 ± 4.6	30.9 ± 2.0	30.7 ± 1.9	30.8 ± 1.8	30.5 ± 2.3
Gestational age calculation method										
Fundal height, n (%)	0 (0)	0 (0)	1 (0.6)	12 (4.3)	1 (0.4)	90 (18.0)	100 (20.0)	263 (52.6)	140 (28.6)	249 (99.2)
Last menstrual period, n (%)	201 (76.4)	36 (57.1)	113 (64.9)	107 (38.8)	139 (62.1)	220 (44.0)	346 (69.3)	181 (36.2)	32 (6.5)	2 (0.8)
Ultrasound, n (%)	62 (23.6)	27 (42.9)	56 (32.2)	156 (56.5)	84 (37.5)	190 (38.0)	53 (10.6)	56 (11.2)	318 (64.9)	0 (0)
Other: Last menstrual period + ultrasound, n (%)	0 (0)	0 (0)	4 (2.3)	0 (0)	0 (0)	0 (0)	0 (0)	0 (0)	0 (0)	0 (0)
Women having other children under care										
n (%)	151 (57.4)	42 (66.7)	92 (52.9)	183 (66.3)	132 (58.9)	304 (60.8)	286 (57.3)	278 (55.6)	217 (44.3)	182 (72.5)
Women caring for other children with alternative childcare provider available										
n (%)	147 (97.4)	37 (88.1)	79 (85.9)	162 (88.5)	124 (93.9)	304 (100)	284 (99.3)	277 (99.6)	215 (99.1)	179 (98.4)

N number of women per group, *n (%)* number (percentage) of women in each category, *SD* standard deviation

informed consent. Following a protocol amendment, the gestational age eligibility window was modified to be consistent with recommendations from the GBS scientific committee specifying that the investigational GBS vaccine should be administered in pregnancy between 28 and 34 weeks of gestation. The new criterion for gestational age was only implemented at three sites from South Africa and the site in Mozambique (SA_2, SA_3, SA_4, and MO_1) because the others had already completed enrolment or were nearing completion at the time of the protocol amendment.

Data were collected from women at each of the three study visits (enrolment, delivery, and infant follow-up visit) by means of questionnaires (Additional file 1). The follow-up visit occurred when the infants reached 90 days of age, which is the upper age limit used to define late-onset GBS infection [12]. The questions were intended to identify the barriers that may hinder access to health-care or participation in a future clinical trial for pregnant women in each of the settings. Questions asked at all three visits were: duration, cost and type of transportation to the study site, access to a telephone, and availability of care for other children. Specific questions at the enrolment visit (prenatal) were gestational age and its method of estimation, estimated delivery date, and details of the clinic for the woman's well-child visit (immunisation). At the delivery visit, the time and place of delivery, labour onset, pregnancy outcome, health status of infant, and day of discharge were recorded. Women not delivering at the study site were asked to provide this information telephonically or by completing the non-study site delivery questionnaire. If needed, a home visit was undertaken as per local practice. Additional time points for data collection were the well-child visit (within 21 days after the estimated delivery date) or the 90-day follow-up visit. At the infant follow-up visit (90 days after delivery), the following information was recorded: the health status of the infant, the well-child visit attendance, and whether the infant was sick during the first 90 days of life (in which case further information was recorded on whether medical care was sought or not, where medical care was sought, or the reasons for not seeking medical care). Education about signs and symptoms of potential sepsis in infants was provided to nearly all women (97.3%) at enrolment and at delivery. Women were counselled to seek urgent medical care if their infant developed any symptom of sepsis. Potential GBS infections could be detected if enrolled women identified these specific sepsis symptoms in their child. Investigators recorded all study data on electronic case report forms stored in a secure electronic data capture system for validation.

The study sample size was driven by the enrolment capacity of the sites. Summary statistics were calculated for all recorded questionnaire data, and were presented as frequencies and percentages. Means and standard deviations were presented for continuous variables (e.g. age, gestational age). Analyses were performed on overall data, by region (Latin America or Africa), by country, and by study site. Statistical testing was used only for descriptive purposes, and no multiplicity adjustments were performed.

Stepwise logistic regressions were performed on all enrolled women and on those who provided data after enrolment. Formula and details on odds ratios (ORs) calculation are given in Supplementary Methods (Additional file 2).

To evaluate factors that might influence whether pregnant women would return to study site for delivery, pregnant women were categorised into two groups: those who returned to a study site to deliver and those who did not. Pregnant women whose delivery status was unknown were grouped with those who delivered at a non-study site. To explore the seeking of medical attention, only women with a sick newborn or infant were included for the first occurrence of illness. The predictor variables included in the logistic regressions were: country of study site; age of pregnant woman; gestational age of pregnancy at enrolment; mode, duration, and cost of transportation to the study site; and alternative childcare (no children, children but with no alternative childcare, children with alternative childcare). The stepwise method was used with p-values to enter factors set at 0.05 and p-values to remove factors set at 0.06. All 95% confidence intervals (CIs) were calculated using the Clopper-Pearson method. All statistical analyses were performed using Statistical Analysis System version 9.1 or a later version.

Results

Study participants

In total, 3614 women were approached for enrolment. Of these, 300 (8.3%) women did not give consent, 67 (1.9%) were not eligible for enrolment, and 4 (0.1%) were not enrolled for other reasons (Fig. 1). Reasons for not participating in the study varied by site; overall, gestational age outside eligibility window was the most common reason. Other reasons included language difficulties, relocation or living outside the study area, family reasons, and lack of interest in participating. Of the 3243 enrolled women, 3069 (94.6%) completed the study. Reasons for premature withdrawal were loss to follow-up ($n = 90$), no live birth ($n = 41$), infant death ($n = 26$), withdrew consent ($n = 13$), signed wrong version of consent form ($n = 3$),

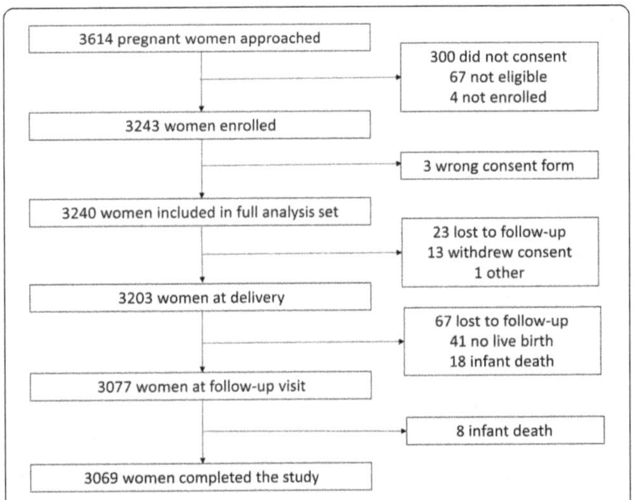

Fig. 1 Participant flow diagram

and other ($n = 1$). Of note, the proportion of women who withdrew because they had no live birth was higher in Africa (38 [1.7%; range across sites: 1.0–2.4%]) than in Latin America (3 [0.3%; range across sites: 0.0–0.6%]), and among the 26 women prematurely withdrawn from the study for infant death, 4 (0.4%; range across sites: 0.0–0.7%) were in Latin America and 22 (1.0%; range across sites: 0.2–2.0%) in Africa.

The mean age and gestational age of enrolled women were similar across sites (Table 1). The method to determine gestational age varied by site and/or country. Fundal height was predominant in Mozambique (99.2% of women) and at one site in South Africa (site SA_3: 52.6%), compared with last menstrual period (LMP) or ultrasound at the other sites. An alternative childcare provider was available at enrolment for 96.8% (range across sites: 85.9–100%) of women caring for other children.

Most women were contactable by phone at all sites for each study visit (range across sites: 75.7–100%). Of those contactable, 99.4–100% of women in Mozambique were contactable by personal mobile phone for the three visits. Personal mobile phone use was also high in South Africa (range across sites: 96.9–99.8%), but slightly lower in the Dominican Republic and Panama (75.8–84.0% and 85.2–96.6%, respectively). No women in Mozambique were contactable by home phone. Home phone access was also low in South Africa (0.2–5.2%), but was higher in the Dominican Republic (18.2–27.8%) and Panama (29.3–44.4%).

Factors influencing delivery at study site

Among the 3229 enrolled women with delivery information, 2053 (63.6%) delivered at the study site, and 1115 (34.5%) delivered at a non-study healthcare facility (Table 2). There were large differences in percentages of women

Table 2 Study site and non-study site deliveries for women included in full analysis set with available delivery information

	Panama			Dominican Republic		South Africa				Mozambique
	PA_1	PA_2	PA_3	DR_1	DR_2	SA_1	SA_2	SA_3	SA_4	MO_1
	N = 263	N = 63	N = 174	N = 272	N = 224	N = 497	N = 499	N = 497	N = 489	N = 251
Delivery location										
Study site, n (%)	203 (77.2)	43 (68.3)	126 (72.4)	249 (91.5)	91 (40.6)	422 (84.9)	126 (25.3)	414 (83.3)	161 (32.9)	218 (86.9)
Non-study healthcare facility, n (%)	57 (21.7)	18 (28.6)	48 (27.6)	21 (7.7)	132 (58.9)	68 (13.7)	357 (71.5)	79 (15.9)	315 (64.4)	20 (8.0)
Home, n (%)	0 (0)	2 (3.2)	0 (0)	0 (0)	0 (0)	3 (0.6)	7 (1.4)	2 (0.4)	3 (0.6)	7 (2.8)
Other, n (%)	0 (0)	0 (0)	0 (0)	0 (0)	0 (0)	2 (0.4)	5 (1.0)	1 (0.2)	2 (0.4)	1 (0.4)
Unknown, n (%)	3 (1.1)	0 (0)	0 (0)	2 (0.7)	1 (0.5)	2 (0.4)	4 (0.8)	1 (0.2)	8 (1.6)	5 (2.0)
Reason for non-study site delivery										
Labour too fast, n (%)	28 (49.1)	14 (70.0)	8 (16.7)	7 (33.3)	5 (3.8)	15 (20.6)	12 (3.3)	8 (9.6)	8 (2.5)	10 (35.7)
Did not want to deliver at site, n (%)	5 (8.8)	1 (5.0)	7 (14.6)	1 (4.8)	7 (5.3)	10 (13.7)	5 (1.4)	9 (10.8)	1 (0.3)	0 (0)
Family did not allow, n (%)	1 (1.8)	0 (0)	1 (2.1)	0 (0)	0 (0)	5 (6.9)	4 (1.1)	15 (18.1)	8 (2.5)	0 (0)
No direct transportation to site, n (%)	0 (0)	2 (10.0)	19 (39.6)	0 (0)	0 (0)	0 (0)	1 (0.3)	2 (2.4)	0 (0)	3 (10.7)
No money for transportation, n (%)	0 (0)	2 (10.0)	10 (20.8)	0 (0)	0 (0)	2 (2.7)	1 (0.3)	0 (0)	0 (0)	0 (0)
No childcare available for other children, n (%)	0 (0)	0 (0)	0 (0)	0 (0)	1 (0.8)	0 (0)	1 (0.3)	0 (0)	0 (0)	1 (3.6)
Other[a], n (%)	25 (43.9)	1 (5.0)	3 (6.3)	14 (66.7)	120 (90.9)	41 (56.2)	349 (94.6)	48 (57.8)	305 (95.3)	14 (50.0)

N number of women per group, *n (%)* number (percentage) of women in each category
[a]Other: includes another hospital or healthcare centre was closer, women had a healthcare insurance coverage or a relative working at another healthcare facility, no free beds at study site, pregnancy complications/emergencies, away from area at time of labour

returning to the study site for delivery, ranging from 25.3–91.5% across sites. Reasons for a non-study site delivery were multiple (categorised as "other") for most women (79.9%; range across sites: 5.0–95.3%), but the most common reason given was "labour too fast" (10.0%; range across sites: 2.5–70.0%) (Table 2).

Both mean age and gestational age were significant factors influencing whether a woman delivered at the study site, with older women and women at later gestational age at enrolment being more likely to deliver at the study site. With every year increase in the woman's age and with every week increase in the gestational age, the participant was more likely to deliver at the study site (ORs = 1.02 [95% CI: 1.01, 1.04] and 1.01 [95% CI: 1.01, 1.01], respectively) (Table 3).

Mode of transportation at enrolment or delivery was similar (data shown for delivery) for all sites within each country, but varied between countries (Table 4). At the delivery visit, the most common modes of transportation in Panama and South Africa were minibus/taxi (43.2% [range across sites: 31.2–62.1%] and 34.3% [19.0–44.8%], respectively) and private car (35.6% [26.4–41.1%] and 38.5% [34.2–44.9%], respectively), while public transport (40.4% [32.1–47.1%]) and minibus/taxi (35.6% [22.5–51.8%]) were most common in the Dominican Republic and walking (53.4%) in Mozambique. When compared to other modes of transportation and holding all other variables constant in the model, women who used minibus/taxi (OR = 1.26 [95% CI: 1.05, 1.50]) at enrolment and those who used public transportation (OR = 1.39 [95% CI: 1.07, 1.80]) or walking (OR = 2.56 [95% CI: 1.62, 4.04]) at delivery were more likely to deliver at the study site, while those reaching the study site by ambulance for delivery (OR = 0.23 [95% CI: 0.18, 0.30]) were less likely to deliver there (Table 3).

Within a country, travel times to the study site were similar (Table 4). In Mozambique, most women travelled 30–59 min (67.8%) to reach the study site for delivery. The majority in the three other countries travelled less than 45 min (66.4% in the Dominican Republic, 66.0% in Panama, and 85.7% in South Africa). A short duration of transportation at delivery was positively associated with women returning to the study site for delivery. When comparing women with 15–29 min of transportation to reach the study site for delivery, those with less than 15 min were more likely (OR = 1.52 [95% CI: 1.15, 2.02]) and those with 30–44 min less likely (OR = 0.50 [95% CI: 0.41, 0.61]) to deliver at the study site (Table 3).

The mean direct cost of transportation at delivery was similar at the sites in Panama, the Dominican Republic, and South Africa ($3.6–$5.9), but much lower in Mozambique ($0.3). With every unit increase in cost of transportation (in

Table 3 Predictor variables included in the logistic regression model for study site delivery and follow-up visit

	Parameter estimate	Odds ratio (95% CI)	*p*-value
Factors influencing delivery at the study site (full analysis set)			
Country of study site			
Dominican Republic vs South Africa	−0.61	1.15 (0.87, 1.52)	<0.0001
Mozambique vs South Africa	1.19	6.96 (4.14, 11.69)	<0.0001
Panama vs South Africa	0.17	2.50 (1.93, 3.23)	0.1391
Age of the pregnant women	0.02	1.02 (1.01, 1.04)	0.0008
Gestational age	0.01	1.01 (1.01, 1.01)	<0.0001
Mode of transportation			
Minibus/Taxi - Visit 1 (Yes vs No)	0.11	1.26 (1.05, 1.50)	0.0123
Public transportation - Visit 2 (Yes vs No)	0.16	1.39 (1.07, 1.80)	0.0124
Walk - Visit 2 (Yes vs No)	0.47	2.56 (1.62, 4.04)	<0.0001
Ambulance - Visit 2 (Yes vs No)	−0.73	0.23 (0.18, 0.30)	<0.0001
Duration of transportation to study site (Visit 1)			
< 15 min vs 15–29 min	−0.35	0.73 (0.58, 0.92)	0.0131
30–44 min vs 15–29 min	−0.06	0.98 (0.79, 1.21)	0.6716
45–59 min vs 15–29 min	0.33	1.43 (1.03, 1.99)	0.0477
60–89 min vs 15–29 min	0.19	1.26 (0.88, 1.80)	0.2515
90–120 min vs 15–29 min	−0.11	0.93 (0.50, 1.73)	0.6957
> 120 min vs 15–29 min	0.03	1.06 (0.31, 3.66)	0.9592
Duration of transportation to study site (Visit 2)			
< 15 min vs 15–29 min	0.70	1.52 (1.15, 2.02)	<0.0001
30–44 min vs 15–29 min	−0.42	0.50 (0.41, 0.61)	0.0007
45–59 min vs 15–29 min	−0.09	0.69 (0.52, 0.93)	0.5444
60–89 min vs 15–29 min	0.04	0.79 (0.56, 1.12)	0.8159
90–120 min vs 15–29 min	0.23	0.96 (0.50, 1.85)	0.4259
> 120 min vs 15–29 min	−0.74	0.36 (0.11, 1.18)	0.1507
Cost of transportation to study site (Visit 1)	0.08	1.09 (1.02, 1.16)	0.0133
Factors influencing return to the study site for follow-up visit (full analysis set with live-born infants)			
Country of study			
Dominican Republic vs South Africa	2.40	19.20 (10.16, 36.27)	<0.0001
Mozambique vs South Africa	−1.32	0.46 (0.32, 0.67)	<0.0001
Panama vs South Africa	−0.52	1.03 (0.82, 1.29)	<0.0001
Mode of transportation to study site			
Walk - Visit 2 (Yes vs No)	0.31	1.85 (1.21, 2.81)	0.0042
Cost of transportation to study site at Visit 2	−0.01	0.99 (0.97, 1.00)	0.0257
Alternative Childcare at Visit 1			
Alternative care available vs No other children	0.21	1.35 (1.14, 1.60)	0.1115

CI confidence intervals, *Visit 1* enrolment, *Visit 2* delivery

United States dollar [USD]) at enrolment, the women were 1.09 (95% CI: 1.02, 1.16) times more likely to deliver at the study site (Table 3).

Outcome at the 90-day infant follow-up visit

In total, 97.8% of women with live-born infants (3077/3145) provided 90-day infant follow-up information, but only 2121 of them (68.9%) returned to the study site for this visit. The overall percentage of women returning to the study site was similar in Mozambique, Panama, and South Africa (62.2–68.2%), but much higher in the Dominican Republic (98.0%), with significant inter-site differences within countries (Fig. 2). At the 90-day infant follow-up visit, information was available for 3106 infants,

Table 4 Transportation to site/healthcare facilities at delivery for women included in the full analysis set

	Panama			Dominican Republic		South Africa				Mozambique
	PA_1	PA_2	PA_3	DR_1	DR_2	SA_1	SA_2	SA_3	SA_4	MO_1
	N = 263	*N* = 63	*N* = 174	*N* = 276	*N* = 224	*N* = 500	*N* = 499	*N* = 500	*N* = 490	*N* = 251
Mode of transportation[a]										
Ambulance, n (%)	13 (4.9)	10 (15.9)	3 (1.7)	0 (0)	0 (0)	69 (13.8)	35 (7.0)	32 (6.4)	174 (35.5)	11 (4.4)
Minibus/taxi, n (%)	82 (31.2)	26 (41.3)	108 (62.1)	62 (22.5)	116 (51.8)	224 (44.8)	173 (34.7)	192 (38.4)	93 (19.0)	5 (2.0)
Private car, n (%)	108 (41.1)	24 (38.1)	46 (26.4)	64 (23.2)	26 (11.6)	189 (37.8)	224 (44.9)	171 (34.2)	182 (37.1)	44 (17.5)
Public transportation, n (%)	60 (22.8)	4 (6.3)	19 (10.9)	130 (47.1)	72 (32.1)	1 (0.2)	44 (8.8)	75 (15.0)	5 (1.0)	41 (16.3)
Walk, n (%)	8 (3.0)	0 (0)	0 (0)	41 (14.9)	12 (5.4)	11 (2.2)	16 (3.2)	10 (2.0)	16 (3.3)	134 (53.4)
Other, n (%)	0 (0)	0 (0)	0 (0)	24 (8.7)	5 (2.2)	0 (0)	1 (0.2)	7 (1.4)	0 (0)	4 (1.6)
Duration of travel										
< 15 min, n (%)	13 (4.9)	5 (7.9)	39 (22.4)	17 (6.2)	26 (11.6)	76 (15.2)	41 (8.2)	73 (14.6)	46 (9.4)	7 (2.8)
15–29 min, n (%)	85 (32.3)	23 (36.5)	54 (31.0)	59 (21.4)	83 (37.1)	209 (41.8)	219 (43.9)	295 (59.0)	199 (40.6)	20 (8.0)
30–44 min, n (%)	61 (23.2)	11 (17.5)	39 (22.4)	71 (25.7)	76 (33.9)	133 (26.6)	170 (34.1)	80 (16.0)	163 (33.3)	85 (33.9)
45–59 min, n (%)	23 (8.7)	7 (11.1)	16 (9.2)	49 (17.8)	19 (8.5)	65 (13.0)	35 (7.0)	27 (5.4)	38 (7.8)	85 (33.9)
60–89 min, n (%)	61 (23.2)	14 (22.2)	16 (9.2)	56 (20.3)	14 (6.3)	8 (1.6)	20 (4.0)	8 (1.6)	17 (3.5)	30 (12.0)
90–120 min, n (%)	11 (4.2)	1 (1.6)	6 (3.4)	17 (6.2)	4 (1.8)	3 (0.6)	7 (1.4)	3 (0.6)	2 (0.4)	9 (3.6)
> 120 min, n (%)	4 (1.5)	0 (0)	3 (1.7)	1 (0.4)	0 (0)	0 (0)	0 (0)	1 (0.2)	2 (0.4)	3 (1.2)
Cost ($)										
mean ± SD	5.4 ± 6.5	5.9 ± 6.0	5.2 ± 4.5	3.6 ± 3.8	4.8 ± 3.1	5.1 ± 6.7	3.8 ± 6.6	5.0 ± 6.8	4.9 ± 7.0	0.3 ± 1.0

N number of women per group, *n (%)* number (percentage) of women in each category, *SD* standard deviation
[a]The women participating in the study were allowed to indicate more than 1 way of transportation, the most frequent combination was "public transportation & walk"

of whom 3089 (99.5%) attended at least one well-child visit at the study site or another healthcare facility.

Women who walked to the site for delivery were significantly more likely to return to the study site for the infant follow-up visit (OR = 1.85 [95% CI: 1.21, 2.81]). Cost of transportation calculated at delivery was also a significant factor influencing whether women returned to the study site for the infant follow-up visit. With every unit increase in cost of transportation (in USD) at delivery, the women were 0.99 (95% CI: 0.97, 1.00) times less likely to return to the study site for their follow-up visit (Table 3).

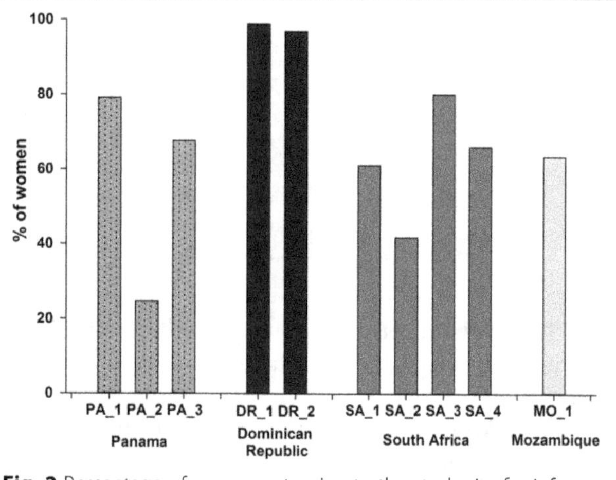

Fig. 2 Percentage of women returning to the study site for infant follow-up visit, 90 days post-delivery

Alternative childcare availability was very high (96.8%; range across sites: 85.9–100%) (Table 1), and women with alternative childcare provider availability at enrolment, representing women with children, were more likely to return to the study site for follow-up than those without other children (OR = 1.35 [95% CI: 1.14, 1.60) (Table 3).

Sick child reporting and medical care

Of the 3199 live born infants, 218 (6.8%; range across sites: 2.0–19.3%) newborns were reported sick before discharge. Overall, the highest percentage of newborns reported sick was in Panama (16.3%) and the lowest in Mozambique (2.1%), but this percentage varied across sites within each country. At the 90-day infant follow-up visit, 666/3106 (21.4%; range across sites: 3.7–68.8%) infants were reported sick during the first 90 days of life; this percentage was lower in Africa (11.3%) compared to Latin America (43.3%). Of these 666 infants, 94.3% (range across sites: 82.2–100%) were taken to a healthcare facility, and 41.9% (range across sites: 4.9–77.3%) were taken to the study site (Table 5). The most common

Table 5 Medical assistance for infants reported sick within 90 days post-delivery

	Panama			Dominican Republic		South Africa				Mozambique
	PA_1	PA_2	PA_3	DR_1	DR_2	SA_1	SA_2	SA_3	SA_4	MO_1
	$N = 254$	$N = 61$	$N = 176$	$N = 269$	$N = 221$	$N = 487$	$N = 480$	$N = 485$	$N = 441$	$N = 232$
Infant reported sick in first 90 days										
n (%)	127 (50.0)	32 (52.5)	121 (68.8)	104 (38.7)	41 (18.6)	18 (3.7)	41 (8.5)	43 (8.9)	73 (16.6)	66 (28.5)
Sick infant taken to										
Study site, n (%)	58 (45.7)	12 (37.5)	77 (63.6)	27 (26.0)	27 (65.9)	7 (38.9)	2 (4.9)	13 (30.2)	5 (6.9)	51 (77.3)
Infant's hospital/immunisation clinic, n (%)	2 (1.6)	6 (18.8)	7 (5.8)	10 (9.6)	3 (7.3)	10 (55.6)	13 (31.7)	10 (23.3)	21 (28.8)	13 (19.7)
Other, n (%)	65 (51.2)	14 (43.8)	34 (28.1)	61 (58.7)	8 (19.5)	1 (5.6)	22 (53.7)	15 (34.9)	34 (46.6)	0 (0)
Not taken to healthcare facility, n (%)	2 (1.6)	0 (0)	3 (2.5)	6 (5.8)	3 (7.3)	0 (0)	4 (9.8)	5 (11.6)	13 (17.8)	2 (3.0)
Reasons for not taking sick infant to healthcare facility										
Newborn did not appear seriously ill, n (%)	0 (0)	0 (0)	3 (100)	4 (66.7)	3 (100)	0 (0)	3 (75.0)	4 (80.0)	13 (100)	1 (50.0)
Lack of money, n (%)	1 (50.0)	0 (0)	0 (0)	1 (16.7)	0 (0)	0 (0)	0 (0)	0 (0)	0 (0)	0 (0)
Lack of transportation, n (%)	0 (0)	0 (0)	0 (0)	0 (0)	0 (0)	0 (0)	0 (0)	0 (0)	0 (0)	0 (0)
No alternative childcare available, n (%)	0 (0)	0 (0)	0 (0)	0 (0)	0 (0)	0 (0)	0 (0)	0 (0)	0 (0)	0 (0)
Other, n (%)	1 (50.0)	0 (0)	0 (0)	1 (16.7)	0 (0)	0 (0)	1 (25.0)	1 (20.0)	0 (0)	1 (50.0)

N infants with information available at 90 days follow-up, *n (%)* number (percentage) of subjects in each category

reason for the sick infant not being taken to a healthcare facility was that the infant did not appear seriously ill (31/38 infants, 81.6%). Other factors were lack of money and "other" (e.g. infant already hospitalised, infant died before reaching healthcare).

Discussion

This study identified factors influencing whether pregnant women would enrol in clinical trials, and would return to study sites for delivery, infant follow-up visits, or to seek medical assistance for their sick infant. By identifying restrictions to maternal/infant healthcare access in potential clinical sites, this study provided a potential platform for improving compliance and retention for future phase 3 clinical efficacy studies of investigational GBS vaccines. Apart from greater efficiency in clinical trials, there is evidence that ante- and post-partum visits improve maternal and infant health, and increase perinatal infant survival rates by offering opportunities for education and medical interventions. A greater understanding of predictors of pregnant women access to healthcare services may therefore also have programmatic implications for the improvement of healthcare utilisation.

Out of all pregnant women who were approached, 10% were not eligible for the study and could not participate. The reasons for not participating were estimated with the most common being lower than required gestational age. Proportions of ineligible women and reasons for ineligibility will be useful in the operational planning of clinical trials enrolling pregnant women, e.g. women with too low gestational age at screening could potentially participate if they return later during pregnancy.

Women at later gestational age at enrolment were more likely to deliver at the study site. In clinical trials, the gestational age is estimated to identify the appropriate time for maternal vaccination to ensure optimum placental antibody transfer to the infant [13]. Here, methods of estimating gestational age varied among sites, the most common being ultrasound or LMP in Latin America and South Africa, and fundal height in Mozambique. Ultrasound is considered the most accurate method, but is less available in resource-limited settings [13–15]. The LMP method can be universally applied, but relies on self-assessment and reporting, and is potentially unreliable [14]. The fundal height method is routinely used in many resource-limited countries [16].

Older women were also more likely to return to study sites for delivery. This observation is in line with previous studies suggesting that women in their 30s attended antenatal healthcare more frequently than younger or older women, but contrasts with other studies suggesting that age had no effect on antenatal healthcare utilisation [17]. Another finding was that women with other children were more likely to return to study site for follow-up visits. A potential explanation for this unexpected finding could be that multiparous women often return to the site of their previous delivery for antenatal visits and are therefore more likely to return to the same site for delivery and follow-up visits.

Additionally, we identified factors that may hinder access to healthcare facilities for pregnant women and their infants. Mode, duration, and cost of transportation had a significant influence on whether women would return to study site for delivery and follow-up visits. Transportation was previously identified as a barrier for access to obstetric care in low- and middle-income countries, with increasing cost, distance, and travel time reducing the likelihood of returning [17–20]. Surprisingly, we found that increased transportation costs at enrolment, which were lower than transportation costs at delivery, were associated with increased likelihood of women returning to study sites for delivery. This observation suggests that women who can afford to pay for transportation to antenatal visits are more likely to return to the same site for delivery. Another potential explanation could be that women living further from the study site may stay nearby when their due date was coming closer, which would then decrease the transportation costs at delivery. In contrast, lower transportation costs at delivery were associated with an increased likelihood of women returning to the study site for follow-up visits. Our results suggest that transportation cost is a barrier for routine follow-up visits, but not for hospital delivery, which is an important finding to consider when preparing clinical trials on maternal immunisation. In Africa, this finding should be interpreted with caution considering the differences in minimum salary in the respective countries [21].

Over 90% of women sought medical care at the study site or another healthcare facility for their sick infant, suggesting that the probability to detect potential GBS infections was high. However, more widespread efforts are needed to collect detailed follow-up information since only two thirds of live born infants were brought to the study site for the 90-day follow-up visits. Each site from a clinical study should establish surveillance in surrounding facilities where sick infants may be seen.

The study had a number of limitations. Although education about signs and symptoms of sepsis was provided to nearly all women, the study failed to clearly define what "sick" or "illness" meant, allowing thresholds for considering a child as ill that could differ by country. In addition, the incidence and causes of disease in infants were not collected as the majority of sick children were not assessed at the study site. When choosing sites for potential phase 3 trials on investigational maternal GBS vaccines, it is important to understand the neonatal invasive GBS disease incidence in the area; however, these estimates are lacking for many low- and middle-income countries [22]. The low proportion of women younger than 18 years of age (0.2%) was another potential limitation. Indeed, 16% of pregnant women in sub-Saharan Africa are under 19 years [23]; these young women are often at higher risk for GBS due to a lack of sexual health education [24] and a lower level of natural immunity against colonisation. Young pregnant women are an important group to study because they are often underrepresented in clinical trials due to legal or logistical reasons. This study was also limited by the fact that only healthcare sites large enough to conduct phase 3 clinical trials were used. These were in large urban areas, except the semirural site in Mozambique. Therefore, factors influencing whether women would return to healthcare facilities may vary for rural areas and smaller healthcare sites. The absence of data on the following variables was a further limitation of this study: the mode of delivery, the occurrence of complications during delivery, and the quality of the antenatal and birthing experience, which may all impact the likelihood of returning for a follow-up visit. Finally, failure to collect information on the impact of other important factors, such as education, parity, and income, was another limitation [25, 26].

Conclusions

In this prospective, multi-centre, observational study, older pregnant women and those at later gestational age at enrolment were more likely to deliver at the study site. Women with other children were more likely to return to study site for follow-up visits. While heterogeneities were observed at site level, shorter travel time at delivery and increased transportation costs at enrolment were associated with increased likelihood of women returning to study site for delivery. Lower transportation costs at delivery were associated with increased likelihood of women returning to study site for follow-up visits. Although high retention was observed from enrolment through 90 days after delivery, post-partum surveillance should be broadened beyond the study sites and an additional follow-up visit should be planned within the first month of life, the most vulnerable time for a child's survival. The factors influencing maternal/infant access to healthcare facilities and the issues identified in this study should be taken into consideration in planning future clinical studies on maternal immunisation in low- and middle-income countries.

Additional files

Additional files 1: Survey Questionnaires. Survey questionnaires completed at enrolment, delivery (at study site or outside of study site) and infant 90-day follow-up visit.

Additional files 2: Supplementary Methods. Formula and details on odds ratios calculation.

Abbreviations

CI: Confidence interval; GBS: Group B *Streptococcus*; LMP: Last menstrual period; OR: Odds ratio; USD: United States dollar

Acknowledgements

The authors thank all women who enrolled in the study. They thank the principal investigators, collaborators and the staff members of the study centres for their contributions to the study, in particular: Anthonet Koen, Lisa Jose, Clare Cutland, Suzette Fourie, Lee-Anne Stotelkamp, Livhuwani Farisani, Emma Kalk, Coreen Ellis, Marchalaine Hendricks, Jacqueline Martin in South

Africa; Ivonne Abadía, Rodolfo Brandao, Olga Tinajeros, Digna Wong, Osvaldo Reyes, Laura Chen in Panama; Sonia Maculuve, Lola Madrid, Azucena Bardaji, Quique Bassat in Mozambique; and Sonia Mazara in the Dominican Republic. They also thank Lisa Bedell for assistance with statistical analysis. For the preparation of this manuscript, the authors thank Jennifer Engelmoer (Novartis Vaccines) for editorial assistance and writing support, Stéphanie Deroo (XPE Pharma & Science c/o GSK) for publication management, Claire Verbelen (XPE Pharma & Science) and Maria Cornelia Maior (XPE Pharma & Science) for medical writing services.

Funding

The study was initiated and sponsored by the Novartis Vaccines Division, whose sponsorship later transferred to GlaxoSmithKline Biologicals SA; on March 2, 2015 Novartis' non-influenza Vaccines Business was acquired by the GlaxoSmithKline group of companies. The Novartis Vaccines Division designed the study and provided support until March 2, 2015. GlaxoSmithKline Biologicals SA was involved in the analysis and interpretation of the data, and took responsibility for all costs associated with the development and publishing of the present manuscript.

Authors' contributions

SM, LR, XSL, CM, DK, ML, RC, SB and MR designed the study. SM, LR, XSL, CM, NCG, MC, ML, RC and MR acquired the data. SM, LR, XSL, CM, NCG, DK, ML, SB and MR analysed the data. SM, LR, XSL, NCG, MC, ML, RC and MR contributed to the conduct of the study. All reviewed and revised the manuscript, and approved the final manuscript as submitted.

Competing interests

RC and MR were employees of the Novartis Vaccines Division at the time of the study. DK was an employee of the GSK group of companies. ML is an employee of the GSK group of companies. SB is a consultant statistician for the GSK group of companies GBS project. SM, XSL and MC declare having received grants from the Novartis Vaccines Division and the GSK group of companies for the work under consideration. Outside the work under consideration, SM declares having received grants from Pfizer, Novartis, Minervax and the Bill and Melinda Gates foundation for the conduct of clinical trials and personal fees for educational material from Medscape, MC declares having received grants from BMS, Gilead, VPM, Novavax, PATH, NIH and Penta for several pharmaceutical and vaccine studies and personal fees from ViiV and MSD for contribution to workshop and symposium. All other authors have no conflicts of interest to declare. On 2 March 2015 Novartis' non-influenza Vaccines Business was acquired by the GSK group of companies.

Author details

[1]Medical Research Council: Respiratory and Meningeal Pathogens Research Unit, University of the Witwatersrand, Johannesburg, South Africa. [2]Department of Science and Technology/National Research Foundation: Vaccine Preventable Diseases, University of the Witwatersrand, Johannesburg, South Africa. [3]National Institute for Communicable Diseases: a division of National Health Laboratory Service, Centre for Vaccines and Immunology, Johannesburg, South Africa. [4]Hospital Universitario Maternidad Nuestra Señora De La Altagracia Perinatology Department, Gazcue, Santo Domingo, Dominican Republic. [5]Hospital del Niño "Dr. José Renán Esquivel", Infectious Disease Department, Panama City, Panama. [6]National System of Investigators (SNI), National Research of the National Secretariat for Science, Technology and Innovation of Panama (SENACYT), Panama City, Panama. [7]Barcelona Institute of Global Health (ISGlobal), Hospital Clinic of Barcelona, Universitat de Barcelona, Barcelona, Spain. [8]Manhiça Health Research Center (CISM), Manhiça, Mozambique. [9]Setshaba Research Centre, Soshanguve, South Africa. [10]Department of Paediatrics and Child Health, Stellenbosch University and Tygerberg Children's Hospital, Cape Town, South Africa. [11]GSK, Bryanston, South Africa. [12]GSK (formerly employee of Novartis Vaccines Division), Cambridge, MA, USA.

References

1. United Nations Inter-agency Group for Child Mortality Estimation. Levels & trends in child mortality. Report 2015. Available at: http://www.childmortality.org/files_v20/download/IGME%20Report%202015_9_3%20LR%20Web.pdf. Accessed 1 Aug 2017.
2. Liu L, Oza S, Hogan D, Chu Y, Perin J, Zhu J, Lawn JE, Cousens S, Mathers C, Black RE. Global, regional, and national causes of under-5 mortality in 2000-15: an updated systematic analysis with implications for the sustainable development goals. Lancet. 2016;388:3027–35.
3. World Health Organization. Newborns: reducing mortality. Fact sheet no. 333. http://www.who.int/mediacentre/factsheets/fs333/en/. Accessed 1 Aug 2017.
4. Akseer N, Lawn JE, Keenan W, Konstantopoulos A, Cooper P, Ismail Z, Thacker N, Cabral S, Bhutta ZA. Ending preventable newborn deaths in a generation. Int J Gynaecol Obstet. 2016;131:S43–8.
5. World Health Organization. Maternal Mortality. Fact sheet no. 348. http://www.who.int/mediacentre/factsheets/fs348/en/. Accessed 1 Aug 2017.
6. World Health Organization. Maternal Immunization against tetanus. Standards for Maternal and Neonatal Care 2006. http://www.who.int/reproductivehealth/publications/maternal_perinatal_health/immunization_tetanus.pdf. Accessed 1 Aug 2017.
7. Sakala IG, Honda-Okubo Y, Fung J, Petrovsky N. Influenza immunization during pregnancy: benefits for mother and infant. Hum Vaccin Immunother. 2016;12:3065–71.
8. Cherry JD. Editorial commentary: tetanus-diphtheria-pertussis immunization in pregnant women and the prevention of pertussis in young infants. Clin Infect Dis. 2015;60:338–40.
9. Safadi MAP. Control of pertussis in infants: time has finally come? Expert Rev Vaccines. 2015;14:781–3.
10. Donders GGG, Halperin SA, Devlieger R, Baker S, Forte P, Wittke F, Slobod KS, Dull PM. Maternal immunization with an investigational trivalent group B streptococcal vaccine: a randomized controlled trial. Obstet Gynecol. 2016;127:213–21.
11. Heyderman RS, Madhi SA, French N, Cutland C, Ngwira B, Kayambo D, Mboizi R, Koen A, Jose L, Olugbosi M, et al. Group B *Streptococcus* vaccination in pregnant women with or without HIV in Africa: a non-randomised phase 2, open-label, multicentre trial. Lancet Infect Dis. 2016;16:546–55.
12. Heath PT, Schuchat A. Perinatal group B streptococcal disease. Best Pract Res Clin Obstet Gynaecol. 2007;21:411–24.
13. Cutland CL, Cunnington M, Olugbosi M, Jones SA, Hugo A, Maharajah K, Slobod K, Madhi SA. Lessons learnt from enrolment and follow up of pregnant women and their infants in clinical trials in South Africa, a low-middle income country. Vaccine. 2015;33:6406–12.
14. Committee on Obstetric Practice, the American Institute of Ultrasound in Medicine, and the Society for Maternal-Fetal Medicine. Committee Opinion No 700: Methods for Estimating the Due Date. Obstet Gynecol. 2017;129(5):e150–4.
15. Jones CE, Munoz FM, Spiegel HML, Heininger U, Zuber PLF, Edwards KM, Lambach P, Neels P, Kohl KS, Gidudu J, et al. Guideline for collection, analysis and presentation of safety data in clinical trials of vaccines in pregnant women. Vaccine. 2016;34:5998–6006.
16. White LJ, Lee SJ, Stepniewska K, Simpson JA, Dwell SL, Arunjerdja R, Singhasivanon P, White NJ, Nosten F, McGready R. Estimation of gestational age from fundal height: a solution for resource-poor settings. J R Soc Interface. 2012;9:503–10.
17. Simkhada B, Teijlingen ER, Porter M, Simkhada P. Factors affecting the utilization of antenatal care in developing countries: systematic review of the literature. J Adv Nurs. 2008;61:244–60.
18. Gage AJ. Barriers to the utilization of maternal health care in rural Mali. Soc Sci Med. 2007;65:1666–82.
19. Some DT, Sombie I, Meda N. What prevent women for a sustainable use of maternal care in two medical districts of Burkina Faso? A qualitative study. Pan Afr Med J. 2014;18:43.
20. Atuoye KN, Dixon J, Rishworth A, Galaa SZ, Boamah SA, Luginaah I. Can she make it? Transportation barriers to accessing maternal and child health care services in rural Ghana. BMC Health Serv Res. 2015;15:333.

21. Bhorat H, Kanbur R, Stanwix B. Minimum wages in Sub-Saharan Africa: a primer. IZA Discussion Paper 9204, 2015. http://ftp.iza.org/dp9204.pdf. Accessed 1 Aug 2017.
22. Edmond KM, Kortsalioudaki C, Scott S, Schrag SJ, Zaidi AKM, Cousens S, Heath PT. Group B streptococcal disease in infants aged younger than 3 months: systematic review and meta-analysis. Lancet. 2012;379:547–56.
23. Hervish A, Clifton D. Status Report: Adolescents and young people in Sub-Saharan Africa. Opportunities and challenges. 2012. www.prb.org/pdf12/status-report-youth-subsaharan-Africa.pdf. Accessed 1 Aug 2017.
24. Akoh CC, Pressman EK, Cooper E, Queenan RA, Pillittere J, O'Brien KO. Prevalence and risk factors for infections in a pregnant adolescent population. J Pediatr Adolesc Gynecol. 2017;30:71–5.
25. Kruk ME, Hermosilla S, Larson E, Vail D, Chen Q, Mazuguni F, Byalugaba B, Mbaruku G. Who is left behind on the road to universal facility delivery? A cross-sectional multilevel analysis in rural Tanzania. Tropical Med Int Health. 2015;20:1057–66.
26. Tsegay Y, Gebrehiwot T, Goicolea I, Edin K, Lemma H, Sebastian MS. Determinants of antenatal and delivery care utilization in Tigray region, Ethiopia: a cross-sectional study. Int J Equity Health. 2013;12:30.

8

Stakeholders' perspectives on facilitators of and barriers to the utilisation of and access to maternal health services in Eritrea

Chol Chol[1*], Cynthia Hunter[2], Berhane Debru[3], Berhana Haile[4], Joel Negin[5] and Robert G. Cumming[6]

Abstract

Background: Wars affect maternal health services by destroying health systems. Eritrea experienced two wars with neighbouring Ethiopia. Despite this, the maternal mortality ratio (MMR) in Eritrea fell by 69% from 1590 per 100,000 live births in 1990 to 501 in 2015. This study aimed to examine facilitators of and barriers to the utilisation of and access to maternal health services in Eritrea.

Methods: Using in-depth interviews and field observations for data collection, this qualitative study was conducted in five healthcare facilities in Asmara, the capital of Eritrea, in February and March 2016. The participants were: women ($n = 40$), husbands ($n = 5$), healthcare providers ($n = 10$), and decision makers ($n = 5$).

Results: There were two perceived facilitators of utilisation of and access to maternal health services: health education (related to the WHO health service delivery building blocks) and improvement in gender equality driven by the role played by Eritrean women as combatants during the War of Independence (1961–1991). The only perceived barrier was poor quality of care due to lack of ultrasound machines, short clinic opening hours, and shortage of healthcare workers (related to the WHO health workforce building block).

Conclusion: This study assessed women and their husbands/partners' perceptions and the possible effects of contemporary Eritrean culture and the history of war on the utilisation of and access to maternal health services in the country. As well, we examined healthcare providers' and decision makers' perspectives. The two key facilitators of women's utilisation of and access to maternal health services were health education and women's empowerment driven by their role as combatants during the War of Independence. One main barrier was poor quality of care due to lack of ultrasound machines, short clinic opening hours, and a shortage of healthcare workers. As only a limited number of qualitative studies have been published about maternal health services in war-affected sub-Saharan African countries, our findings regarding health education and women's empowerment could be considered in other war-affected countries similar to Eritrea. Nevertheless, further research is needed to investigate our findings – particularly regarding female empowerment driven by women's role in combat in relation to their maternal health.

Keywords: Health system, Health system building blocks, Maternal health services, Gender equality, Female empowerment, Armed conflict, War

* Correspondence: ccho0230@uni.sydney.edu.au; cholc97@gmail.com
[1]School of Public Health, The University of Sydney, Sydney, Australia
Full list of author information is available at the end of the article

Background

Wars destroy the health systems responsible for promoting, restoring and maintaining delivery of healthcare and provision of maternal health services [1–5]. Recent studies have shown that between 1989 and 2011, Africa and particularly sub-Saharan Africa (SSA) experienced 46 armed conflicts, more conflicts than in any other region in the world [6, 7]. As well, in 2015 SSA had the highest maternal mortality ratio (MMR) world-wide [8].

Eritrea is one of the SSA countries that have experienced a long history of war, and it also has a high MMR [8–11]. Eritrea experienced two wars with neighbouring Ethiopia: during 1961–1991 (the War of Independence) and 1998–2000 [9, 10]. Women formed 33% of the combatants during the War of Independence [12]. After independence, Eritrea had a very high MMR of 1590 which was reduced to 501 by 2015: a 69% reduction [8]. This MMR reduction could be a result of numerous policies such as the Post-Independence Macro Economic Policy Framework which included a vision to improve access to healthcare facilities [13–15]. As a result of this policy, the number of hospitals increased from 16 to 28, health centres from four to 56, and the number of health stations increased from 106 to 188 during 1990–2013 [13, 14].

Eritrea attempted to solve the shortage of healthcare workers by increasing the number of nurses and by encouraging task shifting. Between 2002 and 2012, the number of nurses increased from 846 to 1253 and associate nurses (diploma and certificate) from 1488 to 2537 [13]. Task shifting to solve shortage of healthcare workers also involved combining midwifery and nursing training as well as employing foreign doctors from countries such as Cuba [13, 16, 17].

Challenges still exist in Eritrea's health system. Only a small percentage of women deliver in health facilities [14]. Despite 57% of Eritrean women having the WHO recommended four antenatal care (ANC) visits by 2015 (compared to SSA average of 48%), only 34% of women delivered in health facilities in 2010 compared to 17% in 1995 – below the SSA average of 48% [18–20]. Moreover, there is a large gap in facility based deliveries between urban and rural areas. In 2010, 73% of women living in urban areas delivered in a health facility compared to only 27% of rural women [18–20].

This study aimed to examine stakeholders' perspectives on facilitators of and barriers to the utilisation of and access to maternal health services in Eritrea, focusing particularly on women's perspectives. The objectives were: (1) to assess women and their husbands/partners' perceptions about the facilitators of and barriers to the utilisation of and access to maternal health services; (2) to examine the possible effect of Eritrean culture on utilisation of and access to maternal health services; (3) to explore how the two wars (1961–1991, 1998–2000) have influenced women's status and affected their utilisation of and access to maternal health services; and (4) to investigate perspectives of healthcare providers and decision makers regarding maternal health services.

Methods

Setting and sampling

This study was conducted over a three-week period during February and March 2016 in Asmara, the capital of Eritrea, in four ANC clinics and one maternity ward. Asmara was chosen because its health facilities receive the largest number of outpatient visits in the country [13]. The four selected ANC clinics were located in Godaief Community Hospital, Edget Health Centre, Freesalam Clinic and Akreya Clinic. The maternity ward was located in Orotta Teaching Hospital. These health facilities were purposively selected based on their demographic characteristics. Edget Health Centre was chosen because it is located in a predominantly Muslim area, and thus could aid investigation into whether religion [21] and polygamy [22] hinder women's utilisation of and access to maternal health services. Freesalam Clinic was selected because it is in an affluent area and Akreya Clinic was chosen because it is in a socially disadvantaged area. Godaief Community Hospital was selected because it is a zobal (regional) hospital and receives patients from health stations and health centres in rural areas. Finally, Orotta Teaching Hospital maternity ward receives high risk women and complicated maternal cases.

The health system in Eritrea is divided into three levels [23]. Primary level healthcare is provided by community hospitals, health centres, and health stations. Community hospitals provide preventive and curative services and receive referrals from health centres and health stations in rural areas. Secondary level healthcare is provided by zobal (regional) referral hospitals which provide inpatient and outpatient services for the whole zoba and receive referrals from primary level health facilities. This level is also responsible for community mobilisation. Finally, tertiary level healthcare is provided by the national referral hospitals located in the capital Asmara: Orotta Teaching Hospital, Halibet Hospital, Berhan Eye Hospital, and St Mary's Psychiatric Hospital. Until 2014 there was private healthcare in the country [24]. However, by 2016, when this research was conducted, the government had abolished privately owned clinics and replaced them with its own out-of-pocket private health services within the public healthcare system.

Participants selection

The majority of our participants were women aged between 15 and 49 years who were pregnant at the time of the research, or had given birth between February and March 2016 (Tables 1 and 2). "Women or female participant" in

Table 1 Characteristics of women participants ($n = 40$)

Characteristic		Number
Ethnicity	Tigrigna	39
	Saho	1
Age (years)	15–16	1
	17–24	11
	25–34	25
	35–49	3
Education	Primary school (grades 0–7)	9
	Middle school (grades 8–10)	15
	Secondary school (grades 11–14)	14
Occupation	Unemployed	35
	Employed	5
Religion	Orthodox Christian	23
	Other Christian	5
	Muslim	8
Marital status	Never married	1
	1st wife	36
	2nd wife	2
	3rd wife	1
Parity (the number of times a female is or has been pregnant (gravidity) and carried the pregnancies to a viable gestational age)	0	13
	1	1
	2–3	9
	4–7	11
Number of abortions		7

the quotes hereafter, refers only to women who used maternal health services in our sample excluding female decision makers and healthcare providers. The second group of our participants were husbands/partners. They were included because their role has been found elsewhere in SSA to have an impact on women's utilisation of and access to maternal health services [25]. Finally, we interviewed healthcare providers and decision makers as key informants to highlight any health system challenges. They were recruited using purposive sampling based on their expertise, involvement in and knowledge of maternal health services [26].

All women and their husbands/partners were approached for recruitment in the general waiting areas and courtyards (that is, away from any of the healthcare providers) to avoid coercion. The lead researcher (CSC), with the help of research assistants, selected the women invited to participate within this cohort. Interviews with the women usually took place in private rooms or quiet courtyards within the health facilities. Although all 40 women were given the option to be interviewed after their consultations, 12 women chose to be interviewed in waiting rooms. These were large rooms where healthcare providers conducted consultations with other women and also contained multiple desks and partitions. We conducted the interviews with the 12 women on benches positioned so that women's privacy was maintained, being far away from healthcare providers so that they could not hear the interviews. Husbands/partners were recruited and interviewed in ANC clinics' courtyards while their wives/partners were having their ANC consultations. Finally, healthcare providers and decision makers were selected as key informants by the lead researcher. Interviews with healthcare providers were conducted in the health facilities early in the morning or at the end of the day to avoid busy consultation hours. Decision makers were interviewed by the lead researcher in their offices at the Ministry of Health at the national headquarters.

Table 2 Characteristics of husbands, healthcare providers and decision makers

Location		Husbands ($n = 5$)	Healthcare providers ($n = 10$)		Decision makers ($n = 5$)
			Nurses/midwives ($n = 9$)	Doctors[a] ($n = 1$)	
Healthcare facilities	Freesalam Clinic	1	2		
	Akreya Clinic	2			
	Edget Health Centre	2	2		
	Godaief C. Hospital		4		
	Orotta Teaching Hospital		1	1	
Ministry of Health	Family planning				1
	Human resources				1
	Research				1
	Data management				1
	FGM[b] programme				1

[a]Head of gynaecology department [b]Female genital mutilation

Conceptual framework

There are many factors that have been found to affect women's utilisation of and access to maternal health services. However, the focus of this study was factors associated with the WHO six health system building blocks, as well as an additional three factors [27–29], as shown in Fig. 1. The WHO six health system building blocks are broad indicators used to measure health system performance: (1) health services delivery; (2) health workforce; (3) health information system; (4) essential medicines; (5) health finance system; and (6) leadership and governance [27]. The six health system building blocks are also concerned with how stakeholders' perspectives and satisfaction could be used to measure health services delivery [27].

Figure 1 shows our adapted framework based on the WHO framework with an additional three factors not incorporated in the WHO framework: cultural beliefs, gender equality, and war. Cultural beliefs and gender equality were added because they have been found to affect women's health [28, 29]. War was added to the framework because it was one of our study objectives and has been found to negatively affect women's utilisation of and access to maternal health services [30–32].

Data collection

To generate knowledge about maternal health services in Eritrea, we collected data through in-depth interviews and field observations. For the in-depth interviews, identical open-ended questions were used for each group of participants (see supplementary material for our interview guidelines). The lead researcher conducted interviews with all healthcare providers and decision makers in English. The rest of the interviews were conducted with help from or by local research assistants – a male and two females in their seventh year of medical school who had had prior experience in conducting qualitative research. Research assistants who were fluent in both English and the main language spoken in the country (Tigrigna) were coached by the lead researcher about conducting qualitative research face to face. Research assistants then used the Tigrigna language to explain the selection criteria, confidentiality, disclosure of information and the aim of the study to participants before obtaining their consent.

All interviews were conducted one-on-one. As participants did not want the interviews to be recorded using a voice recorder, extensive note taking was used to record the interviews. Each interview lasted between 20 and 45 min, and stopped when no new ideas emerged. For the field observations, the lead researcher used extensive note taking that included documenting healthcare providers' interactions with women such as the consultation process, how healthcare providers recorded patients' information, and the general environment of the health facilities – such as their level of cleanliness.

Data analysis

Data analysis proceeded in several stages. First, when possible, the transcripts were read multiple times by the lead researcher and discussed face-to-face with research assistants on the same day as the interviews. During these daily discussions between the lead researcher and research assistants, field observation notes were also used to cross examine and interpret our in-depth interviews [33]. The

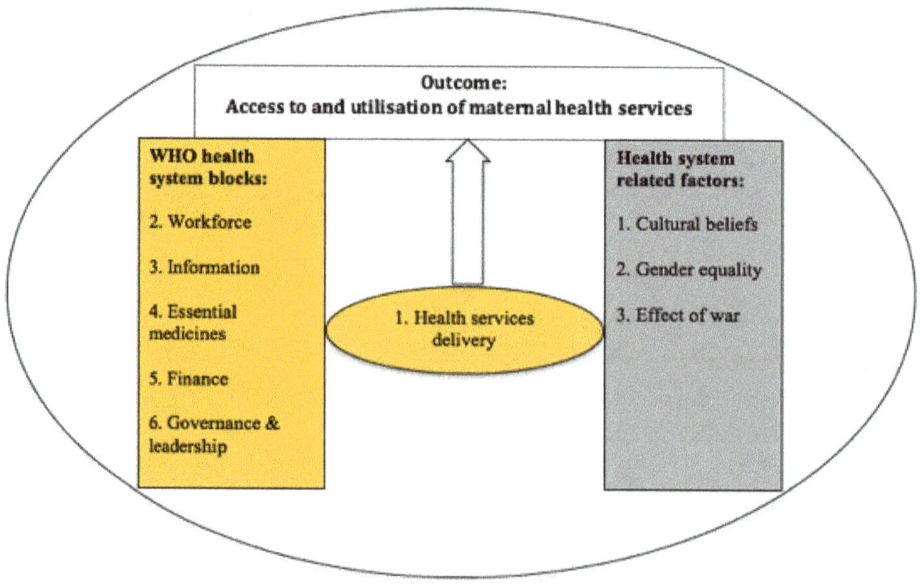

Fig. 1 Conceptual framework: Factors affecting women's utilisation of and access to maternal health services in Eritrea

aim of this stage of the process was to better understand the cultural context of the quotes beyond the obvious meaning or direct translation. Second, the qualitative information that was collected was subsequently used to inductively generate theory from the raw data (using Microsoft Excel) about health system performance and maternal health services [34, 35].

During the second stage of analysis, themes were inductively generated in three steps. First, a unique colour was assigned to words and/or phrases with similar meanings (codes) that were linked to the study objectives and prior knowledge of the literature review about Eritrea. Second, codes were assigned to each segment of the transcript in order to categorise the main concepts and link emerging data to research objectives while keeping the original phrases and context [34, 36–38]. Third, repeated codes were grouped into themes, examined for consistency, and discussed with co-author (CH). Finally, themes were grouped under the appropriate category and used for the final interpretation of the data.

Ethical approval and consent to participate

Ethics approval was obtained from the Health Research and Ethics Committee, Ministry of Health, The State of Eritrea. The Ethics Committee approved either written or oral consent to be obtained from the participants including minors' guardian. As our study included a 16 year old participant, her mother gave an oral consent for her participation and to use her quotes in this study. All participants gave oral consent for this study and were recorded by their initials only. No incentives or any form of financial compensation was given to any of the participants. This was explained to all participants during the recruitment process.

Results

In this study, 60 in-depth interviews were conducted: women ($n = 40$); husbands/partners ($n = 5$); healthcare providers ($n = 10$) (nine females and a male); and decision makers ($n = 5$) (three females and two males). Characteristics of participants are shown in Tables 1 and 2. Table 3 shows perceived facilitators of and barriers to women's utilisation of and access to maternal health services in Eritrea.

Table 3 Women's perspectives regarding perceived facilitators of and barriers to maternal health services in Eritrea ($n = 40$)

Facilitators	Barriers
Health education:	Perception of quality of care:
Information related to:	A call for private healthcare:
• Importance of delivering in a health facility	Reasons:
• Danger signs (fever, vomiting, bleeding, discharge, persistent headache and/or dizziness)	• To have access to ultrasound scans (no ultrasound scans were performed on pregnant women who participated in this study in all antenatal care clinics we visited except in Orotta Teaching Hospital maternity ward)
• Breast check during shower for any lumps	
• Vaccination	
	• To decrease the workload on the public clinics and avoid crowdedness of the health facilities. Therefore, less waiting time.
	• To avoid short opening hours in the public clinics
Improvement in gender equality:	Previous hospital experience:
• Role of Eritrean women as combatants during the War of Independence	Reasons for dissatisfaction:
	• Staff shortage
• Improvement in men's attitude towards maternity care	• Lack of sympathy
	• Poor treatment by healthcare providers
	• Not enough information in the postnatal period (6 weeks after childbirth)

Our study revealed two perceived facilitators of maternal health services in Eritrea: health education and improvement in gender equality. One major perceived barrier was women's perception of poor quality of care (Table 3).

Health education

We investigated the level of satisfaction expressed by women and their husbands/partners with the health information provided to them during their ANC visits. Thirty-four of the 40 women and all five husbands/partners we interviewed were satisfied. Women mentioned that they were encouraged to visit a health facility if they felt any of the danger signs during pregnancy: fever, vomiting, bleeding, discharge, persistent headache and/or dizziness (Table 3). The lead researcher observed that all five health facilities we visited had educational sessions each morning. These sessions were conducted by nursing cadres in the health facility courtyards, and provided an opportunity for nurses to discuss and answer health questions from pregnant women, husbands/partners and other family members. The lead researcher also observed that health education involved use of posters and signs raising awareness about maternal health issues in all healthcare facilities we visited.

> *"It is helpful* [health education] *in a way that it encourages you to follow up your health situation"*
> **Female participant from Edget Health Centre**

> *"Information about variety of tests, about how to support women physically and mentally and supporting them to come to the clinic has big role"*
> **Husband from Freesalam Clinic**

However, six women wanted more health-related information. A mother who had given birth 2 days prior at Orotta Teaching Hospital maternity ward, complained about lack of information given to her in the hospital. One of the six women also complained about the lack of reinforcement of the information each time they visited ANC clinics.

> *"No information was given about childbirth"* **Female participant from Orotta Teaching Hospital maternity ward**

> *"My experience could have been better if the information given to pregnant women was given several times"* **Female participant from Edget Health Centre**

Although all five husbands/partners were satisfied overall with the health information given to them in the courtyard sessions, some of them complained that they were not able to accompany their wives/partners during their consultations with nurses/midwives. This was confirmed by the lead researcher who observed that during all ANC visits, women were seen separately from their husband/partner. The only exception observed was during the first trimester, when women and their husbands/partners are consulted together and tested for HIV and other infectious diseases.

> *"Better if I learn more here* [at the ANC clinic] *with my wife, but I learn a lot by reading books"* **Husband from Akreya Clinic**

We investigated how contemporary cultural beliefs affect women's utilisation of and access to maternal health services in the country. Although the government health education strategy to combat negative cultural practices such as Female Genital Mutilation (FGM) involves use of mass media, some participants mentioned that mass media could be improved to enhance the distribution of health messages. Of the 40 women we interviewed, 38 women indicated that contemporary culture in Eritrea encourages them to access and utilise maternal health services. One example that seems to indicate a degree of cultural change was the account told to us by a 16 year old mother interviewed in Orotta Teaching Hospital maternity ward about her decision to access health services. She spoke of her hesitation to attend an ANC clinic because of her extramarital pregnancy at a young age. However, she eventually gave birth in a healthcare facility and was supported by both her mother and her boyfriend.

> *"Our culture and families motivate us to come to the clinic and follow our pregnancy"* **Female participant from Akreya Clinic**

> *"I was afraid to come to antenatal clinic because I was not married and became pregnant...my mam and my culture motivated me to access maternal health services"* **Female participant from Orotta Teaching Hospital maternity ward**

> *"During the war, we tried to stop FGM even during the war by putting policies in place.... our position as women is much better than before the war. We have more rights"* **Decision maker (female) from Ministry of Health**

> *"FGM is practised by all ethnic groups regardless of religion. It is punishable by law with jail time and fine of 10,000 nakfa* [Eritrean currency]. *It is higher among Muslims compared to Christians. The reasons among Muslims is for cleanliness and among Christians is to maintain virginity"* **FGM programme decision maker (male) from Ministry of Health**

> *".... mass media needs to increase the awareness and improve the knowledge of men about pregnancy... It is not well understood that men have to support women, because society lacks awareness but I believe that I need to support my wife"* **Husband from Edget Health Centre**

Even though the majority of the participants indicated that contemporary cultural beliefs in the country encourage women's utilisation of and access to maternal health services, some disagreed. For example, one woman indicated that the cultural preference is for women to deliver at home but that she prefers to deliver in hospital.

> *"I believe cultural beliefs prefer that women deliver at home but I personally prefer to deliver in a hospital and go to a clinic while I am pregnant"* **Female participant from Godaief Community Hospital**

Community mobilisation – that is, community-driven activities where communities make autonomous decisions to improve their own health [39, 40] – was mentioned by a decision maker as being one of the factors that helped influence women's utilisation of and access to maternal health services. However, our study could not substantiate this claim since no community driven health activities were observed or mentioned by most of the participants.

"Community mobilization and making information available to them [women] *is one of the most effective health policy strategies that helps reduce maternal mortality here"* **Decision maker (female) from Ministry of Health**

Improvement in gender equality

Role of Eritrean women during the war of independence (1961–1991)

Women were asked how the history of wars affected women's status and their utilisation of and access to maternal health services. All women mentioned that war helped to improve gender equality in the country. This improvement was mainly driven by their role as combatants during the War of Independence. For example, a former combatant now working as a nurse/midwife was interviewed, and showed the lead researcher marks of five healed bullet wounds in her lower limbs. She spoke of how she suffers from a permanent hip injury from the war and about her fighting experience alongside men during the War of Independence.

"I was a fighter and a field doctor at the same time. First, I was shot twice during the war and while recovering, I gave birth to my eldest son in a mobile clinic. Women used to hide their pregnancies so they could be in the field fighting with men. When they were about to give birth, they were provided with a place to give birth and stay with their babies for one year and a half but some women sometimes chose to leave early to fight. After I gave birth to my son I used to look after other women's children while they were fighting. I left my son after a year with the Sewera brigade [revolution brigade responsible for looking after other women's children while they are in the field fighting]. *After I went back to the war, I was again shot three times and suffered a permanent hip injury... and my husband was killed during the war* [emotional]...*I still believe in helping women to give birth safely...I agree with the government for men to pay if they do not come with their wives for check-up. We are the same now because we fight together. I struggled in the war like them* [men]*"* **Nurse/midwife (female) from Godaief Community Hospital. A former freedom fighter who also worked as a field doctor (nurse/midwife) during the War of Independence.**

"The role of Eritrean women during the war was an important factor for gender equality in Eritrea...." **Decision maker (female) from Ministry of Health**

"My mother fought as a freedom fighter to make it better for me now. My husband helps me with cooking now because he knows we are the same. No difference now between a girl and a boy" **Female participant from Freesalam Clinic**

"During the war mothers were not able to get access to health centres as there were no adequate hospitals, medical supplies and workforce.... I am the same with my man now. My mother and my father liberated the country fighting together. Because of this we are the same now with my husband [putting both index fingers alongside each other meaning equal]*"* **Female participant from Edget Health Centre**

"After the war, women are more aware [of their rights] *and free to go to hospitals and get service. There are more health centres* [now] *and better service"* **Female participant from Edget Health Centre**

Role of men during pregnancy and child delivery

We asked the participants about men's role during pregnancy and childbirth. Twenty-three women would like their husbands/partners to help with housework and 13 women said they would like their husbands/partners to support them by being there during childbirth. All five husbands/partners who were interviewed agreed that men should support their wives/partners.

The involvement of men in their wives/partners' maternity care has been addressed by the government through community education programmes [41]. For example, men are required to accompany their wives/partners in the first trimester to check for infectious diseases. In addition, men are required not to divorce their wives/partners during pregnancy.

"It has been made compulsory for fathers to attend in the 1st trimester with their wives to check for STDs [sexually transmitted diseases] *and HIV. Men are obligated to stay with their wives during this period of pregnancy and not to divorce"* **Nurse/midwife (female) from Freesalam Clinic**

"My husband helps me a lot with housework and heavy lifting, he motivates me and he is here now. He learns with me" **Female participant from Akreya Clinic**

"Men should help women during pregnancy and when giving birth. My boyfriend helped me a lot during my pregnancy and now after I gave birth" **A young**

unmarried female participant from Orotta Teaching Hospital maternity ward

"During pregnancy men should support mothers morally and help them with housework. During delivery men should stand beside mothers and share their pain" **Female participant from Akreya Clinic**

"Continue to increase awareness that a man needs to come to the clinic with his wife" **Husband from Edget Health Centre**

Quality of care

Preference for private healthcare (unexpected finding)

Privately owned health clinics existed in Eritrea until 2014, but by the time this research was conducted in 2016 they had been abolished by the government. Instead, the government provided its own out-of-pocket private health services within the public healthcare system. Our initial interview guidelines did not include a question concerning private healthcare because we were not aware of the demand for this service. However, a question about private healthcare was added when the issue emerged during our first interview when the first woman we interviewed said she would like private healthcare due to the lack of ultrasound machines in the government ANC clinics.

We asked women if they would like to see private healthcare reinstated, the reason for their choice, and whether they could afford it. Of the 40 women we interviewed, 31 expressed dissatisfaction with some aspects of the government services and stated that they would like private clinics reinstated. Their dissatisfaction was due to three reasons: lack of ultrasound machines, short clinic opening hours, and a shortage of healthcare workers. A lack of ultrasound machines was observed by the lead researcher: none of the five ANC clinics we visited had an ultrasound machine. The lead researcher also observed that most of the ANC clinics did have short opening hours as well as having long wait times: they opened at 7 o'clock each morning and closed at midday, with the average waiting time of 40 min. Finally, shortage of healthcare workers was observed by the lead researcher as a particularly significant concern in one of the ANC clinics, which had only one nurse/midwife (former freedom fighter) attending to 34 pregnant women on the day the clinic was visited.

"It would be nice if there is private clinics to have ultrasound [scan] *and I could afford it"* **Female participant from Freesalam clinic**

"It is really good [to have private healthcare]. *I would have been able to get a better concept about the health of my child, like doing ultrasound* [scan]*"* **Female participant from Godaief Community Hospital**

"It is good that the private clinic exists, because it is better with timing and you can access it at any time" **Female participant from Akreya Clinic**

"Increase the workforce as this nurse is lone and has very big workload" **Female participant from Edget Health Centre**

Although 31 women wanted private health care, nine women disagreed. They were satisfied with the current public services and they believed that private healthcare would be a waste of resources that could otherwise be spent to improve the existing public health services. They also mentioned that they would not be able to afford to pay for private health care.

"No need [for private healthcare]. *Because it is waste of time and money as the health professionals are more helpful and supportive at this health centre"* **Female participant from Godaief Community Hospital**

"No, I don't think private clinics should be available. It would be better to just improve the services given in the [current] *clinics and hospitals"* **Female participant from Edget Health Centre**

"Private clinics are quite expensive and it is hard to afford financially. So, I do not prefer private clinics..." **Female participant from Godaief Community Hospital**

Previous hospital experience

Women were asked to describe their previous hospital experiences and their treatment by healthcare providers during childbirth or any maternal complications. This question was answered by 23 of the 40 women we interviewed. Seventeen women were excluded – four chose not to comment and 13 women had no comments to make as it was their first pregnancy. Fifteen women had had a positive previous hospital experience and eight women had had a negative experience. The dissatisfaction of the latter group of women was due to shortage of healthcare workers, poor treatment by healthcare providers, and long waiting times.

"It is important that I went to the health centre to follow my pregnancy and I am so happy to deliver in this hospital" **Female participant from Akreya Clinic**

"The last visit was good. If it had not been for them [healthcare providers], *I would not have delivered a healthy baby because my baby had an abnormal presentation and the staff managed to help"* **Female participant from Freesalam Clinic**

"We need health professional help during pregnancy and labour. Women should get access to delivery at hospitals" **Female participant from Godaief Community Hospital**

"I had a caesarean section. I could have given birth naturally if I had received adequate support. There were not enough health professionals around in the evening" **Female participant from Edget Health Centre**

"My delivery was successful but the midwives were not following my labour properly" **Female participant from Akreya Clinic**

"It is better that the health service providers understand that we have children to take care of at home, so better to manage the time and accessibility" **Female participant from Freesalam Clinic**

Discussion

This study set out to explore stakeholders' perspectives (particularly women's) on facilitators of and barriers to the utilisation of and access to maternal health services in Eritrea. Two major perceived facilitators that emerged were: health education and improvement in gender equality based on the Eritrean women's role forming 33% of the armed forces during the War of Independence. One perceived barrier was poor quality of care, mainly due to lack of ultrasound machines, short clinic opening hours, and shortage of healthcare workers.

Out study revealed two findings related to the WHO health service delivery and health workforce building blocks. Health education – as a component of health promotion – was one of the facilitators we found related to the health service delivery building block. The second finding related to the health workforce building block was shortage of healthcare workers as a barrier. It is interesting that the majority of women did not mention affordability as a barrier to the use of maternal health services when they called for private healthcare to be reinstated in the country after it was abolished by the government in 2014. As well, they did not mention task shifting to solve shortage of healthcare workers or possible barriers associated with family composition, their financial situation or distance from healthcare centres.

Perceived facilitators of maternal health services

Health education

We assessed the perceptions held by women and their husbands/partners regarding the facilitators of and barriers to maternal health services in Eritrea (objective 1). Health education (a component of health promotion) was the only facilitator related to the WHO health service delivery building block [27, 42]. Health promotion forms an essential part of comprehensiveness which is one of eight key characteristics of the health service delivery building block [27]. It is defined as "the process of enabling people to increase control over their health and its determinants, and thereby improve their health." [42].

Health education in Eritrea takes two forms: education provided through health facilities and education enabled through the use of mass media. Health education in health facilities mainly involves sessions in the morning targeting women and their families. These sessions were acknowledged by 34 of the 40 women we interviewed as being effective in encouraging them to access and utilise maternal health services. Furthermore, 34 women expressed satisfaction with the health information given to them at the health facilities which encouraged them to visit a health facility if they experienced the five danger signs. Health education could also be one of the reasons for the increase in the percentage of women attending an ANC clinic at least four times – an attendance pattern recommended by the WHO as an essential requirement for maternal mortality reduction [18]. During 1995–2015, the percentage of Eritrean women attending an ANC clinic four or more times increased from 41% to 57%, compared to SSA average of 48% [18, 19]. However, although the percentage of women who deliver in health facilities increased from 17% to 34% during 1995–2010, facility-based deliveries in Eritrea remain below the SSA average of 48% [18, 19].

We examined the possible effect of Eritrean culture on women's utilisation of and access to maternal health services (objective 2). We found that Eritrea uses mass media to target negative aspects of traditional cultural beliefs and practices. One of the female decision makers from the Ministry of Health mentioned FGM as one of the negative aspects of traditional cultural practices that the government has been attempting to eradicate. The lead researcher interviewed a decision maker from the Ministry of Health responsible for implementing FGM policies. His task is to conduct regular visits to ANC clinics to remind pregnant women and families about the media campaigns which are conducted by the government which includes a warning that FGM is punishable by law with imprisonment and a 10,000 nakfa (Eritrean currency) fine. Another example that could indicate the effectiveness of mass media in this study is that most of the women who had had a previous pregnancy reutilised maternal health services despite their dissatisfaction with some aspects of the government health services.

Another example of the traditional cultural beliefs that influence the degree to which women access and utilise maternal health services is related to some traditional practices such as belief in the traditional birth attendants (TBAs) [28]. For example, in Ethiopia, it was found that even though 71% of women attended ANC services, 42% believed that seeking facility-based delivery was not necessary, due to influence of TBAs [28]. Although in our study 38 of the 40 women stated that contemporary culture in Eritrea encourages them to access and utilise maternal health services, the country has a relatively low rate of facility based deliveries and home birth is still common [18, 19]. This suggests that belief in traditional cultural practices still exists in Eritrea and more efforts are needed to increase women's awareness about the significance of childbirth in a health facility.

Improvement in gender equality (role of Eritrean women during the two wars with Ethiopia (1961–1991, 1998–2000))

We explored how the two wars in Eritrea (1961–1991, 1998–2000) have influenced women's status and affected their utilisation of and access to maternal health services (objective 3). We found that Eritrean women's role as combatants during the War of Independence was mentioned by women as being a major factor in their empowerment, in improving women's status, and thereby enhancing gender equality. This is significant because empowering women through gender equality has been found to be associated with improvement in maternal health outcomes [43, 44]. In addition, two indicators that could suggest improvement in gender equality were males' involvement in maternity care and related government regulations that discourage men from divorcing their wives/partners during pregnancy.

Women's empowerment has been found in countries like Uganda and Burkina Faso to be associated with men's involvement in their wives/partners attendance at ANC clinics [25]. In our study, all five husbands/partners interviewed indicated that their role is crucial in supporting their wives/partners during pregnancy and childbirth. Government policy that requires men to accompany their wives/partners to ANC clinics during the first trimester for infectious diseases testing as mentioned by some participants could be an indicator of female empowerment.

Women's political participation and the female labour participation rate are two other indicators that could also explain the improvement in gender equality and women's empowerment in Eritrea. After independence, Eritrean women gained significant status and formed 50% of the Constitutional Commission during the 1997 ratification process of the constitution [45]. The equal male and female involvement in the ratification process could be due to Eritrean women's important role as combatants during the War of Independence, during which they made up 33% of the armed forces [12]. Another indicator of women's empowerment is the labour participation rate [46]. In 2014, the labour participation rate among Eritrean females aged 15 and older was 85% compared to 70% for SSA overall [47].

Quality of care as a potential barrier to women's utilisation of and access to parts of maternal health services

Our estimation of quality of care – a difficult issue to assess – is based on the WHO patient-centred approach which focuses on whether or not healthcare providers listen to patients' concerns as well as the perception of the services provided [27, 48]. For example, we used the lack of ultrasound machines in ANC clinics and the observed shortage of healthcare workers as factors in determining women's perception of poor quality of care. Shortage of healthcare workers has elsewhere been identified as one of the factors contributing to poor quality of care in Eritrea [17]. Short clinic opening hours, a lack of ultrasound machines and shortage of healthcare workers were the three major reasons why women called for private healthcare independent from that run within the public sector by the government (Table 3). This finding also supports the estimation of Eritrea's maternal healthcare system as offering a low quality of care.

Although the perception that health care is of poor quality appears to be a barrier to women's utilisation of and access to maternal health services in Eritrea, a recent study in Eritrea found improvements in quality of care [17]. Women's reutilisation of government healthcare facilities for consecutive pregnancies also suggests an improvement in quality of care and that poor quality was not a total barrier to women's utilisation of and access to maternal health services in Eritrea. For example, 11 women who previously delivered in health facilities or had hospital experience related to maternity care reported a positive experience which could be one of the reasons they reutilised the health services.

To our knowledge this study is the first to explore maternal health services in Eritrea while also taking into account the influence of the country's history of wars. This study has some limitations. First, it is not representative of the whole country since we only interviewed women who lived in Asmara and had access to government health facilities. Second, women who did not utilise maternal health services were not interviewed for this study. Third, there are several factors – such as distance to healthcare facilities and transport – that are likely to have had an effect on women's utilisation of and access to maternal health services but which are beyond the conceptual framework of this study. Fourth, our interviews with healthcare providers and decision makers did not provide us with information on barriers to maternal health. During those interviews, the comments from most interviewees focused mainly on the facilitators of maternal health services such as improvement in gender equality. This could be due to two reasons: either they have low level of awareness of the barriers mentioned by women or they know about the barriers but chose not to address it as a sensitive issue. Finally, although most of the healthcare providers and decision makers experienced the War of Independence, most of the women did not address the effect of war on utilisation of and access to maternal health services. This is because most of the women were not born or were very young during the War of Independence that ended in 1991. Nevertheless, they acknowledged the improvement in gender equality in the country driven mainly by their mothers and female fighters during the War of Independence.

Conclusion

This study assessed women and their husbands/partners' perceptions and the possible effect of contemporary Eritrean culture and the history of war on the utilisation of and access to maternal health services in the country. As well, we examined healthcare providers' and decision makers' perspectives. The two key facilitators of women's utilisation of and access to maternal health services were health education and women's empowerment driven by their role as combatants during the War of Independence. One main barrier was poor quality of care due to lack of ultrasound machines, short clinic opening hours, and a shortage of healthcare workers. As only a limited number of qualitative studies have been published about maternal health services in war-affected sub-Saharan African countries, our findings especially regarding health education and women's empowerment could be considered in other war-affected countries similar to Eritrea. Nevertheless, further research is needed to investigate our findings – particularly regarding female empowerment driven by women's role in combat in relation to their maternal health.

Abbreviations

ANC: Antenatal care; FGM: Female genital mutilation; MMR: Maternal mortality ratio; SSA: Sub-Saharan Africa; STD: Sexually transmitted disease

Acknowledgements

This analysis is a part of CSC thesis to fulfil the requirement for a PhD at School of Public Health, the University of Sydney. We are deeply grateful to all the Eritrean participants in this study and to the Eritrean research assistants who assisted with interviews and initial discussions of data. We acknowledge the assistance of the staff of the Consulate General of the State of Eritrea in Melbourne Australia and Ministry of Health of the State of Eritrea for their support. We also thank Shannon McKinn from School of Public Health, the University of Sydney and Georgina Crisp for providing feedback on the final draft of the manuscript.

Funding

None.

Authors' contributions

CSC: Conceptualised the study, collected and analysed the data, and drafted the first manuscript; CH: participated in the design, data interpretation, and provided substantial input into the data analysis. BD, BH and JN: participated in study design, data interpretation and in reviewing the manuscript. As a member of the ethics committee, BD also helped in obtaining ethics clearance for the study, but to avoid conflict of interest, BD did not participate in any decision or meetings which resulted in the ethics approval of this study. RGC: participated in the study design, and provided crucial input into the data interpretation and reviewing the manuscript. All authors reviewed and approved the final manuscript.

Competing interests

The authors declare that they have no competing interests.

Author details

[1]School of Public Health, The University of Sydney, Sydney, Australia. [2]Senior Lecturer, School of Public Health, The University of Sydney, Sydney, Australia. [3]Director General of Research and Human Resource Development, Ministry of Health, Asmara, Eritrea. [4]Director of Family and Community Health, Ministry of Health, Asmara, Eritrea. [5]School of Public Health, The University of Sydney, Sydney, Australia. [6]School of Public Health, The University of Sydney, Sydney, Australia.

References

1. Garfield RM. War-related changes in health and health services in Nicaragua. Soc Sci Med. 1989;28(7):669–76.
2. Busza J, Lush L. Planning reproductive health in conflict: a conceptual framework. Soc Sci Med. 1999;49(2):155–71.
3. World Health Organization. The world health report 2000. Health systems: improving performance. Geneva: WHO; 2000.
4. Price JI, Bohara AK. Maternal health care amid political unrest: the effect of armed conflict on antenatal care utilization in Nepal. Health Policy Plan. 2013;28(3):309.
5. Chi PC, Bulage P, Urdal H, Sundby J. Perceptions of the effects of armed conflict on maternal and reproductive health services and outcomes in Burundi and northern Uganda: a qualitative study. BMC Int Health Hum Rights. 2015;15(1):7.
6. Strand H, Wilhelmsen L, Gleditsch N, International Peace Research Institute Oslo (PRIO). Armed conflict dataset codebook. Uppsala: PRIO; 2003.
7. Themnér L, Wallensteen P. Armed conflicts, 1946–2011. J Peace Res. 2012; 49(4):565–75.
8. WHO, UNICEF, UNFPA, The World Bank, United Nations Population Division. Trends in maternal mortality: 1990 to 2015. Geneva: WHO; 2015.
9. Murphy SD, editor The Eritrean-Ethiopian War (1998-2000). The Eritrean-Ethiopian war (1998–2000). George Washington University Legal Studies Conference. Washington, DC: Oxford University Press; 2016.
10. Bernal V. Eritrea goes global: reflections on nationalism in a transnational era. Cult Anthropol. 2004;19(1):3–25.

11. World Health Organization. Beyond the numbers: reviewing maternal deaths and complications to make pregnancy safer. Geneva: WHO; 2004.
12. The United Nations. Women's anti-discrimination committee takes-up report of Eritrea; told gender equality efforts hindered by stereotypes, poverty, war. New York: UN; 2006.
13. The State of Eritrea Ministry of Health. Eritrea annual health service activity report of year 2012. Asmara: Eritrea Ministry of Health; 2013.
14. UNDP. Innovations driving health MDGs in Eritrea. UNDP Eritrea: Asmara; 2014.
15. The State of Eritrea Ministry of Health. National health policy. Asmara: Eritrea Ministry of Health; 2010.
16. Holzgreve W, Greiner D, Schwidtal P. Maternal mortality in Eritrea: improvements associated with centralization of obstetric services. Int J Gynecol Obstet. 2012;119(SUPPL.1):S50–S4.
17. Sharan M, Ahmed S, Ghebrehiwet M, Rogo K. The quality of the maternal health system in Eritrea. Int J Gynaecol Obstet. 2011;115(3):244.
18. World Health Organization. World health statistics 2015. Geneva: WHO; 2015.
19. The State of Eritrea Ministry of Health, ORC Macro. Eritrea Demographic and Health Survey 2002. Asmara: Eritrea Ministry of Health, Bureau of Statistics, and Calverton, MD, USA: ORC Macro; 2002.
20. The State of Eritrea National Statistics Office (NSO), Fafo Institute for Applied International Studies (AIS). Eritrea Population and Health Survey 2010. Eritrea population and health survey 2010. Asmara: Eritrea Ministry of Health; 2013.
21. Austin A, Fapohunda B, Langer A, Orobaton N. Trends in delivery with no one present in Nigeria between 2003 and 2013. Int J Womens Health. 2015; 7:345–56.
22. Mugo N, Dibley M, Agho K. Prevalence and risk factors for non-use of antenatal care visits: analysis of the 2010 South Sudan household survey. BMC Pregnancy Childbirth. 2015;15(1):68.
23. The State of Eritrea Ministry of Health. Second national integrated monitoring and evaluation framework 2012–2016. Asmara: Eritrea Ministry of Health; 2012.
24. Habtom GK, Ruys P. The choice of a health care provider in Eritrea. Health Policy. 2007;80(1):202–17.
25. Jennings L, Na M, Cherewick M, Hindin M, Mullany B, Ahmed S. Women's empowerment and male involvement in antenatal care: analyses of demographic and health surveys (DHS) in selected African countries. BMC Pregnancy Childbirth. 2014;14(1):297.
26. Bowling A. Research methods in health: investigating health and health services. Maidenhead: McGraw-Hill Education; 2014.
27. World Health Organization. Monitoring the building blocks of health systems: a handbook of indicators and their measurement strategies. Geneva: WHO; 2010.
28. Shiferaw S, Spigt M, Godefrooij M, Melkamu Y, Tekie M. Why do women prefer home births in Ethiopia? BMC Pregnancy Childbirth. 2013;13(1):5.
29. Langer A, Meleis A, Knaul FM, Atun R, Aran M, Arreola-Ornelas H, et al. Women and health: the key for sustainable development. Lancet. 2015; https://doi.org/10.1016/ S0140-6736(15)60497-4.
30. Sidel V, Levy B. The health impact of war. Int J Inj Control Saf Promot. 2008; 15(4):189–95.
31. Sondorp E. A new tool for measuring the brutality of war. PLoS Med. 2008; 5(12):e249.
32. Chi PC, Bulage P, Urdal H, Sundby J. A qualitative study exploring the determinants of maternal health service uptake in post-conflict Burundi and northern Uganda. BMC Pregnancy Childbirth. 2015;15:18.
33. Kawulich BB. Participant observation as a data collection method. Qualitative forum: qualitative social research; 2005. https://doi.org/10.17169/fqs-6.2.466.
34. Thomas DR. A general inductive approach for analyzing qualitative evaluation data. Am J Eval. 2006;27(2):237–46.
35. El-Jardali F, Adam T, Ataya N, Jamal D, Jaafar M. Constraints to applying systems thinking concepts in health systems: a regional perspective from surveying stakeholders in eastern Mediterranean countries. Int J Health Policy Manage. 2014;3(7):399–407.
36. Miles MB, Huberman AM. Qualitative data analysis: a sourcebook of new methods. California: Sage Publications; 1984. Report No: 0803922744; 9780803922747
37. Gale NK, Heath G, Cameron E, Rashid S, Redwood S. Using the framework method for the analysis of qualitative data in multi-disciplinary health research. BMC Med Res Methodol. 2013;13:117.
38. Braun V, Clarke V. Using thematic analysis in psychology. Qual Res Psychol. 2006;3:77–101.
39. Howard-Grabman L, Snetro G. How to mobilize communities for health and social change. Maryland: Management Science for Health; 2003.
40. Rosato M, Laverack G, Grabman LH, Tripathy P, Nair N, Mwansambo C, et al. Community participation: lessons for maternal, newborn, and child health. Lancet. 2008;372(9642):962–71.
41. Turan JM, Tesfagiorghis M, Polan ML. Evaluation of a community intervention for promotion of safe motherhood in Eritrea. J Midwifery Womens Health. 2011;56(1):8–17.
42. World Health Organization. Ottawa charter for health promotion. Geneva: WHO; 1986.
43. Frenk J, Gómez-Dantés O, Langer A. A comprehensive approach to women's health: lessons from the Mexican health reform. BMC Womens Health. 2012;12(1):42.
44. Singh K, Bloom S, Brodish P. Gender equality as a means to improve maternal and child health in Africa. Health Care Women Int. 2015;36(1):57–69.
45. The United Nations. Implementation of the Beijing platform for action and the outcome douments of the twenty-third special session of the general assembly. New York: UN; 2004.
46. Elborgh-Woytek K, Newiak M, Kochhar K, Fabrizio S, Kpodar K, Wingender P, et al. Women, work, and the economy: macroeconomic gains from gender equity. IMF Staff Discussion. Washington DC: IMF; 2010.
47. The World Bank. Labor force participation rate. Washington DC: World Bank; 2016.
48. Cleary PD, McNeil BJ. Patient satisfaction as an indicator of quality care. Inquiry. 1988;25(1):25–36.

Uptake of intermittent preventive treatment for malaria during pregnancy with Sulphadoxine-Pyrimethamine (IPTp-SP) among postpartum women in Zomba District, Malawi

Steven Chifundo Azizi[1,2*], Gershom Chongwe[1], Helen Chipukuma[3], Choolwe Jacobs[1], Jessy Zgambo[1] and Charles Michelo[1]

Abstract

Background: Malaria in pregnancy causes adverse birth outcomes. Intermittent preventive treatment of malaria during pregnancy with sulphadoxine-pyrimethamine (IPTp-SP) is recommended as a chemoprevention therapy. Zomba district IPTp uptake falls far below the national average. The study was conducted to assess determinants of IPTp-SP uptake during pregnancy among postpartum women in Zomba district after adoption of new IPTp-SP policy in 2014.

Methods: This was a cross-sectional survey. Two public health facilities (HFs) were randomly selected from urban and rural areas in Zomba district. Study participants were postpartum women selected by using exit poll method from HFs. A total of 463 postpartum women were interviewed using structured questionnaire. Bivariate and multiple logistic regression was used in data analysis.

Results: Out of all the enrolled participants ($n = 463$), 92% women had complete information for analysis. Of these, ($n = 426$) women, 127 (29.8%, 95% CI: 25.6%–34.3%) received three or more doses of SP, 299 (70.2%, 95% CI: 65.7%–74.4%) received two or less doses. Women receiving SP from rural HF were less likely to get at least three doses of SP than urban women, (AOR = 0.31, 95% CI 0.13–0.70); Others less likely were those with three or few antenatal care (ANC) visits versus four or more visits (AOR = 0.29, 95% CI 0.18–0.48); not taking SP under direct observation therapy (DOT) (AOR = 0.18, 95% CI (0.05–0.63).

Conclusions: There is low utilisation of at least three doses of SP in this population and this seems to be associated with the number of ANC visits and use of DOTs. These determinants may therefore be important in shaping interventions aimed at increasing the uptake of IPTp in this district. In addition, the rural urban differential suggests the need for further research to understand the barriers and enablers of uptake in each context in order to improve the health of the community.

Keywords: Pregnancy, Intermittent preventive treatment, Sulphadoxine-pyrimethamine, Malaria, Uptake, Postpartum, Malawi

* Correspondence: steve_aziz@hotmail.com
[1]Department of Epidemiology and Biostatistics, School of Public Health, University of Zambia, Post Box 50110, Lusaka, Zambia
[2]Malawi Defence Force, Malawi Military Health Services, Kamuzu Barracks, Private Bag 43, Lilongwe, Malawi
Full list of author information is available at the end of the article

Background

Malaria in pregnancy (MiP) is a significant cause of maternal morbidity and poor birth outcomes yet is preventable and treatable [1–4]. Women are particularly predisposed to adverse effects of malaria during their first and second pregnancies [5]. Globally, it is estimated that 125 million pregnant women are at risk of malaria infection each year and 30 million come from sub-Saharan Africa [6]. Furthermore, 75,000–200,000 infants and 10, 000 women deaths are estimated annually and the deaths are attributed to MiP [6, 7]. Particularly, *Plasmodium falciparum* infections in pregnancy contributes to approximately 11% (100, 000) of neonatal deaths due to low birth weight in areas of Africa where malaria is endemic (LBW) [7–9]. Infection with malaria in pregnancy predisposes women to increased risk of severe anaemia, intra-uterine growth retardation, intrauterine death, stillbirth, pre-term delivery, low birth weight (LBW), maternal death and placental malaria; and there is increased risk to unborn baby from miscarriage, stillbirth and LBW [10–12].

World Health Organisation (WHO) recommends three-pronged approach in stable malaria transmission areas for malaria prevention and control in pregnancy, which are Intermittent Preventive Treatment of malaria during pregnancy with sulphadoxine-pyrimethamine (IPTp-SP) , use of insecticides treated nets (ITNs), and prompt diagnosis and effective treatment. In the IPTp-SP interventional regimen, each dose contains three tablets of sulphadoxine/pyrimethamine and each tablet contains 500 mg/25 mg SP [13, 14]. Although in 2004, WHO recommended a minimum of two doses of IPTp-SP during pregnancy [15, 16], in October 2012 this policy was updated to "at least three doses during pregnancy and to be administered at least 1 month apart at each scheduled antenatal care (ANC) visit, beginning from second trimester under direct observational therapy" [17, 18]. Malawi adopted the updated policy in 2013 [19]. WHO envisage the policy would increase IPTp-SP uptake as it also recommends at least four ANC visits during the second and third trimesters of pregnancy under the Focused antenatal care (FANC) model [17, 20]. Roll Back Malaria set a target of 100% utilization of at least two doses of IPTp-SP by 2015 [21]. Antenatal Care is the main point of contact of pregnant women with the health system [7]. ANC clinics are used as a vehicle of coverage of health interventions against malaria and other adverse conditions. Thus, the uptake of IPTp-SP would depend on attendance of pregnant women and delivery of the intervention at a health facility [16, 22].

Studies that estimated proportions of uptake of at least three doses of IPTp-SP and identified factors associated with it among pregnant women are few since WHO updated the IPTp-SP policy. However, previous studies revealed that, successful uptake of at least two doses of IPTp-SP is determined by the number of ANC visits [4, 18, 23–28], directly observed therapy (DOT) [4, 29, 30], residential area [18, 31], age of woman [31], education level and socioeconomic status [4, 32], parity [4, 31], timing of initial ANC visit [4, 33], knowledge about malaria/IPTp [4] and stockouts of the commodity [4]. This study envisages to contribute to identifying obstacles to completion of recommended doses of SP during pregnancy using the updated policy in order to develop a robust and multidisciplinary implementation approach for IPTp-SP intervention in resource limited settings. The aims of the study were to estimate the proportion of and identify factors determining the uptake of at least three doses of IPTp-SP among pregnant women in Zomba district, Malawi.

Methods

Study design and study settings

A cross sectional study was conducted in two health facilities in Zomba district, which is located in the southern region of Malawi between November 23, 2016 and January 27, 2017. Zomba district was purposively chosen because it was among the districts that had the lowest IPTp uptake in Malawi [34].

Study population

The target population was all pregnant women and the study population was all postpartum women aged 15–49 who had just delivered (< 48 h) and those that delivered at home but visited the health facility for check-up at a randomly sampled Government-owned health facility in Zomba district.

Inclusion and exclusion criteria

The study included postpartum women of the ages between 15 to 49 years who delivered at Government Health facility (HF), or delivered at home but brought a baby to HF within 48 h for check-up to minimise recall bias. They had singleton pregnancy, absence of reported antimalarial treatment other than SP in the previous 1 month. On the other hand, complicated cases of pregnancy, postpartum women on cotrimoxazole prophylaxis during their pregnancy because of increased risk of adverse drug reactions when taken together with SP were excluded from the study [14, 35].

Variables

Guided by literature review, the study included the following variables that had been theoretically and empirically linked to malaria in pregnancy and uptake of IPTp-SP. The outcome was IPTp-SP uptake (≤2 doses versus 3+ doses) and. Explanatory variables were age, marital status, residence (location of the health facility), level of education, occupation, religion, tribe, knowledge about malaria transmission, knowledge about dangers of malaria in pregnancy, parity, number and timing of antenatal clinic visits, taking SP each time under directly observed therapy, distance to health facility, need for spouse's escort to ANC, worried no health care provider and drugs at health facility and gravida (Table 1).

Sampling and sample size determination

The district was divided into two sites according to residential settings: rural and urban. All Government owned health facilities that offered maternity and antenatal services were included in the stratified sampling frame. There were seven public health facilities out of 15 that were offering maternity and antenatal services in rural. Only two public health facilities among five offered maternity and antenatal services in urban. One health facility was selected from each stratum using simple random sampling drawn from Excel spreadsheet "RAND()" command.

Sample size was determined using a single population proportion estimation formula and calculated using Epi Info 7 with 43.5% proportion [34], 5% of decision precision, 95% confidence interval and non-response rate of 20%. The calculated overall sample size was 454.

Since the number of deliveries varies for different health facilities, a proportionate method was used for determining the sample size for each facility. The sample for each facility was calculated by weighting the total sample size required with the relative proportion of clients (total deliveries for each facility, as reported by the heads of the facilities) for the week prior to beginning of data collection as numerator; and the sum of deliveries in all the facilities as denominator [36]. Systematic sampling was employed to choose postpartum women as they existed from the labour ward at a specified interval by using the estimate of the average clinic deliveries to calculate sampling interval. The first participant was

Table 1 Variables used in the study

Variable	Definition	Measurement scale
IPTp-SP uptake (Primary outcome)	Two or less (≤2) doses is incomplete and three or more (3+) is optimal	Nominal/binary
Explanatory variable		
Age group	Age of a woman	Nominal
Marital status	Marital status of a woman	Nominal
Residence (Zone)	Type of woman's residence	Nominal/binary
Education	Level of education of woman	Nominal
Occupation	Woman's occupation	Nominal
Religion	Woman's religion	Nominal
Tribe	Woman's tribe	Nominal
First pregnancy	Woman's first pregnancy	Nominal/binary
Parity	Number of birth that a woman had after 20 weeks gestation	Nominal
Timing of 1st ANC visit	Age of the pregnancy a first time a woman visited antenatal care clinic (ANC)	Nominal
ANC visits	Number of antenatal care visits a pregnant woman made during her gestation period	Nominal
Gravida	Total number of confirmed pregnancies that a woman had regardless of the outcome	Nominal
Knowledge of malaria transmission	Three items (sugarcane, mosquito, witchcraft). If only mosquito is selected as the an agent of transmission, then the person is knowledgeable, otherwise inadequate knowledge	Nominal/binary
Knowledge of dangers of malaria in pregnancy	Three items (abortion, still birth, low birth weight) indicated knowledgeable of consequences of malaria in pregnancy. Otherwise, inadequate knowledge	Nominal/binary
Took SP under DOT each time	Whether a woman took SP under direct observation therapy (DOT) strategy or not	Nominal/binary
Permission to go to HF	Seeking permission from spouse to visit health facility (HF) for ANC	Nominal/binary
Distance to HF	Distance to health facility from a woman's residence	Nominal/binary
Transport to HF	Transportation to heath facility	Nominal/binary
Need for spouse escort to HF	Spouse escort to health facility	Nominal/binary
Worried no health provider at HF	Worried that there would be no health care provider	Nominal/binary
Worried no drugs at HF	Worried that there might be no drugs at clinic	Nominal/binary

enrolled at random. The random selection was done by entering all the names of women discharged at a particular day in Excel spreadsheet and executed RAND() command.

Data collection and quality management

A total of six public nurses were recruited and trained in data collection methods and management for 2 days, followed by one-day fieldwork. This was done to ensure the data collected were consistent across data collectors, complete and valid. The investigator monitored and supervised the data collectors throughout the data collection exercise.

The study used a structured interviewer-administered questionnaire with some questions adapted from 2014 Malawi Malaria Indicator Survey and 2010 Malawi Demographic and Health Survey [34, 37] (Additional file 1). The questionnaire solicited data on demographic, number of IPTp-SP doses a woman received during pregnancy, knowledge about malaria and IPTp-SP, number of and timing of antenatal clinic visits, parity and gravida. Number of ANC visits, number of IPTp-SP doses received, date of the first ANC visit, and woman's age were the data that were obtained from the questionnaire and triangulated by women's ANC cards and health facility records. The cards and records were used to verify verbal reports and whenever there was information discordance, the cards and records data were collected.

The questionnaire was administered by trained nurses (interviewers). The English version questionnaire was translated into Chichewa, which is a local language by a multilingual person. Another individual with knowledge of both English and Chichewa translated the Chichewa version back to English to check consistency in meaning. The questionnaire was pre-tested on 30 postpartum women from peri-urban health facility. Results from the pre-test exercise were discussed among the research team and a revised version of the questionnaire was adopted to be used in data collection. During data collection process, the investigator checked 15% of the completed questionnaires for completeness and consistency and where necessary provided feedbacks to data collectors.

A template of the questionnaire was prepared using EpiData 3.1 (CDC, Atlanta, GA, USA) and data were entered into the software and validated by a second data entry (double entry). The data were then exported into Stata version 14.2 (Stata Corp, College Station, Tx, USA) for further cleaning and analysis.

Data analysis

Data were summarised in the form of proportions and frequencies for categorical variables. Means with their respective standard deviations were used to summarise the data if the variables were continuous and normally distributed, otherwise median and respective interquartile range were used.

Bivariate binary logistic regression analysis was performed to determine the presence or absence of association between outcome and respective explanatory variables by generating crude odds ratios (OR). All explanatory variables with $p < 0.20$ in the bivariate analysis were included in both automated and investigator-led backward-stepwise multiple binary logistic regression analysis to further examine the association between the outcome and each explanatory variable while controlling the effects of other explanatory variables by calculating adjusted odds ratios (AOR) The level of significance used was 5% (0.05), two-tailed at 95% confidence interval (CI). The CI for proportions were calculated using logit transformation, which is a default option in Stata.

Assessment of goodness of fit of the models

The goodness of fit of the models was tested using likelihood ratio (LR), and Homsmer and Lemeshow tests. The full model consisting of all the independent variables was compared with the model created by backward stepwise regression at 5% significant level. Test result with significant level above 5% was interpreted as a model with fewer independent variables and better than the full model. The classification ability of the models was evaluated using Receiver Operating Characteristics (ROC) curve. The ROC value above 0.5 meant that a model classification was not due to chance.

The Likelihood ratio (LR) chi-square with 22° degrees of freedom was 14.09, p-value = 0.898. This means the model with fewer (nine) explanatory variables was better model than the one with 21 variables. The Hosmer-Lemeshow goodness-of-fit test was found to be not significant ($\chi^2 = 8.39$, $df = 8$, $p = 0.396$). Thus we do not have enough evidence to reject the null hypothesis that the model fitted the data well. Furthermore, ROC value for the selected model as shown in Fig. 1 is 0.77, which suggests that classification is not due to chance as ROC value is close to 1 than 0.5.

Ethical approval and consent to participate

Ethics approval was obtained from National Health Sciences Research Committee in Malawi (issued September 12, 2016, protocol number 1656) and University of Zambia Biomedical Research Ethics Committee in Zambia (issued August 3, 2016, reference number 017–06-16). Written permission to conduct the study in the health facilities (Matawale and Likangala) was obtained from Zomba District Health Office health facilities involved in the study. Informed written consents and assents were obtained from study participants whose age was 18 years and above and below 18 years respectively. Willingness to participate in the study and parental permission was

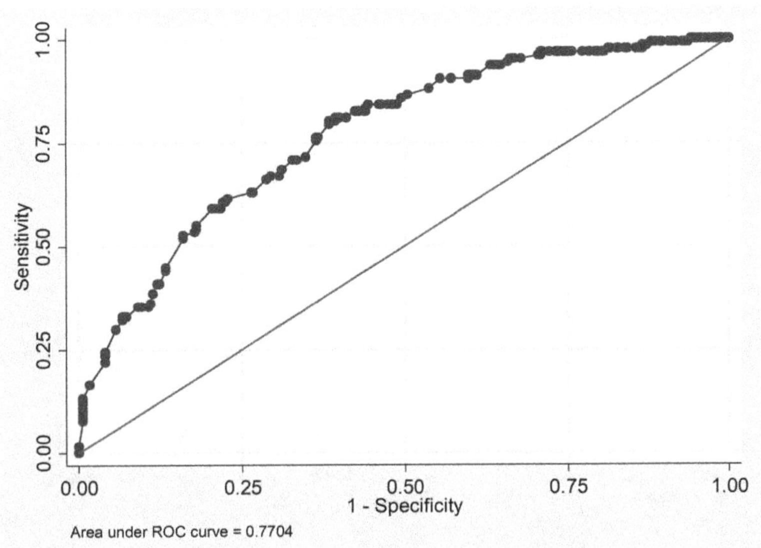

Fig. 1 Receiver Operating Characteristic (ROC) curve

confirmed by signing (finger print for illiterates) on the informed consent sheet.

Results

Prevalence of IPTP-SP uptake

A total of 463 women were enrolled into the study. Out of this, 426 (92%) women with complete information had their data analysed to investigate the determinants of IPTp-SP uptake. Of 426 women, 127 (29.8%, 95% CI: 25.6%–34.3%) received three (optimal) or more doses of SP, 299 (70.2%, 95% CI: 65.7%–74.4%) received two or less doses (poor uptake or suboptimal).

Sociodemographic characteristics of participants

Out of 426 women, 55% delivered at urban health facility and 45% delivered at the rural health facility. Of 233 women who delivered at urban health facility, 40% took three or more doses and 60% received two or less doses of SP during pregnancy. Among 193 delivering women at rural health centre, 17% received three or more doses while 83% took two or less doses of SP. More than half (232, 54%) of participants had completed at least senior primary school. Pregnant women in the age group 25–35 had the highest uptake of optimal SP doses compared to the rest of the women. Women who were divorced or separated or widowed had highest percentage of taking optimal SP doses (Table 2).

Cultural characteristics

Women who had problems with spouses' escort to ANC clinic had higher percentage (42%) of receiving three or more doses than those who had no problem with escorts (23%). Participants with a small problem in getting permission from their spouse to visit HF had a slight higher percentage (30%) of completing SP doses than women who had a big problem with seeking permission (25%). Women who first visited ANC in first trimester had the highest percentage of completing the recommended doses (Table 3).

Individual characteristics

The percentages for completing SP doses were similar for both primigravida and multigravida (29.9% vs 29.5% respectively). At least four ANC visits a pregnant woman made was associated with higher proportion of taking three or more SP doses than three or less visits. Both groups of women who were knowledgeable and partially knowledgeable about malaria transmission had similar percentages of taking three or more doses of SP (29.8% vs 30%). However, those women who were aware of dangers of malaria in pregnancy had higher percentage (32%) of completing recommended SP doses than those with inadequate knowledge (25%) (Table 4).

Structural factors (access to health facility and provider readiness) faced by participant

Pregnant women who took SP under Direct Observation Therapy (DOT) each time had higher percentage of completing three or more doses than those who did not take SP under DOT each time they visited ANC (33% vs 6%). Participants who had problems with long distance and lack of transport to health facility had lower percentage of completing the recommended doses. The women who worried most that there would be no health provider at HF had lower percentage (20%) of completing the recommended

Table 2 Sociodemographic characteristics of participants by IPTp uptake

Characteristic	*N* (Total = 426)	% of women who took IPTp			
		≤2 doses[a] n (%)	95% CI	3+ doses[b] n (%)	95% CI
Zone					
Urban	233	139 (59.7)	53.2–65.8	94 (40.3)	34.2–46.8
Rural	193	160 (82.9)	76.9–87.6	33 (17.1)	12.4–23.1
Education					
No formal education/junior primary	194	130 (67.0)	60.0–73.3	64 (33.0)	26.7–39.9
Senior primary	125	97 (77.6)	69.4–84.1	28 (22.4)	15.9–30.
Secondary/tertiary	107	72 (67.3)	57.8–75.6	35 (32.7)	24.4–42.2
Age group					
15–24	201	146 (72.6)	66.0–78.4	55 (27.4)	21.6–33.9
25–34	176	114 (64.8)	57.4–71.5	62 (35.2)	28.5–42.6
35+	49	39 (79.6)	65.9–88.7	10 (20.4)	11.3–34.1
Occupation					
Unemployed	307	228 (74.3)	69.1–78.9	79 (25.7)	21.1–30.9
Self-employed	104	64 (61.5)	51.8–70.4	40 (38.5)	29.6–48.2
Employed	15	7 (46.7)	23.4–71.5	8 (53.3)	28.5–76.6
Marital status					
Married	382	272 (71.2)	66.4–75.5	110 (28.8)	24.5–33.6
Divorced/separated/widowed	19	10 (52.6)	30.5–73.8	9 (47.4)	26.2–69.5
Never married	25	17 (68.0)	47.3–83.4	8 (32.0)	16.6–52.7
Religion					
CCAP[c]/7th day[d]/Baptist	112	70 (62.5)	53.1–71.0	42 (37.5)	28.9–46.9
Other Christian	134	102 (76.1)	68.1–82.6	32 (23.9)	17.4–31.9
Catholic/Anglican	93	65 (69.9)	59.8–78.4	28 (30.1)	21.6–40.2
Muslim/other religions	87	62 (71.3)	60.8–79.8	25 (28.7)	20.2–39.2
Tribe					
Nyanja	106	85 (80.2)	71.4–86.8	21 (19.8)	13.2–28.6
Chewa	107	69 (64.5)	54.9–73.0	38 (35.5)	26.9–45.1
Lomwe	102	75 (73.5)	64.1–81.2	27 (26.5)	18.8–35.9
Other	111	70 (63.1)	53.7–71.6	41 (36.9)	28.4–46.3

[a]uptake of two or less doses of IPTp-SP
[b]uptake of three or more doses of IPTp-SP
[c]Church of Central Africa Presbyterian
[d]Seventh Day Adventist

doses against 35% for participants who felt otherwise (Table 5).

Determinants of uptake of IPTp-SP

Bivariate analysis

Bivariate logistic regression results showed that 12 out of 21 predictor variables were significantly associated with completion of the recommended doses of SP during pregnancy (Table 6). Significant barriers to completion of recommended SP doses by a pregnant women: Attending ANC from health facility in rural setting compared to urban setting (OR = 0.30, 95% CI: 0.19–0.48, $p < 0.001$), women who attained senior primary school education than women without formal or junior primary education (OR = 0.58, 95% CI: 0.35–0.98, $p = 0.043$), being a member of other Christian denomination than a member of Church of Central Africa Presbyterian (CCAP) or Seventh Day Adventist or Baptist (OR = 0.52, 95% CI: 0. 30–0.91, $p = 0.021$), commencing ANC in third trimester than in second trimester (OR = 0.26, 95% CI: 0.09–0.67, $p = 0.005$), three or less number of ANC visits against four or more visits (OR = 0.31, 95% CI: 0.19–0.49, $p < 0.001$), not taking SP doses under direct observation of health care provider (OR = 0.13, 95% CI: 0.04–0.43, $p = 0.001$),

Table 3 Cultural characteristics by IPTp uptake

Characteristic	N (Total = 426)	% of women who took IPTp			
		≤2 doses	95% CI	3+ doses	95% CI
Permission to go to HF[a]					
Small problem	410	287 (70.0)	65.3–74.3	123 (30.0)	25.7–34.6
Big problem	16	12 (75.0)	48.2–90.6	4 (25.0)	9.4–51.8
Need for spouse escort to HF					
Small problem	276	212 (76.8)	71.4–81.4	64 (23.2)	18.6–28.6
Big problem	150	87 (58)	49.9–65.7	63 (42.0)	34.3–50.1
Timing of 1st ANC visit					
2nd trimester	284	198 (69.7)	64.1–74.8	86 (30.3)	25.2–35.9
1st trimester	92	56 (60.9)	50.5–70.4	36 (39.1)	29.6–49.5
3rd trimester	50	45 (90.0)	77.9–95.8	5 (10.0)	4.2–22.1

[a]Heath Facility

distance to health facility (OR = 0.37, 95% CI: 0.19–0.71, $p = 0.003$), transport problem to health facility (OR = 0. 42, 95% CI: 0.23–0.78, $p = 0.006$), and worried that there would be no drugs at health facility (OR = 0.54, 95% CI: 0.34–0.84, $p = 0.006$).

The enabling determinants significantly associated with a pregnant woman to more likely to complete recommended doses were: being self-employed woman versus unemployed women (OR = 1.80, 95% CI: 1.13–2.89, $p = 0.014$), being employed against unemployed (OR = 3.30, 95% CI: 1.15–9.39, $p = 0.025$), being Chewa tribe than Nyanja tribe (OR = 2.23, 95% CI: 1.19–4.15, $p = 0.011$), being of other tribe rather than Nyanja (OR = 2.37, 95% CI: 1.28–4.38, $p = 0.006$), and having problems with spouse escort to health facility (OR = 2.40, 95% CI: 1.56–3.68, $p < 0.001$).

Multivariable analysis

In multiple binary logistic regression results, six out of nine explanatory variables were significantly associated with a pregnant woman receiving at least three doses of SP. Only two enablers were significantly associated with a pregnant woman completing at least recommended SP

Table 4 Clinical characteristics and level of knowledge among participants by IPTp uptake

Characteristic	N (Total = 426)	% of women who took IPTp			
		≤2 doses n (%)	95%CI	3+ doses n (%)	95% CI
First pregnancy					
No	304	213 (70.1)	64.7–75.0	91 (29.9)	25.0–35.3
Yes	122	86 (70.5)	61.8–77.9	36 (29.5)	22.1–38.2
Parity					
One child	121	85 (70.3)	61.5–77.8	36 (29.8)	22.2–38.5
Two children	111	72 (64.9)	55.5–73.2	39 (35.1)	26.8–44.5
3+ children	194	142 (73.2)	66.5–78.9	52 (26.8)	21.0–33.5
ANC visits					
4+	234	140 (59.8)	53.3–65.9	94 (40.2)	34.1–46.6
Three or less	192	159 (82.8)	76.8–87.5	33 (17.2)	12.5–23.2
Gravida					
multigravida[a]	194	141 (72.7)	65.9–78.5	53 (27.3)	21.5–34.1
Secundigravida[b]	110	72 (65.4)	56.0–73.8	38 (34.6)	26.2–43.9
primigravida[c]	122	86 (70.5)	61.8–77.9	36 (29.5)	22.1–38.2
Knowledge of malaria transmission					
knowledgeable	386	271 (70.2)	65.4–74.6	115 (29.8)	25.4–34.6
Inadequate Knowledge	40	28 (70.0)	54.0–82.3	12 (30.0)	17.7–46.0
Knowledge of dangers of malaria in pregnancy					
Knowledgeable	303	207 (68.3)	62.8–73.3	96 (31.7)	26.7–37.2
Inadequate knowledge	123	92 (74.8)	66.3–81.7	31 (25.2)	18.3–33.7

[a]a woman that has been pregnant for at least a second time
[b]a woman in her second pregnancy
[c]a woman who is pregnant for the first time

Table 5 IPTp uptake against factors that affect access to health facility and health provider DOT adherence

Characteristic	N (Total = 426)	% of women who took IPTp			
		≤2 doses	95%CI	3+ doses	95% CI
Took SP under DOT[a] each time					
Yes	376	252 (67.0)	62.1–71.6	124 (32.9)	28.4–37.9
No	50	47 (94.0)	82.8–98.1	3 (6.0)	1.9–17.2
Distance to HF					
Small problem	348	233 (67.0)	61.8–71.7	115 (33.1)	28.3–38.2
Big problem	78	66 (84.6)	74.7–91.1	12 (15.4)	8.9–25.3
Transport to HF					
Small problem	344	231 (67.2)	61.9–71.9	113 (32.9)	28.1–38.0
Big problem	82	68 (82.9)	73.1–89.7	14 (17.1)	10.3–26.9
Worried no health provider at HF					
Small problem	280	183 (65.4)	59.6–70.7	97 (34.6)	29.3–40.4
Big problem	146	116 (79.5)	72.1–85.3	30 (20.0)	14.7–27.9
Worried no drugs at HF					
Small problem	263	172 (65.4)	59.4–70.9	91 (34.6)	29.1–40.6
Big problem	163	127 (77.9)	70.8–83.6	36 (22.1)	16.3–29.1

[a]Direct Observation Therapy

doses. First, being in the age group 25–34 compared to age group 15–24 (AOR = 1.72, 95% CI: 1.06–2.78, $p = 0.028$). Second, pregnant women with problem of spouse escort to health facility (AOR = 2.03, 95% CI: 1.26–3.26, $p = 0.004$).

The following determinants made a pregnant woman less likely to complete at least the recommended doses of SP after adjusting for other independent variables. Pregnant women who attended ANC from health facility in rural setting than those from urban settings (AOR = 0.31, 95% CI: 0.13–0.70, $p = 0.005$), pregnant women who had three or less ANC visits (AOR = 0.29, 95% CI: 0.18–0.48, $p < 0.001$), women who did not take doses of SP under direct observations of health care provider (AOR = 0.18, 95% CI: 0.05–0.63, $p = 0.007$), and being a Catholic or Anglican member compared to a member of Church of Central Africa Presbyterian (CCAP) or Seventh Day Adventist (AOR = 0.53, 95% CI: 0.28–0.97, $p = 0.041$). The results are presented in Table 6.

Discussion

The WHO new recommended doses of IPTp-SP uptake was very low in the study population when comparing to Roll Back Malaria (RBM) benchmark target for all pregnant women in areas with moderate-to-high transmission in Africa [7]. Some of the factors associated with the low uptake that the study found were attending ANC clinic in rural area, three or less ANC visits, not taking SP under DOT.

Health facility location/women's residential area setting has been found in this study to be related to uptake of IPTp-SP. Women who attended rural health facility were less likely to complete the recommended SP doses during pregnancy. This finding is similar to a study done in Geita district, Tanzania [18] and Nigeria [36]. To the best knowledge of the authors, the Geita-Tanzania study was the only study that evaluated uptake of IPTp-SP, categorised into less than three doses versus three or more doses of SP, at the time of writing this paper. This observation might either indicate that rural health facility had lower stock levels of SP than urban health facility because of poor supply chain from district health office (DHO) due to challenges in transportation of the commodity or understaffing [4] which leads to high client-to-staff ratios and subsequently long queues and waiting times. This could prompt some pregnant women not make further ANC visits. Kibusi et al. [31] reported that being a resident of Eastern Zone (urban) in Tanzania was associated with completing two or more doses of SP. This implies that Zomba District Health Office (ZDHO) should strive to strength the rural health systems and achieve equity. On the other hand, there is need for further investigation into the rural-urban differential to understand the real barriers and enablers of uptake in each context in order to improve the health of the community.

This study has shown that receipt of at least three doses of SP was higher among pregnant women making four or more ANC clinic visits than those making three or less visits. The finding is consistent with a study conducted in Tanzania [18, 24], in Ghana [27], in Burkina Faso [25], and in Mali [26, 28] in Cameroon, and in Benin [23]. ANC clinic is the vehicle that carries the intervention from the healthcare provider to the pregnant woman, hence the more visits a pregnant woman makes to ANC clinics the higher the number of SP doses she would receive as long as the visits are scheduled at least 1 month apart beginning from second trimester. Out of 426 women, 234 (55%) made at least four ANC visits but only 94 out of 234 (40%) received optimal doses of SP. This suggests a missed opportunity to provide the recommended doses of SP to women who attended WHO recommended number of at least four scheduled ANC visits, as two-thirds (284 out of 426) of the women commenced ANC clinic in the second trimester. The mismatch between percentage of four or more ANC visits and percentage of receipt of three or more doses could occur in part because of intermittent

Table 6 Factors associated with uptake of three or more doses of IPTp-SP among postpartum women, $N = 426$

Characteristics	N	Crude Odds Ratio (95%CI)	Unadjusted *p*-value[a]	Adjusted Odds Ratio (95%CI)	Adjusted *p*-value[b]
Zone					
Urban	233	1		1	
Rural	193	0.30 (0.19–0.48)	< 0.001	0.31 (0.13–0.70)	0.005
Education					
No formal education/junior primary	194	1			
Senior primary	125	0.58 (0.35–0.98)	0.043		
Secondary/tertiary	107	0.99(0.60–1.63)	0.961		
Age group					
15–24	201	1		1	
25–34	176	1.44 (0.93–2.23)	0.100	1.72 (1.06–2.78)	0.028
35+	49	0.68 (0.32–1.46)	0.322		
Occupation					
Unemployed	307	1			
Self-employed	104	1.80 (1.13–2.89)	0.014		
Employed	15	3.30 (1.15–9.39)	0.025		
Marital status					
Married	382	1		1	
Divorced/separated/widowed	19	2.23 (0.88–5.63)	0.091	2.58 (0.90–7.39)	0.078
Never married	25	1.16 (0.49–2.77)	0.733		
Religion					
CCAP/7th day/Baptist	112	1		1	
Other Christian	134	0.52 (0.30–0.91)	0.021	0.61 (0.35–1.05)	0.075
Catholic/Anglican	93	0.72 (0.40–1.29)	0.267	0.53 (0.28–0.97)	0.041
Muslim/other religions	87	0.67 (0.37–1.23)	0.195		
Tribe					
Nyanja	106	1			
Chewa	107	2.23 (1.19–4.15)	0.011		
Lomwe	102	1.46 (0.76–2.79)	0.256		
Other	111	2.37 (1.28–4.38)	0.006		
First pregnancy					
No	304	1			
Yes	122	1.04 (0.65–1.64)	0.883		
Parity					
One child	121	1			
Two children	111	1.28 (0.74–2.23)	0.382		
3+ children	194	0.86 (0.52–1.43)	0.571		
Timing of 1st ANC visit					
2nd trimester	284	1			
1st trimester	92	1.48 (0.91–2.41)	0.116		
3rd trimester	50	0.26 (0.09–0.67)	0.005		
ANC visits					
4+	234	1		1	
Three or less	192	0.31 (0.19–0.49)	< 0.001	0.29 (0.18–0.48)	< 0.001

Table 6 Factors associated with uptake of three or more doses of IPTp-SP among postpartum women, $N = 426$ *(Continued)*

Characteristics	N	Crude Odds Ratio (95%CI)	Unadjusted *p*-value[a]	Adjusted Odds Ratio (95%CI)	Adjusted *p*-value[b]
Gravida					
multigravida	194	1			
Secundigravida	110	1.40 (0.85–2.32)	0.187		
primigravida	122	1.11 (0.67–1.84)	0.674		
Knowledge of malaria transmission					
knowledgeable	386	1			
Inadequate Knowledge	40	1.01 (0.50–2.06)	0.978		
Knowledge of dangers of malaria in pregnancy					
Knowledgeable	303	1			
Inadequate knowledge	123	0.73 (0.45–1.17)	0.186		
Took SP under DOT each time					
Yes	376	1		1	
No	50	0.13 (0.04–0.43)	0.001	0.18 (0.05–0.63)	0.007
Permission to go to HF					
Small problem	410	1			
Big problem	16	0.78 (0.25–2.46)	0.669		
Distance to HF					
Small problem	348	1		1	
Big problem	78	0.37 (0.19–0.71	0.003	0.49 (0.23–1.06)	0.070
Transport to HF					
Small problem	344	1			
Big problem	82	0.42 (0.23–0.78)	0.006		
Need for spouse escort to HF					
Small problem	276	1		1	
Big problem	150	2.40 (1.56–3.68)	< 0.001	2.03 (1.26–3.26)	0.004
Worried no health provider at HF					
Small problem	280	1			
Big problem	146	0.49 (0.30–0.78)	0.003		
Worried no drugs at HF					
Small problem	263	1		1	
Big problem	163	0.54 (0.34–0.84)	0.006	1.84 (0.82–4.12)	0.140

[a]Bivariate logistic regression
[b]Multiple logistic regression

shortage of SP in the health facility, poor fidelity in implementation of IPTp-SP by individual healthcare providers as recommended in WHO policy brief [38], and women's negative attitudes towards the use of the drug during pregnancy [4, 18, 26, 39]. This implies that health care providers and community leaders have to collaborate to aggressively promote optimal ANC attendance among pregnant women and make sure that every eligible pregnant woman who attends ANC at scheduled visit receives a dose of SP. This will maximise the opportunity of optimal SP uptake in the district for those who make four or more ANC visits.

In regards to direct observation therapy (DOT), the study has revealed that pregnant women who did not take doses of SP under DOT had less likelihood of completing the recommended number of doses. GM Mubyazi, P Magnussen, C Goodman, IC Bygbjerg, AY Kitua, OE Olsen, J Byskov, KS Hansen and P Bloch [40] observed that uptake of SP was low among the study participants especially when women were allowed to take the SP at home. There are many reasons why healthcare providers allowed women to take the drug home such as shortages of clean water and cups [40], high client-to-staff ratios which reduces consultation times resulting in poor or no observation [4, 30]. Taking doses of SP under direct observation therapy (DOT) of healthcare provider is one of the strategies in implementation of IPTp-SP with high fidelity [13]. This suggests that health care providers should strive to follow protocols in SP provision. Besides, health facilities' management has to strengthen their efforts in supervising ANC providers and learn about challenges they face in order find solutions of strengthening DOT, which would work in their context. Considering that resources, such as cups and clean drinking water, will never be sufficient, ZDHO and health facility management ought to be pragmatic in overcoming this challenge. One solution might be engaging community leaders to encourage pregnant women to bring with them a cup when on a scheduled ANC visit.

The odds of completing at least three doses of SP was more than 1.72 times higher among pregnant women between age group 25 to 34 than those aged between 15 to 24 years old. This result indicates that young pregnant women were under utilizing the intervention, which is similar result that Kibusi's study revealed [31]. Therefore, there is need to increase awareness of importance of completing recommended doses of IPTp-SP among pregnant women aged between 15 to 24 years as well pregnant women older than 34 years. The study has shown that poor uptake is affected by differentially on women born at different times, which might reflect women's culture of health care utilization at different ages. For instant, teen pregnancies are usually unplanned therefore are less likely to consistently utilize ANC services and subsequently miss out on receiving optimal doses of SP.

Lastly, spouse escort to health facility has shown to be positively associated with good uptake of several interventions offered at ANC [41]. However, pregnant women in the study population who had a problem with spouse escort were more likely to complete the recommended doses of SP. Mostly, these women were either divorced or windowed or on separation, hence they were socially vulnerable and probably took their situation positively by attending ANC clinics and took the recommended SP doses to avoid MiP and its adverse effects. The other possible explanation would be that they had more autonomy in relation to the use of ANC than married women [42]. This might imply that pregnant women with more autonomy are in a position to have confidence in prioritization of health care services.

This study had the following limitations. First, the study participants were recruited from health facility maternity wings and antenatal clinics. In Malawi, according to National Statistical Office (NSO) [Malawi] and ICF Macro [34], 20% of births occur at home and 80% of women who received no antenatal care services deliver at home. Therefore, it would not be representative of the wider population of postpartum women in Zomba district. However, the researcher minimised the limitation by including women who delivered at home and visited the health facility within 48 h for check-up. Only 14% of women age 15–49 giving birth outside health facility received a postnatal check in the first 2 days after delivery [43]. Second, the health systems factors (time and patient flow challenges, integration of services into ANC); Policy and guidance environment, human resource factors, and supply chain factors (SP availability at the facility) also play an important role in the coverage of the intervention. However, this study did not study them because the focus was primarily on pregnant women's perceptive. This limitation would under-or-overestimate the problem understudy when viewed holistically. Third, the study focused on determinants of IPTp-SP uptake in postpartum women from catchment areas of selected Health facilities in Zomba district. Hence, the results would not be generalised to all districts in Malawi because the participating district was purposively sampled because of its low uptake. However, the results could be related to other districts with similar characteristics as the sampled one. Finally, recall bias is an inherent limitation of the survey design. There was a possibility of women reporting past exposures/experiences with varying degree of accuracy. However, some of these recall biases were minimised by using records such as ANC cards and interviewing the women immediately after delivering.

Conclusion

Malaria in pregnancy continues to pose a major public health problem in sub-Saharan Africa and particularly in Malawi. However, there are a number of evidenced-based interventions for preventing MiP and one of them is IPTp-SP. This study was conducted to identify the enablers and barriers of a pregnant woman completing at least three doses of IPTp-SP and estimate the uptake levels in Zomba district. The study demonstrated that there is low utilisation of SP in this population and this seems to be associated with the number of ANC visits, use of DOTs and health facility location. Therefore, community-based health promotion on optimal ANC attendance should be encouraged and antenatal care clinics should strengthen IPTp messages particularly on younger pregnant women. Zomba District Health Office in collaboration with health facilities' management have to strengthen their efforts in supervising ANC providers to enhance DOT. Further research needs to be carry out to understand factors affecting the rural-urban differential IPTp uptake to provide evidence that would address the variance.

Abbreviations
ANC: Antenatal care; FANC: Focused antenatal care; IPTp1: Single dose of IPTp-SP; IPTp2: Two doses of IPTp-SP; IPTp3 +: Three or more doses of IPTp-SP; IPTp-SP: Intermittent preventive treatment in pregnacy with Sulphadoxine Pyrimethamine; ITNs: Insecticides treated nets; MiP: Malaria in pregnancy; SP: Sulphadoxine Pyrimethamine; WHO: World Health Organization

Acknowledgements
We are grateful to the financial support for the training scheme as provided by the UNICEF/UNDP/World Bank/ WHO Special programme for Research and Training in Tropical Diseases (TDR).

Authors' contributions
SCA designed the study, performed the analysis and drafted the manuscript. GC and CM assisted with the study design. SCA, GC, CM, HC, CJ and JZ, contributed to interpretation of findings, edited and reviewed the manuscript. All authors read and approved the final manuscript.

Authors' information
SCA and HC are master's degree candidates and recipients of TDR scholarship under the Postgraduate Training Scheme in Implementation Research at the Department of Epidemiology and Biostatistics and Department of Health Policy and Management respectively, School of Public Health, University of Zambia, Lusaka, Zambia. GC, CJ and JZ are lecturers at Department of Epidemiology and Biostatistics, School of Public Health, University of Zambia, Lusaka, Zambia. CM is Dean of School of Public Health, University of Zambia, Lusaka, Zambia.

Ethics approval and consent to participate
Ethics approval was obtained from National Health Sciences Research Committee in Malawi (issued September 12, 2016, protocol number 1656) and University of Zambia Biomedical Research Ethics Committee in Zambia (issued August 3, 2016, reference number 017-06-16). Written permission to conduct the study in the health facilities was obtained from Zomba District Health Office and clinic-in-charge of each health facility. The research team informed prospective participants about the purpose of the study, procedures required of them if recruited, risks and benefits, and that they had the right to volunteer whether or not to participate in the study. Informed consent was obtained from each participants before administering the questionnaire. For women aged below 18 years, informed assent was obtained from parents or parents in-law, or their husbands if the husbands were above 18 years. The respondents were informed that they had the right to withdraw from the study at any time and without adverse consequences. The respondents were assured of privacy, confidentiality and that no names would appear on the questionnaire. Willingness to participate in the study and parental permission was confirmed by signing (finger print for illiterates) on the informed consent/assent sheet.

Competing interests
The authors declare that they have no competing interests.

Author details
[1]Department of Epidemiology and Biostatistics, School of Public Health, University of Zambia, Post Box 50110, Lusaka, Zambia. [2]Malawi Defence Force, Malawi Military Health Services, Kamuzu Barracks, Private Bag 43, Lilongwe, Malawi. [3]Department of Health Policy and Management, School of Public Health, University of Zambia, Post Box 50110, Lusaka, Zambia.

References
1. Guyatt H, Snow R. The epidemiology and burden of plasmodium falciparum -related anemia among pregnant women in sub-Saharan Africa. Am J Trop Med Hyg. 2001;64:36–44.
2. Menéndez C, D'Alessandro U, ter Kuile FO. Reducing the burden of malaria in pregnancy by preventive strategies. Lancet Infect Dis. 2007;7(2):126–35.
3. Desai M, ter Kuile F, Nosten F, McGready R, Asamoa K, Brabin B, Newman R. Epidemiology and burden of malaria in pregnancy. Lancet Infect Dis. 2007;7: 93–104.
4. Hill J, Hoyt J, van Eijk AM, D'Mello-Guyett L, Ter Kuile FO, Steketee R, Smith H, Webster J. Factors affecting the delivery, access, and use of interventions to prevent malaria in pregnancy in sub-Saharan Africa: a systematic review and meta-analysis. PLoS Med. 2013;10(7):e1001488.
5. WHO. World Health Organization regional Office for Africa. A strategic framework for malaria prevention and control during pregnancy in the African region. Brazzaville: World Health Organization Regional Office for Africa; 2004.
6. Dellicour S, Tatem A, Guerra C, Snow R, ter Kuile F. Quantifying the number of pregnancies at risk of malaria in 2007: a demographic study. PLoS Med. 2010;7:e1000221.
7. Roll Back Malaria Partnership. The contribution of malaria control to maternal and newborn health. In: Progress & impact. Geneva: World Health Organization; 2014.
8. Eisele TP, Larsen DA, Anglewicz PA, Keating J, Yukich J, Bennett A, Hutchinson P, Steketee RW. Malaria prevention in pregnancy, birthweight, and neonatal mortality: a meta-analysis of 32 national cross-sectional datasets in Africa. Lancet Infect Dis. 2012;12(12):942–9.
9. Guyatt H, Snow R. Impact of malaria during pregnancy on low birth weight in sub-Saharan Africa. Clin Microbiol Rev. 2004;17:760–9.
10. Rogerson SJ, Mwapasa V, Meshnick SR. Malaria in pregnancy: linking immunity and pathogenesis to prevention. Am J Trop Med Hyg. 2007;77(6 Suppl):14–22.
11. Steketee R, Nahlen B, Parise M, Menendez C. The burden of malaria in pregnancy in malaria-endemic areas. Am J Trop Med Hyg. 2001;64(1):28–35.
12. Lagerberg RE. Malaria in pregnancy: A literature review. J Midwifery Womens Health. 2008;53(3):209–15.
13. WHO: World Health Organization, WHO policy brief for the implementation of intermittent preventive treatment of malaria in pregnancy using Sulfadoxine-Pyrimethamine (IPTp-SP), April 2013 (rev. January 2014). 2013. Available from http://www.who.int/malaria/publications/atoz/Policy_brief_IPTp-SP_implementation_11april2013.pdf.pdf. Access on 5 Dec 2015.
14. Peters PJ, Thigpen MC, Parise ME, Newman RD. Safety and toxicity of Sulfadoxine/ Pyrimethamine: implications for malaria prevention in pregnancy using intermittent preventive treatment. Drug Saf. 2007;30(6): 481–501.
15. WHO: Malaria in pregnancy guidelines for measuring key monitoring and evaluation indictors. 2007. http://whqlibdoc.who.int/publications/2007/9789241595636_eng.pdf Accessed on 24 Nov 2015.
16. Andrews KG, Lynch M, Eckert E, Gutman J. Missed opportunities to deliver intermittent preventive treatment for malaria to pregnant women 2003-2013: a systematic analysis of 58 household surveys in sub-Saharan Africa. Malar J. 2015;14:1–10.
17. WHO. Updated WHO policy recommendation: intermittent preventive treatment of malaria in pregnancy using sulfadoxine-pyrimethamine (IPTp-SP). Geneva: World Health Organization; [accessed on Nov 20, 2015]. Geneva: World Health Organization; 2012. Available from http://www.who.int/malaria/publications/atoz/who_iptp_sp_policy_recommendation/en/
18. Mpogoro FJ, Matovelo D, Dosani A, Ngallaba S, Mugono M, Mazigo HD. Uptake of intermittent preventive treatment with sulphadoxine-pyrimethamine for malaria during pregnancy and pregnancy outcomes: a cross-sectional study in Geita district, north-western Tanzania. Malar J. 2014; 13(1):455.
19. Mwendera CA, Jager C, Longwe H, Phiri K, Hongoro C, Mutero CM. Changing the policy for intermittent preventive treatment with sulfadoxine–pyrimethamine during pregnancy in Malawi. Malar J. 2017; 16(1):84.
20. WHO. Provision of effective antenatal care, integrated management of pregnancy and childbirth (IMPAC). Standards for maternal and neonatal

care. Geneva: World Health Organization; 2006. Available from http://www.who.int/reproductivehealth/publications/maternal_perinatal_health/effective_antenatal_care.pdf. Accessed on 26 Nov 2015
21. Roll Back Malaria Partnership. The contribution of malaria control to maternal and newborn health. Geneva: World Health Organization; 2012. Report No 10. Available from http://rbm.who.int/ProgressImpactSeries/docs/report17-en.pdf. Access on 22 Nov 2015
22. van Eijk AM, Hill J, Larsen DA, Webster J, Steketee RW, Eisele TP, ter Kuile FO. Coverage of intermittent preventive treatment and insecticide-treated nets for the control of malaria during pregnancy in sub-Saharan Africa: a synthesis and meta-analysis of national survey data, 2009-11. Lancet Infect Dis. 2013;13(12):1029–42.
23. d'Almeida TC, Agboton-Zoumenou MA, Garcia A, Massougbodji A, Briand V, Imorou Y, Cottrell G. Field evaluation of the intermittent preventive treatment of malaria during pregnancy (IPTp) in Benin: evolution of the coverage rate since its implementation. Parasit Vectors. 2011;4:108.
24. Exavery A, Mbaruku G, Mbuyita S, Makemba A, Kinyonge IP, Kweka H. Factors affecting uptake of optimal doses of sulphadoxine-pyrimethamine for intermittent preventive treatment of malaria in pregnancy in six districts of Tanzania. Malar J. 2014;13(1):13–22.
25. Gies S, Coulibaly SO, Ky C, Ouattara FT, Brabin BJ, D'Alessandro U. Community-based promotional campaign to improve uptake of intermittent preventive antimalarial treatment in pregnancy in Burkina Faso. Am J Trop Med Hyg. 2009;80(3):460–9.
26. Hill J, Kayentao K, Touré M, Diarwara S, Bruce J, Smedley J, Doumbo OK, Kuile FO, Webster J. Effectiveness of antenatal clinics to deliver intermittent preventive treatment and insecticide treated nets for the control of malaria in pregnancy in Mali: a household survey. PLoS One. 2014;9(3):1–13.
27. Hommerich L, von Oertzen C, Bedu-Addo G, Holmberg V, Acquah PA, Eggelte TA, Bienzle U, Mockenhaupt FP. Decline of placental malaria in southern Ghana after the implementation of intermittent preventive treatment in pregnancy. Malar J. 2007;6:144.
28. Leonard N, Eric FB, Judith AK, Samuel W. Factors associated to the use of insecticide treated nets and intermittent preventive treatment for malaria control during pregnancy in Cameroon. Arch Public Health. 2016;74:5.
29. Mubyazi GM, Bygbjerg IC, Magnussen P, Olsen O, Byskov J, Hansen KS, Bloch P. Prospects, achievements, challenges and opportunities for scaling-up malaria chemoprevention in pregnancy in Tanzania: the perspective of national level officers. Malar J. 2008;7:135.
30. Pell C, Straus L, Andrew EVW, Meñaca A, Pool R. Social and cultural factors affecting uptake of interventions for malaria in pregnancy in Africa: a systematic review of the qualitative research. PLoS One. 2011;6(7):e22452.
31. Kibusi SM, Kimunai E, Hines CS. Predictors for uptake of intermittent preventive treatment of malaria in pregnancy (IPTp) in Tanzania. BMC Public Health. 2015;15(1):540.
32. Mwandama D, Gutman J, Wolkon A, Luka M, Jafali J, Ali D, Mathanga DP, Skarbinski J. The use of intermittent preventive treatment in pregnancy and insecticide-treated bed nets for malaria prevention by women of child-bearing age in eight districts in Malawi. Malar J. 2015;14(1):1–10.
33. Launiala A, Honkasalo M-L. Ethnographic study of factors influencing compliance to intermittent preventive treatment of malaria during pregnancy among Yao women in rural Malawi. Trans R Soc Trop Med Hyg. 2007;101(10):980–9.
34. National Statistical Office (NSO) [Malawi] and ICF Macro. Malawi demographic and health survey 2010. Zomba and Calverton: NSO and ICF Macro; 2011.
35. WHO. Evidence review group: intermittent preventive treatment of malaria in pregnancy (IPTp) with sulfadoxine–pyrimethamine (SP). Geneva: World Health Organization; 2012. Available from http://www.who.int/malaria/mpac/sep2012/iptp_sp_erg_meeting_report_july2012.pdf
36. Onoka CA, Hanson K, Onwujekwe OE. Low coverage of intermittent preventive treatment for malaria in pregnancy in Nigeria: demand-side influences. Malar J. 2012;11:82.
37. National Malaria Control Programme (NMCP) [Malawi] and ICF International. Malaria Indicator survey (MIS) 2014. Lilongwe and Rockville: NMCP and ICF International; 2015.
38. WHO. World Health Organization, WHO policy brief for the implementation of intermittent preventive treatment of malaria in pregnancy using Sulfadoxine-Pyrimethamine (IPTp-SP), 2013: World Health Organization; 2013. http://www.who.int/malaria/publications/atoz/Policy_brief_IPTp-SP_implementation_11april2013.pdf.pdf. Accessed 22 Nov 2015.
39. Bausell L, Wolf K. Treatment uptake and availability of antimalarialdrugs for intermittent preventative treatment in pregnant women in Malawi. Arlington, Va: USAID DELIVER PROJECT; 2015. Task Order 7
40. Mubyazi GM, Magnussen P, Goodman C, Bygbjerg IC, Kitua AY, Olsen OE, Byskov J, Hansen KS, Bloch P. Implementing intermittent preventive treatment for malaria in pregnancy: review of prospects, achievements, challenges and agenda for research. Open Trop Med J. 2008;1:92–100.
41. Tweheyo R, Konde-Lule J, Tumwesigye NM, Sekandi JN. Male partner attendance of skilled antenatal care in peri-urban Gulu district, northern Uganda. BMC Pregnancy Childbirth. 2010;10(1):53.
42. Simkhada B, Teijlingen ER, Porter M, Simkhada P. Factors affecting the utilization of antenatal care in developing countries: systematic review of the literature. J Adv Nurs. 2008;61(3):244–60.
43. National Statistical Office (NSO) [Malawi] and ICF. Malawi demographic and health survey 2015–16. Zomba and Rockville: NSO and ICF; 2017.

The fourth delay and community-driven solutions to reduce maternal mortality in rural Haiti

Tonya MacDonald[1*], Suzanne Jackson[2], Marie-Carmèle Charles[3], Marius Periel[4], Marie-Véna Jean-Baptiste[4], Alex Salomon[4] and Éveillard Premilus[4]

Abstract

Background: In Haiti, the number of women dying in pregnancy, during childbirth and the weeks after giving birth remains unacceptably high. The objective of this research was to explore determinants of maternal mortality in rural Haiti through Community-Based Action Research (CBAR), guided by the delays that lead to maternal death. This paper focuses on socioecological determinants of maternal mortality from the perspectives of women of near-miss maternal experiences and community members, and their solutions to reduce maternal mortality in their community.

Methods: The study draws on five semi-structured Individual Interviews with women survivors of near-misses, and on four Focus Group Discussions with Community Leaders and with Traditional Birth Attendants. Data collection took place in July 2013. A Community Research Team within a resource-limited rural community in Haiti undertook the research. The methods and analysis process were guided by participatory research and CBAR.

Results: Participants identified three delays that lead to maternal death but also described a fourth delay with respect to community responsibility for maternal mortality. They included women being carried from the community to a healthcare facility as a special example of the fourth delay. Women survivors of near-miss maternal experiences and community leaders suggested solutions to reduce maternal death that centered on prevention and community infrastructure. Most of the strategies for action were related to the fourth delay and include: community mobilization by way of the formation of Neighbourhood Maternal Health/Well-being Committees, and community support through the provision/sharing of food for undernourished women, offering monetary support and establishment of a communication relay/transport system in times of crisis.

Conclusions: Finding sustainable ways to reduce maternal mortality requires a community-based/centred and community-driven comprehensive approach to maternal health/well-being. This includes engagement of community members that is dependent upon community knowledge, political will, mobilization, accountability and empowerment. An engaged/empowered community is one that is well placed to find ways that work in their community to reduce the fourth delay and in turn, maternal death. Potentially, community ownership of challenges and solutions can lead to more sustainable improvements in maternal health/well-being in Haiti.

Keywords: CBAR, Maternal mortality, Fourth delay, Near-miss maternal experiences

* Correspondence: tmacdonald2@laurentian.ca
[1]School of Midwifery, Health Sciences Building, Laurentian University, 935 Ramsey Lake Road, Sudbury, ON P3E 2C6, Canada
Full list of author information is available at the end of the article

Background

The United Nation's fifth Millennium Development Goal aimed to reduce global maternal mortality by three-quarters between 1990 and 2015 [1]. Haiti is a low-income country where approximately 37% of births are attended by Skilled Health Personnel [2], 64% of births take place at home [3], less than 10% occur in a health facility for women of the lowest wealth quintile [4], and where the maternal mortality ratio is unacceptably high. According to 2015 WHO data, Haiti's maternal mortality ratio indicated 359 [range 236–601] maternal deaths per 100,000 live births [4] although these data lack complete registration of maternal deaths. Recent literature shows Haiti's poor progress towards reducing inequalities in reproductive health compared to other Latin American and Caribbean countries, and points to the need for renewed actions to bridge gaps in maternal health [5].

Determinants of maternal mortality have been described and discussed extensively in the literature. In 1991 Thaddeus and Maine introduced the Three Delays framework to describe obstetric obstacles that lead to maternal death [6]. Maternal death can result from the delay: (1) to seek appropriate medical help for an obstetric emergency; (2) to reach an appropriate obstetric facility; and (3) to receive adequate care at the facility [6–9].

In a comprehensive review of literature from 1980 to 2011, Pacagnella and group critiqued the Three Delays model for its retrospective approach, neglect to consider underlying factors that contribute to maternal death and lack of consideration for preventative care that reduces maternal mortality [9]. They and others have suggested that there might be a fourth delay related to community factors [9, 10].

In terms of literature specific to delays and maternal health in Haiti, Barnes-Josiah et al. applied Thaddeus and Maine's Three Delays framework to understand the social and medical circumstances surrounding Haitian maternal mortalities [7]. They found that while most maternal deaths occur due to the first delay, that the third delay (to receive adequate care at an obstetric facility) was the most significant [7]. Barnes-Josiah and colleagues concluded that improving the maternity care system would most greatly impact maternal mortality in Haiti [7]. Furthermore, White et al.'s examination of health-seeking behaviours of pregnant women in rural Haiti found the first delay to be most significant in this community [11]. These authors emphasized that most interviewed participants lacked a certain awareness of their healthcare needs and relied on their partner's/husband's and/or mother's advice regarding seeking care [11]. This highlights the need for culturally competent health promotion campaigns targeted at women and other key players in their social networks [11]. This study also considered how the socioecological context contributed to the delay to reach an appropriate obstetric facility [11]. Several researchers have investigated the determinants of institutional delivery in Haiti. Babalola, for example, investigated antenatal services and Skilled Birth Attendants to conclude that maternal health service use in Haiti must especially consider the needs of multiparous women, women with little or no education and must take into account accessibility of services for the poor and the "distance-decay" phenomenon in reaching services [12]. Babalola brings to light the importance of considering community mobilization efforts; these efforts allow a community to self-identify service-use norms and expectations within the community's context [12]. No other literature about maternal health in Haiti was found where specific reference was made regarding this second delay of the Three Delays framework.

Literature on personal accounts of "near-miss", community (user) perspectives, and community engagement to reduce maternal mortality in Haiti is limited. In terms of near-misses, women survivors of maternal experiences are a proxy group that often shares common characteristics with those who died "on the road of death" [9]. While these survivors have a unique perspective on maternal mortality that may contribute to insight on reducing maternal death [9], no studies were located that considered personal accounts of near-misses. Conversely, a few studies examined community views of Haitian women and healthcare workers as they relate to contraceptive needs in Northern Haiti [13], and a maternal/child health needs assessment [14] to help inform program development in maternal/child health. One study, by Small and colleagues in rural Haiti, highlighted the importance of community members' engagement in maternal mortality reduction activities [15]. Small and team concluded that maternal mortality would be best addressed through systematic evaluation of hospital-based practices in collaboration with community-based strategies and driven by engaged community members [15].

A conceptual framework, Maternal Mortality in a Community in Rural Haiti (Fig. 1) was developed for our study as a visual representation of causal linkages together with their effects and impacts [16]. Our framework is underpinned by Social Constructivism and overlaps with theories of empowerment, participatory communication, social change, socioecology and public health. The framework represents a proximal focus- of causal linkages that correspond to community perspectives on why women die in pregnancy, during birth and the 42 days after giving birth in this rural Haitian community, and what can be done to reduce maternal mortality in the community; it links individual and micro-level factors that play a role and are influenced by modifying and confounding environmental and social factors that work at multiple levels [16].

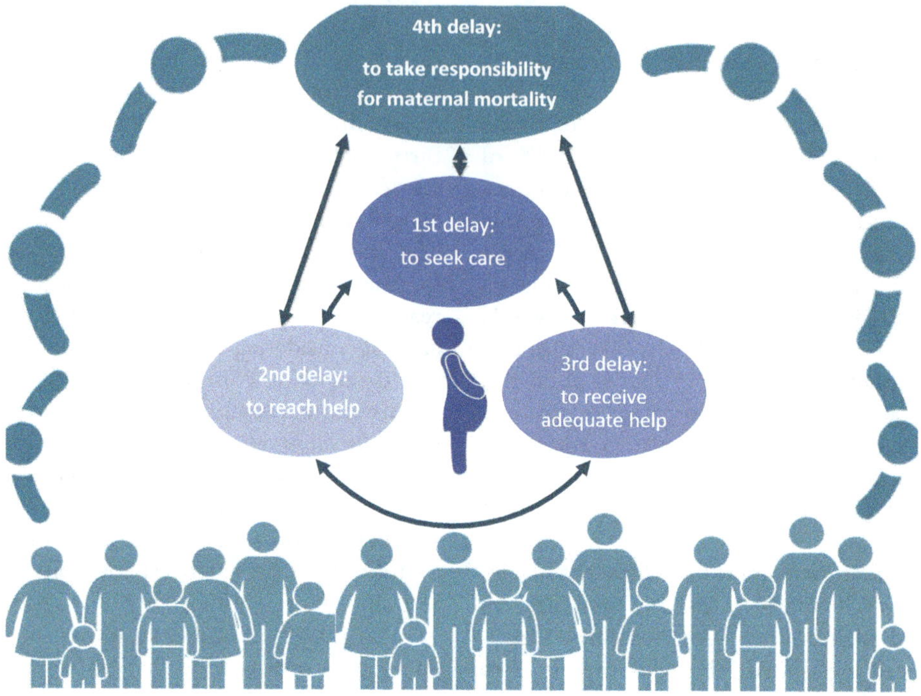

Fig. 1 Maternal Mortality in a Community in Rural Haiti

In our conceptual framework, the large outer circle represents a community in rural Haiti, dispersed geographically, and impoverished by way of availability and accessibility to water, food, electricity, employment, healthcare, and transportation (to name a few). This community is made up of women, men, and many youth and children. The woman (and her maternal health) is at the heart of this rural Haitian community and of the framework. The issue of maternal mortality is greatly influenced by four delays as seen by the incorporation of Thaddeus and Maine's Three Delays Framework, and the (recently added) Fourth Delay. Taken alone, either of the delays can lead to maternal death. Taken in combination or altogether, the four delays also contribute to maternal death. The representation illustrates a direct relationship between these delays and the community. The four delays are embedded within the community, influenced by the community and in turn impact the community as a whole.

The first to fourth delays are influenced by the socioecological determinants of a woman's health, such as status of woman or socioeconomic factors like knowledge, age, economic status, and social support. The community's resources and its engagement likewise impact the delays. Community resources refer to the availability of human and natural resources within the community and the infrastructure to access them. Community "resourcefulness" is affected by the distribution of resources which inevitably also plays a role in the socioecological determinants of maternal health. Community engagement here refers to the concept of community members' collective commitment and involvement regarding the issue of maternal mortality and its reduction.

Finally, our conceptual framework aims to provide an hypothesis of the causal linkages of maternal mortality and their effects and impacts at the individual, family and community levels. In this framework, the fourth delay figures prominently and appears to exert a larger effect on maternal death in this rural Haitian community. The fourth delay represents the delay in which the most potential rests in the community's hands because this delay has the potential to also impact (positively or negatively) the other three delays. Power derived at the community level stands the greatest chance for practical, achievable, immediate and sustainable changes. Positive change is influenced by community members' knowledge of the issue of maternal mortality in their community, political will to bring about change, community efforts to mobilize; it is affected by the degree of accountability toward maternal death, and the community's level of empowerment and belief that they can reduce maternal mortality.

Finally, the objective of this research was to explore maternal mortality in rural Haiti through Community-Based Action Research (CBAR). This paper focuses on the determinants of maternal mortality from the perspectives of women of near-miss maternal experiences and community members, and their solutions to reduce maternal mortality in their community. We hoped that sustainable ways to reduce maternal mortality could be found through a community-based/centred and community-driven comprehensive approach to maternal health/well-being.

Methods

This study took place over three months in 2013, in a resource-limited rural community populated by 22,000 Haitians, many living in mountainous/hard--to-reach villages that line the Artibonite Valley of central Haiti. The community had one clinical dispensary that provided vaccination services, malnutrition screening, maternal healthcare and public health education. The dispensary was run by Hôpital Albert Schweitzer, a nongovernmental hospital serving a population of over 350,000 [11, 15, 17].

This CBAR study directly engaged members of the community to explore perspectives of their own community about maternal mortality. Our study design incorporated an Idealist paradigm in which the world is seen as socially constructed, built upon the thought that individuals interpret their own circumstances and a researcher (or research team) becomes part of the environment. The choice of a CBAR approach was justified by Small and colleagues' study in rural Haiti [15] that highlighted the importance of community members' engagement in maternal mortality reduction activities.

The initial step in our study was the formation of a community research team (the CRT). The CRT consisted of six members, literate in Haitian Creole and/or French, and included two Co-Leads (first author and Haitian (Htn) nurse-midwife) and four community members (health agent coordinator, pastor, homemaker and farmer). A skills training workshop facilitated by the Co-Leads aided the team's acquisition of qualitative research skills and a deeper understanding of maternal mortality and the obstetric delays framework.

A total of 36 participants took part in either focus group discussions (FGD) or individual interviews (II). We convened 31 participants (adult women and men) in four focus groups with half from each of two different geographical parts of the community: two focus groups with Community Leaders (CL) (15 participants), and two focus groups with Traditional Birth Attendants (TBAs) known as 'matwon' (16 participants) (Table 1). The CRT undertook purposive sampling and direct/face-to-face recruitment to recruit 11 women and 4 men Community Leaders, and 12 women and 4 men TBAs. Focus group participants were from a broad range of age (25–65 years), community status and occupation.

We also conducted five semi-structured individual interviews with adult women (W) of near-miss maternal experiences (Table 2) to gather their views about the causes of maternal mortality.

A list of potential interview participants was generated with the help of dispensary staff and CRT from women survivors in the catchment area who ranged in age (20–35 years) and different stages of near-miss experience (i.e. in pregnancy, during birth, and in the first 42 days postpartum). Women on this list were approached by a CRT member and invited to participate in interviews. Five women survivors were recruited.

The focus group discussions/interviews were led by different Haitian members of the CRT (with the first author always present as an active observer) and took place at various secure and convenient locations within the community. Individual interviews took place at or near the participant's home. Participants were asked what they believed were causes of maternal mortality in their community, community impact of maternal death, and proposed solutions to reduce maternal mortality within their community. Similarly, interview participants were asked about their unique, near-miss maternal experiences, challenges encountered, support received, and lessons learned (see Table 3).

Focus groups/interviews lasted between 25 min and 1 1/2 h. With participants' permission, all discussions/interviews were digitally recorded and transcribed verbatim in Haitian Creole by a Creole-French-speaking Haitian with professional experience in transcription. The nine transcripts were independently reviewed by the Co-Leads to ensure accuracy of transcription.

A participatory qualitative analysis group process [18] was adapted and employed by the CRT. The group analysis process (in Haitian Creole) involved four phases:

In Phase 1 (Preanalysis Step), the Co-Leads colour-coded the transcripts by focus group number and cut print-outs of the participants' sentences and/or paragraphs into strips and bundled them into categories corresponding to the three guiding questions: a) Why do women die in pregnancy, during birth and the 42 days after birth in the community? b) What is the impact of maternal death on the community? c) What solutions can be offered to reduce maternal mortality in the community? In Phase 2 (Grouping Data and Identifying Themes) the CRT grouped the strips in each category into themes and subthemes, in relationship to the guiding questions and the study's research questions. In this phase, the CRT also identified key quotes that best illustrated the community's views.

Interview data were similarly analyzed for Phases 1 and 2 using Jackson's group process [17]. The CRT decided to analyze the interviews one at a time, and focused on three themes: a) woman's near-miss maternal experience b) woman's experience of community help and c) woman's proposed solutions to reduce maternal mortality in her community. The CRT used the themes

Table 1 Features and characteristics of focus group discussions

Focus group discussion	Participant features	Participant ratio of women to men	Age range (in years)	Facilitator characteristics
FGD 1 Community Leaders ($n = 7$)	Teacher, volunteer health worker, farmer, pastor, homemakers	4:3	25–50	CRT Htn Co-Lead
FGD 2 Community Leaders ($n = 8$)	Merchant, volunteer health worker, elder, farmer, homemakers	7:1	25–40	CRT Member
FGD 3 Traditional Birth Attendants ($n = 8$)	All with some community training	5:3	35–65	CRT Htn Co-Lead
FGD 4 Traditional Birth Attendants ($n = 8$)	All with some community training	7:1	40–50	CRT Member

and subthemes that emerged from focus groups, and looked for similarities in the interviews. Outlying themes/subthemes were noted. Key quotes were identified for use in the final report for the voices of the individual interview participants to be heard and honoured.

Phases 3 and 4 of Jackson's process [18] required making sense of the themes and making interconnections between and across all data. The Co-Leads completed these phases.

Results

Results are presented under the themes that emerged from data analysis, and guided by the socioecological determinants of (maternal) health and the four delays conceptual framework. The first delay relates to the decision to seek help during an obstetrical emergency; the second- a delay to receive help; the third- a delay to receive adequate help; and fourth- a delay to take responsibility/to be accountable for maternal death.

1st delay: Decision to seek help

In our study participants were very aware that pregnancy hypertension/eclampsia, hemorrhage, anemia and obstructed labour contributed to maternal mortality in their community. According to a woman survivor, maternal mortality is caused by:

> *Eclampsia kills babies and mothers... and when you are pregnant and you don't feel well, go see the doctor; your feet are swollen, go to the doctor; you have a headache, go to the doctor; you have a problem "below", go to the doctor; for all problems you have it's going to the doctor's that will resolve the problems.* – Mother of Two Children (one stillborn and one neonatal death) (W2)

Within focus group discussions, participants introduced the idea of "negligence" and its role in maternal outcomes. They described this concept as a woman's lack of

Table 2 Features and characteristics of individual interviews

Individual interview number	Participant characteristics	Age range (in years)	Interview location features	Interviewer characteristics
II 1	Mother: 1 infant (died at 3 months old) • not partnered • unemployed • literate	20–25	Participant's home, outdoors	CRT Htn Co-Lead
II 2	Mother: 3 living children • partnered • market merchant • illiterate	25–35	Community church, outdoors; several hours walk from participant's home	CRT Member
II 3	Mother: 3 living children + 1 miscarriage • partnered • homemaker • literate	30–35	Participant's home, outdoors	CRT Member
II 4	Mother: 2 living children + 1 stillborn • partnered • homemaker • illiterate	25–35	Participant's home, outdoors	CRT Member
II 5	Mother: 1 stillborn + 1 neonatal death • partnered? • market merchant • illiterate	25–35	Community church, outdoors; within participant's neighbourhood	CRT Member

Table 3 Key questions covered in focus group discussions and individual interviews

Data Collection/Participants	Question Guides
FGD 1 + 2 Community Leaders ($N = 15$)	1. As CLs, what is your understanding of maternal mortality? 2. As CLs, what is your experience of why women in your community die in pregnancy, during birth and in the six weeks following giving birth? 3. From your knowledge and experience, what are the causes for women dying in pregnancy, during birth and in the 42 days after giving birth? 4. How do women in the community know when they are having problems in their pregnancy, during labour/birth or for the weeks following birth? 5. In our community, what does the community do to help women in pregnancy, during labour and birth and after birth? 6. As CLs, what help can you give/do you give for women having these kinds of problems? 7. What is the impact on our community when women die, either in pregnancy, while giving birth, or in the 42 days after having a baby? 8. As CLs, what can you propose for our community as ways to stop women dying at this time in their lives?
FDG 3 + 4 Traditional Birth Attendants ($N = 16$)	1. As TBAs, what is your understanding of maternal mortality? 2. In our community, what do you do to help women in pregnancy, during labour and birth and after birth? 3. When things are not going well in pregnancy, labour and birth or the weeks after having a baby, how does that look? 4. As TBAs, how do you know when women in the community are having problems in their pregnancy, during labour/birth or for the weeks following birth? 5. In our community, as TBAs what do you do to help women in pregnancy, during labour and birth and after birth, when they are having problems? 6. As TBAs, what is your experience of why women in your community die in pregnancy, during birth and in the six weeks following giving birth? 7. What is the impact on our community when women die, either in pregnancy, while giving birth, or in the 42 days after having a baby? 8. What help could the whole community give so women don't die in our community? 9. As TBAs, what can you propose for our community as ways to stop women dying at this time in their lives?
IIs 1–5 Women Survivors of Near-Miss Maternal Experiences ($N = 5$)	1. What was it like for you to be pregnant, to be in labour/give birth, and/or during the days/weeks after you had your baby? 2. What challenges or difficulties did you experience in your pregnancy, during birth or in the weeks after having a baby? 3. How did you know when something wasn't going well for you? 4. What did you do to try to "fix the problem"? 5. What help did you get from those around you? From your community? 6. How did people from your community help you? 7. How do you feel about this experience of pregnancy/birth/weeks after birth? 8. What did you learn from this difficult experience? 9. What advice can you give others (other women, other community members), given the difficult experience you have had?

Legend: *FGD* Focus Group Discussion, *CLs* Community Leaders, *TBAs* Traditional Birth Attendants, *IIs* Individual Interviews

awareness of and/or denial of pregnancy danger signs/symptoms, waiting too long before seeking care for these, or negligence to seek healthcare in pregnancy at all. Participants felt that knowledge impacted maternal death because women (especially youth in the community) lacked knowledge/awareness (of maternal health/well-being, of community prenatal care and social services), were misinformed of pregnancy/birth/afterbirth or were "negligent" in seeking appropriate healthcare advice. These participants also linked youth to having a lesser degree of maternal health knowledge, increased fear/level of stress in pregnancy which included hiding a pregnancy from one's partner/family/friends, lesser degree of partner involvement and reduced ability to make informed choices. Focus group participants identified several concepts that may be related to the first and fourth delays-delays in decisions to seek help and/or in the community's accountability with respect to maternal death where delays have occurred.

Economic status of the woman or her family played a significant role and contributed to different delays in the decision to seek help. One woman related economic means and family planning:

> *It's that you should go to the hospital [to deliver]. Well sometimes you are home and you don't have money to go to the hospital. Your husband doesn't have money for you to go so if you don't go, the baby can get really big in your belly and you don't go to the hospital so you won't know what kind of baby you are having, and if it will die....well I say that problems can happen if you have more children so it's better to use family planning.*
> -Mother of Three Living Children (W1)

Focus group participants discussed socioecological status of the woman and linked these to women's stress of an unwanted pregnancy (by youth and by adults already with children), the decision to conceal or terminate a pregnancy (due to financial worries), and family burden of an additional child. Women's degree of independence was associated with decisions about abortion, seeking care and leaving home for hospital-based care. Women survivors of near-misses felt obliged to await the return of their partners (from the field, another community, the 'boko' (Haitian Voodoo sorcerer) or 'houngan' (Haitian Voodoo male priest) before a critical decision about their health/well-being could be made, leading to serious delays of the first type.

2nd delay: To reach help

Participants directly related maternal death from hemorrhage to the second delay. Many participants described hemorrhage (e.g. from retained products of conception or the use of various folk/spiritual rituals) contributed as a leading cause of mortality in the community. They cited causes of maternal death as distance travelled to reach help, and time taken before receiving adequate care to treat blood loss.

Of the five women survivors of near-misses, one participant had complications due to an incomplete miscarriage that occurred at home in mid-pregnancy. When asked if she could have died from her situation she responded:

> *It is the road to death, yes when you lose a lot of blood and you hemorrhage; now you can die if you lose a lot of blood until you have none left and you die, yes.*
> -Mother of Three Living Children (W1)

For survivors of near-misses, hypertension and eclampsia figured prominently with respect to reaching help. Three of the participants suffered severe complications of hypertension during their pregnancies and were transported to the hospital, each suffering from eclamptic seizures en route. They gave birth at the hospital: one delivered a live infant; the second delivered a live infant by caesarean section but the infant died at three months of age for reasons unknown. The third woman was delivered by caesarean section and her infant died shortly after birth. This participant also reported suffering from hypertensive seizures in the early postpartum period, an incisional infection, and ongoing visual disturbances.

Focus group participants often discussed economic status with respect to age (i.e. being more precarious for pregnant unemployed youth), and related this to the second and third delays. In general, economic instability impacted the ability to have work in the first place, seek or pay for maternal healthcare, eat well/at all, or pay for transportation to a healthcare facility. This is exemplified in a female Community Leader's words:

> *People have economic problems, they don't have money and they can die while somebody gets others to carry her, she can die, she can die because the road is too long to get to the dispensary, and then they don't take care of her. She can die. Those are all the problems we see here.* (CL2)

3rd delay: To receive adequate help

In our study, participants from each focus group made direct ties between community infrastructure and healthcare services at the dispensary or hospital as they related to receiving adequate help. They stated that healthcare services were inadequate, incomplete and inappropriate in their community citing a lack of adequately skilled maternal care providers, which included TBAs and dispensary staff alike. Nonetheless, participants from three of the focus groups regarded the provision of maternal healthcare as a form of community help to women, and encouraged community members to seek healthcare services. For women survivors, maternal healthcare offered by dispensary/hospital staff, in a serious time of need, constituted an important form of community help to them as did care by the matwon, a Traditional Birth Attendant.

Interactions between TBAs and dispensary/hospital staff were brought up by some participants from the matwon focus group as they related to receiving adequate help and care at a critical juncture. Matwon participants described feeling unwelcomed, humiliated and dismissed by healthcare staff upon arrival with a woman in a critical state. These TBAs perceived lack of respect for them and staff disregard for the urgency of the woman's situation. They viewed these as contributing to the third kind of delay.

Another delay: Of community to take responsibility

A community's delay to take responsibility/be accountable for maternal death can also contribute to maternal mortality. For example, the issue of abortion and its complications were discussed by both groups of Community Leaders as they related to community responsibility. Participants spoke passionately about experiences of young women in the community with unwanted pregnancies. They also described women's choices for induced abortion (illegal in Haiti) and related these to a partner's insistence to abort a pregnancy because of a woman's precarious socioeconomic status. They recounted devastating outcomes of hemorrhage and death when common illicit means were used to induce bleeding and terminate pregnancies. These means included self-medication of street drugs or ingestion of medicinal concoctions sold by the local boko (Voodoo sorcerer) or houngan (Voodoo male priest). A female Community Leader (CL3) reflected on maternal mortality as it relates to unwanted pregnancy, abortion and infection. She explained:

> *Sometimes someone gets pregnant but it's not the right time...she doesn't want to tell her parents; she talks to her friends; her friends give her advice to take medicine, medicine that is too strong for her; it forces the baby out and after the baby is born she develops an infection, she doesn't go to the hospital, she dies, she dies from the infection.* (CL3)

The status of the woman within the community and the impact of maternal death also emerged from discussions related to the fourth delay. While this topic was not broached with women survivors of near-miss experiences, it was discussed across four different focus groups: some participants described the coarse effects on motherless children, i.e. children without a father's involvement would become uncared children then orphans and grow up as delinquents. Other participants cited a reduced socioeconomic status when women die since their community depends on women's economic contribution. Many participants' reflections related to community well-being and spoke of profound sadness when women die in their community. One leader described this:

> *It's very sad. Women aren't supposed to die but we see women in our zone, they are pregnant and when the baby dies inside them, they can't deliver the dead baby; after the delivery the woman dies herself; she's not supposed to die, and it's not good that women die because mothers give life and when they give life they aren't supposed to lose their own lives- this is a sad time.* -male Community Leader (CL7)

In addition many focus group and interview participants discussed community social support with respect to the fourth delay. Some interview participants discussed the negative impact that social support might have on maternal outcomes. During discussions participants used examples of social support in which certain cultural/spiritual/religious beliefs had unintended negative impacts on women: A near-miss survivor described cultural beliefs and their effects when she sought the help of a boko leaf doctor in an attempt to relieve abdominal pain. She explained that she found no real help in the healer's leaves, used up valuable resources and delayed getting medical healthcare, thereby negatively impacting her pregnancy outcome. This survivor participant recommended that problems of pregnancy were better left to treatment by a medical doctor. In another example, a woman's partner spent precious money for the advice of a boko that delayed the woman reaching medical help, or obtaining it at all, or left her unable to pay for transportation to obtain essential healthcare services.

Participants also related examples of social support from partners, family members and neighbours which positively impacted maternal well-being. They described practical support as offered food, money or transportation for women. Women survivors appreciated supportive partners during labour or critical decision-making; neighbours who provided transportation; and family/friends who advised them to seek help/treatment (from matwon, traditional healer, healthcare provider). Community Leader participants included TBAs' positive contribution to community responsibility vis-à-vis the fourth delay. They viewed these matwon as a vital link for women, as critical players who connect their community with healthcare providers and whose potential impact on maternal mortality in this community deserves close attention. Women survivors echoed this sentiment of positive support and added appreciation of their matwon who offered them food, tender care, trusted advice and physical/emotional support, and even accompaniment to hospital.

Finally, focus group and interview participants offered solutions to reduce maternal mortality in their community, and ways to reduce the fourth delay. These community solutions centered on prevention, community infrastructure and community mobilization. Participants suggested that prevention strategies should include more community education (for women and men, for teenagers/youth) related to Family Planning and birth spacing: consideration of a woman's past pregnancy outcome(s), her current health, economic and social status, and cover topics such as pregnancy/birth/postpartum care, pregnancy danger signs, and the importance of receiving complete maternal healthcare. The need for more training of TBAs was suggested as another prevention strategy. Other solutions centered on improved community infrastructure including improved transportation infrastructure such as better roads and safer ways to transport women to hospital, and greater access to healthcare in their community which translated to more resources for TBAs/dispensary staff, more skilled dispensary staff and extended access to emergency care at the dispensary level. Participants also suggested community mobilization by way of the formation of Neighbourhood or Community Committees to directly address the problem of maternal mortality, and a coordinated communication relay/transport system (i.e. geographically, strategically-placed community stretchers, headlamps for carriers of women on stretchers fitted with security belts) in times of maternal health crisis.

Participants who survived near-miss maternal experiences offered solutions of a nature specific to the grave maternal circumstances they lived to tell. Their solutions included suggestions to seek appropriate care (i.e. care provided by a medical doctor and the avoidance of care/remedies by the boko or houngan), to seek care without delay (by calling on social support when needed, with the onset of danger signs and "earlier rather than later"), to choose an appropriate place of birth (recognizing that previous birth experiences play an important role in choice of birthplace) and to provide community support to pregnant, labouring and postnatal women (by the provision/sharing of food/financial support and participation of community members when needed for transportation, communication relay etc.).

Being carried: A special example of the fourth delay

Many study participants from focus groups and interviews discussed women being transported on a board/door from their community in times of a maternal health crisis. The challenges of being carried were numerous and not simply a consequence of delays related to an individual's decision to seek help, time to reach help, or provision of adequate care. "Being carried" constituted a particular example of the community's involvement –and of their challenges created by the community's own delay of responsibility for maternal death as they related to political will, mobilization and accountability.

Participants described the physical and logistical difficulties associated with getting a woman to the hospital, several hours walk away. Transportation of a woman (on a door) often involved locating four willing carriers (men), walking amidst challenging conditions and were also impacted by a family's and/or matwon's decisions to seek help from community members in the first place, and the time to reach help given physical and logistical transportation issues which had not been overcome. The scene is described in one male participant's words:

> *Carrying someone on our heads, [the path] isn't wide enough for two people in front of each other to carry the lamp in the bucket so we need to walk one by one so we can see where we are going. Imagine if it is a pregnant woman who is in pain with labour and we drop her; they will both die, you see all of this problem why women die and they shouldn't die because they are supposed to give life. We shouldn't die under conditions like that.* –male Community Leader (CL7)

The timing of when to transport a woman from the community and the terrain that needed to be covered were impacted by community infrastructure. Focus group participants from each focus group and survivors of near-misses alike gave examples to illustrate the impact on maternal outcomes because of poor community infrastructure and lack of community engagement to overcome these obstacles. They suggested that as a community they are isolated because they are in a mountainous, hard-to-reach zone, and their dwellings are mostly distant one from the other.

> *We don't have roads, we don't have roads. If we had roads, when someone has a problem, we could load them [on a vehicle], go to the hospital and then they don't have time to die. But because we don't have roads that means we have to wait until the morning to carry the person on our heads to the hospital...*-female Community Leader (CL6)

One woman survivor associated maternal death to several different delays and summarized it this way:

> *Delays cause death; when you are pregnant you have the right [can] go to the doctor, and with every delay you can get sick; eclampsia can happen; but you might not find anyone to take you to the doctor's; if you don't have good roads they need to bring you on their heads to go to the hospital; delays can cause you to die because the roads aren't made and there aren't vehicles; if you have a [motorcycle] taxi number you can call it to come get you but the delay can cause you to die because you don't have a road and so all you can do is go down the mountain on the carriers' heads [on a door] and you can fall from the mountain when the carriers knock their feet on rocks and you slip with them [off the door*]. –Mother of Two Children (one stillborn and one neonatal death) (W2)

The community's recognition that there has been a delay in their collective engagement to work together to identify ways within the community to improve their ability to transport women in crisis, mobilize resources already available and seek support to reduce poor maternal outcomes is clearly different from the other types of delays.

Discussion

Maternal health and well-being in Haiti requires renewed actions to accelerate a reduction of reproductive health inequalities compared to other Latin American and Caribbean countries [5]. Haiti's push toward safe motherhood continues to have its challenges related to unintended and adolescent pregnancies and abortion [19], provision of maternal health service among rural Haitian women, accessibility to antenatal care and skilled birth attendance and structural inequalities as they relate to socioeconomic determinants of maternal health (e.g. education, parity, distance from services) [12, 20]. Our study focused first on understanding community perspectives as to why women die during pregnancy, childbirth and the days after giving birth, and second on community-driven solutions to reduce maternal mortality in rural Haiti.

The delay in the decision to seek help (first delay) continues to be significant when maternal mortality is considered in rural Haiti. In agreement with prior research [12, 20] participants felt that women's (especially youth) lack of knowledge/awareness, and misinformation about pregnancy/birth/afterbirth impacted maternal death in their community; they also identified the impact of economic status and how the status of the woman plays into maternal outcomes and women's health-seeking behaviours [21]. Our participants connected these to an important community-identified concept of "negligence" and tied them to the first delay. Furthermore, our research overlaps with Weeks and team's work where factors related to socioeconomic determinants of maternal mortality in Uganda were status of the woman, poor health education, limited resources and poor quality community health care [22].

Reaching help (second delay) during a maternal crisis also figured significantly in this rural community. Participants emphasized the need to improve community infrastructure- better roads, safer ways to transport women to hospital, closer access to care. These results support other literature regarding the second delay [11, 12, 22].

With respect to the third delay (to receive adequate care), we found the quality of interactions between the community and its healthcare resources and provision of them, impacted women in terms of receiving adequate help and care, much in alignment with other literature [22, 23]. While women survivors' described positive interactions with matwon and/or dispensary/hospital staff, focus group participants described inadequate/incomplete/inappropriate healthcare services in their community, and viewed negative interactions with dispensary/hospital staff as contributing to a delay of the third kind. There is some overlap between our findings and research done in Ethiopia where community women's and their partners' perspectives were explored regarding decisions to deliver at home versus in health facilities [23]. Emergent themes from their work regarded client-related factors such as dependence on TBAs, and health system factors like poor welcome by staff [23] that contributed to the delay of women receiving adequate care.

Unique to our study, participants offered solutions to the first, second and third delays. Focus groups suggested the importance of community education, complete maternal healthcare, and Family Planning, a key form of maternal death prevention among teenagers/youth, and for other women attempting to use family planning and birth spacing for a variety of reasons. Women survivors of near-misses framed prevention by way of appropriate care, care sought without delay, appropriate choice of birthplace and provision of community support to pregnant, labouring and postnatal women. This aligns well with research on health-seeking behaviours and use of healthcare facilities [24]. Participants highlighted solutions and recommended optimal use of healthcare expertise and resources at the dispensary level and suggested the need for training of TBAs- committed accoucheurs already an integral part of the community whose expertise should be optimized to reduce maternal mortality.

Finally, in our study intimately related issues such as the status of the woman, women's socioeconomic status and the social support of women emerged from discussions relating to maternal death. Participants referred to the community's delay (and not just an individual's delays) to take responsibility for reducing the number of women dying during pregnancy, childbirth and in the 42 days after birth. This seemed to be different from the other three delays and we believe it constitutes a fourth delay. The literature identifies two different types of fourth delay. One type is a delay related to the economic, psychological and physiological repercussions of near-miss maternal events; these repercussions are a consequence of a woman surviving a severe obstetric complication, and result in further maternal health complications and ongoing consequences for the woman and her family [9]. The second type corresponds to a community-based accountability for maternal (and newborn) health, and recognizes that the reduction of maternal mortality "takes a village" in order to affect change [10, 25]. This last type of fourth delay matches our findings most closely. No literature about maternal health in Haiti was located where specific reference was made regarding this notion of a fourth delay. However, it appears that many of this rural community's challenges and participants' solutions address a fourth delay- one that has the potential to impact individuals' first, second and third delays. Together these emphasize the relevance of the community-based accountability type of fourth delay.

In terms of community accountability, focus group participants provided concrete examples of community mobilization as a strategic solution to reduce maternal mortality. In addition, the difficult experiences and practical solutions shared by women survivors of near-miss maternal experiences are valuable and insightful. This kind of proxy group of women, as described by Pacagnella and colleagues, represents a novel maternal group that often shares common characteristics as those who died "on the road of death" [9]. In our study, these novel participants framed community support through provision of food, money, and transportation from community members. Other researchers have also investigated near-misses in different low-middle income settings, and their impact on subsequent pregnancies [26]. They have considered the perspectives of women survivors in terms of women's bodily integrity, household economy and social identity/stability as a result of their near-loss of life experiences [27], and women's fear of dying, loss of their baby and how the quality of care they received could impact future health-seeking behaviour/use of healthcare facilities [24]. In our study the valuable contribution of these women's unique perspectives has provided a better understanding of the socioecological determinants of maternal death and solutions needed to reduce maternal mortality in this rural Haitian community of which most solutions point to the fourth delay.

In terms of maternal wellness, we found this fourth delay to affect the first, second and third delays, and to be impacted by the community's knowledge, political will, accountability, mobilization and empowerment. Through local ownership and engagement in our study we found that community knowledge and awareness of maternal death in the community impacted the political will to mobilize and find solutions to reduce maternal mortality and in turn created a sense of empowerment whereby positive change could be realized.

The CBAR design of our research strengthened this study by way of encouraging community learning, building project integrity and accountability, and bringing about community mobilization. This capacity-building allowed for better understanding of maternal mortality in this rural Haitian community that may provide valuable insight for future interventions that are community-based, community-driven and sustainable.

The study was limited by small sample size and selective inclusion of key community members' perspectives regarding maternal mortality. Consequently, findings from this research are not representative and should not be generalized to all rural (Haitian) communities. Future explorations should include the missed perspectives of under-represented community members such as teenagers/youth, traditional healers, elders of the community, religious leaders, dispensary/hospital staff and administration, and policy makers. The authors must also consider a possible bias in drawing conclusions with respect to the fourth delay as part of our conceptual framework.

Conclusion

This study highlights the indigenous knowledge and experience of members of a rural Haitian community as they relate to maternal mortality in their community. Community perspectives on maternal death are important in Haiti. A deeper exploration regarding the important community-identified concept of negligence is needed in order to better understand the implications of individual and community accountability for maternal health and well-being, and community health at large, and how these overlap the first and fourth delays and potentially impact the other delays as well. Finding sustainable ways to reduce maternal mortality requires a community-based/centred and community-driven comprehensive approach to maternal health/well-being. This includes the engagement of community members that is dependent upon community knowledge, political will, mobilization, accountability and empowerment. An engaged and empowered community is one that is well placed to find ways that work in their community to reduce the fourth delay and in turn maternal death. Potentially, community ownership of the challenges and the solutions can lead to more sustainable improvements in maternal health/well-being in Haiti.

Abbreviations

CBAR: Community-Based Action Research; CL: Community Leader; CRT: Community Research Team; FGD: Focus Group Discussion; Htn: Haitian; II: Individual Interview; TBA: Traditional Birth Attendant; W: Woman (survivor of near-miss maternal experience)

Acknowledgements

TM is thankful for the help, direction and support of the following people and organizations who facilitated the research: Helen McDonald, Nancy Salbach, TM's parents and children Mykelti, Elijah and Maévah, Lydia Kapiriri, St Joseph's Healthcare Hamilton-International Outreach Program, and Hôpital Albert Schweitzer. We are also indebted to the generous women and men participants from this rural Haitian community without whose support this research could not have taken place.

Funding

Funding was supported by St. Joseph's Healthcare Hamilton-International Outreach Program (SJHH-IOP), a University of Toronto Global Health Student Research Award and through a small donor fund-raising campaign by TM. In no way did the funding bodies play a role in the design of this study, collection/analysis/interpretation of data or writing of the manuscript.

Authors' contributions

This study was part of a Master of Public Health field inquiry project carried out by TM. Project conception, research questions, and study outline/implementation, data collection/analysis, interpretation, and manuscript writing/review/revisions were undertaken by TM. SJ provided important direction, mentorship and editorial expertise throughout all stages of the project from conception to manuscript writing. MC was project Co-Lead and was involved with data collection/analysis, interpretation, review and revision of the draft manuscript and approval of the final version. MP undertook participant recruitment, data collection/analysis, interpretation, review and revision of the draft manuscript and approval of the final version. MJ-B was involved with data collection/analysis, interpretation, review and revision of the draft manuscript and approval of the final version. AS was involved with participant recruitment, data collection/analysis, interpretation, review and revision of the draft manuscript and approval of the final version. ÉP undertook participant recruitment, data collection/analysis, interpretation, review and revision of the draft manuscript and approval of the final version.

Authors' information

TM is a Registered Midwife, Assistant Clinical Professor (McMaster University) and Master Lecturer (Laurentian University) of Midwifery. MC is a Haitian Nurse-Midwife currently completing a Registered Nurse bridging program in Montreal, Québec. MP continues to work for Hôpital Albert Schweitzer as Community Health Worker Coordinator. MJ-B is a homemaker and community member in which the research took place, as are, ÉP, a local farmer and AS, a community pastor. SJ is Associate Professor Emerita (University of Toronto).

Competing interests

The authors declare that they have no competing interests.

Author details

[1]School of Midwifery, Health Sciences Building, Laurentian University, 935 Ramsey Lake Road, Sudbury, ON P3E 2C6, Canada. [2]Dalla Lana School of Public Health, Health Sciences Building, University of Toronto, 155 College Street, Suite 526, Toronto, ON M5T 3M7, Canada. [3]Cégep du Vieux Montréal, Montreal, Canada. [4]Hôpital Albert Schweitzer, Deschapelles, Haiti.

References

1. World Health Organization (WHO): Millennium Development Goal 5. http://www.who.int/topics/millennium_development_goals/maternal_health/en/index.html (2015). Accessed 23 Sept 2012.
2. World Health Organization (WHO): World health statistics 2016: monitoring health for the SDGs, sustainable development goals: Annex B, Part 1. Geneva: WHO; 2016.
3. Ministère de la Santé Publique et de la Population (MSPP), Institut Haïtien de l'Enfance (IHE) et ICF International. 2013. L'Enquête Mortalité, Morbidité et Utilisation des Services en Haïti de 2012: Rapport de synthèse. Calverton, Maryland: MSPP, IHE, et ICF International.
4. World Health Organization (WHO): Global Health Observatory (GHO) data, equity country profiles: Haiti. http://www.who.int/gho/health_equity/countries/en/.
5. Restrepo-Méndez MC, Barros AJ, Requejo J, Durán P, Serpa LA, França GV, et al. Progress in reducing inequalities in reproductive, maternal, newborn and child health in Latin America and the Caribbean: an unfinished agenda. In: Rev Panam Salud Publica; 2015. https://www.scielosp.org/pdf/rpsp/2015.v38n1/09-16-en.
6. Thaddeus S, Maine D. Too far to walk: maternal mortality in context. Soc Sci Med. 1994; https://doi.org/10.1016/0277-9536(94)90226-7
7. Barnes-Josiah D, Myntti C, Augustin A. The "three delays" as a framework for examining maternal mortality in Haiti. Soc Sci Med. 1998; https://doi.org/10.1016/S0277-9536(97)10018-1.
8. Ministère de Sante Publique et de la Population (MSPP). L'Infirmière sage-femme dans la communauté: manuel de l'étudiante infirmière sage-femme: cours de santé publique en santé reproductive. 2nd ed. Petite Rivière l'Artibonite: Centre Médical Charles Colimon de Petite Rivière l'Artibonite; 2006.
9. Pacagnella RC, Cecatti JG, Osis MJ, Souza JP. The role of delays in severe maternal morbidity and mortality: expanding the conceptual framework. Repro Health Matters. 2012; https://doi.org/10.1016/S0968-8080(12)39601-8.
10. Saving Lives at Birth https://www.savinglivesatbirth.net/blog/12/02/01/meet-innovator-moi-university-school-medicine.
11. White K, Small M, Frederic R, Joseph G, Bateau R, Kershaw T. Health seeking behavior among pregnant women in rural Haiti. Health Care Women Int. 2006;27(9):822–38.
12. Babalola SO. Factors associated with use of maternal health services in Haiti: a multilevel analysis. In: Rev Panam Salud Publica; 2014. https://www.scielosp.org/scielo.php?pid=S1020-49892014000600001&script=sci_abstract&tlng=es.
13. Lathrop E, Telemaque Y, Goedken P, Andes K, Jamieson DJ, Cwiak C. Postpartum contraceptive needs in northern Haiti. Int J Gynaecol Obstet. 2011; https://doi.org/10.1016/j.ijgo.2010.09.012.
14. Cianelli R, Mitchell E, Albuja L, Wilkinson C, Anglade D, Chery M, Peragallo N. Maternal-child health needs assessment in Haiti. Int J Appl Sci Technol. 2014;4(5):30–8.
15. Small MJ, Kershaw T, Frederic R, Blanc C, Neale D, Copel J, Williams KP. Characteristics of preeclampsia- and eclampsia-related maternal death in rural Haiti. J Matern Fetal Neonatal Med. 2005;18(5):343–8.
16. Earp JA, Ennet ST. Conceptual models in health education research and practice. Health Educ Res. 1991;6:163–71.
17. Hôpital Albert Schweitzer Haiti- origins/mission. https://hashaiti.org/vision/our-network-of-care/.
18. Jackson SF. A participatory group process to analyze qualitative data. Prog Community Health Partnersh. 2008 Summer;2(2):161–70.
19. Huber B. Haiti's push for safe motherhood. Lancet. 2015; https://doi.org/10.1016/S0140-6736(15)61490-8. Accessed 4 Dec 2015
20. Séraphin MN, Ngnie-Teta I, Ayoya MA, Khan MR, Striley CW, Boldon E, Mamadoultaibou A, Saint-Fleur JE, Koo L, Clermont M. Determinants of institutional delivery among women of childbearing age in rural Haiti. Matern Child Health J. 2015; https://doi.org/10.1007/s10995-014-1646-1.
21. Arps S. Threats to safe motherhood in Honduran Miskito communities: local perceptions of factors that contribute to maternal mortality. Soc Sci Med. 2009; https://doi.org/10.1016/j.socscimed.2009.06.005.
22. Weeks A, Lavender T, Nazziwa E, Mirembe F. Personal accounts of 'near-miss' maternal mortalities in Kampala, Uganda. BJOG. 2005; https://obgyn.onlinelibrary.wiley.com/doi/abs/10.1111/j.1471-0528.2005.00703.x.
23. Roro MA, Hassen EM, Lemma AM, Gebreyesus SH, Afework MF. Why do women not deliver in health facilities: a qualitative study of the community perspectives in south Central Ethiopia? BMC Res Notes. 2014; https://doi.org/10.1186/1756-0500-7-556.
24. Tunçalp Ö, Hindin MJ, Adu-Bonsaffoh K, Adanu R. Listening to women's voices: the quality of care of women experiencing severe maternal morbidity, in Accra, Ghana. PLoS One. 2012; https://doi.org/10.1371/journal.pone.0044536.
25. Kc NP, Kc A, Sharma N, Malla H, Thapa N, Aryal K, Vitrakoti R, Bhandari RM. Community participation and mobilization in community-based maternal, newborn and child health programmes in Nepal. J Nepal Health Res Counc. 2011;9(19):101–6.
26. Haddad SM, Cecatti JG, Parpinelli MA, Souza JP, Costa ML, Sousa MH, Surita FG, Silva JL PE, Pacagnella RC, Camargo RS, Bahamondes MV, Zotareli V, Gurgel LT, Say L, Pattinson RC, National Network for the sSurveillance of Severe Maternal Morbidity Group1. From planning to practice: building the national network for the surveillance of severe maternal morbidity. BMC Public Health. 2011; https://doi.org/10.1186/1471-2458-11-283.
27. Storeng KT, Murray SF, Akoum MS, Ouattara F, Filippi V. Beyond body counts: a qualitative study of lives and loss in Burkina Faso after 'near-miss' obstetric complications. Soc Sci Med. 2010;71(10):1749–56.

11

Barriers associated with care-seeking for institutional delivery among rural women in three provinces in Afghanistan

Ariel Higgins-Steele[1,4*], Jane Burke[2], Abo Ismael Foshanji[3], Farhad Farewar[3], Malalai Naziri[1], Sediq Seddiqi[2] and Karen M. Edmond[1]

Abstract

Background: In the past fifteen years, Afghanistan has made substantial progress in extending primary health care. However, coverage of essential health interventions proven to improve maternal and neonatal health outcomes, particularly skilled birth attendance, remains unacceptably low. This is especially true for those in the poorest quintile of the population. This cross-sectional quantitative and qualitative study assessed barriers associated with care-seeking for institutional delivery among rural Afghan women in three provinces.

Methods: The study was conducted from November to December 2016 in 12 districts across three provinces – Badghis, Bamyan, and Kandahar – which are predominately rural. Districts were used as the primary sampling unit with district-level sample sizes reflecting the ratio of that district's population to provincial population. Villages within these districts, the secondary sampling units, were randomly selected. A household survey was used to collect data on: demographics, socio-economic status, childbearing history, health transport and service costs, maternal health seeking behavior and barriers to service uptake. Data on barriers to facility delivery were compared across provinces using chi square tests.

Results: Of the 2479 women of child bearing age interviewed, one-third were from each province (33% $n = 813$ Badghis, 34% $n = 840$ Bamyan, 33% $n = 824$ Kandahar). Among those respondents who had delivered none of their children in a health center, money to pay for services appeared to be most important barrier to accessing institutional delivery (56%, $n = 558$). No transportation available was the second most widely cited reason (37%, $n = 368$), followed by family restrictions ($n = 30\%$, $n = 302$). Respondents in Badghis reported the highest levels of barriers compared to the other two provinces. Respondents in Badghis were more likely to report familial or cultural constraints as the most important barrier to institutional delivery (43%) compared to Bamyan (2%) and Kandahar (12%) ($p < 0.001$).

Conclusions: Despite the socio-demographic and geographic diversity of the three provinces under study, the top barriers to institutional delivery reported in all three areas are consistent with available evidence, namely, that distance, transport cost and transport availability are the main factors limiting institutional delivery. Proven and promising approaches to overcome these barriers to institutional delivery in Afghanistan should be explored and studied.

Keywords: Maternal health, Institutional delivery, Skilled birth attendance, Barriers, Afghanistan

* Correspondence: ahiggins@unicef.org
[1]UNICEF Afghanistan, Kabul, Afghanistan
[4]United Nations Office Complex in Afghanistan (UNOCA), Jalalabad Road, Kabul, Afghanistan
Full list of author information is available at the end of the article

Background

Afghanistan has among the highest maternal (396 per 100,000 live births) and newborn mortality (40 per 1000 live births) rates in the world [1, 2]. However, in the past fifteen years, Afghanistan has made substantial progress in extending primary health care through its 'basic package of health services' (BPHS) [3, 4] including improved availability of public facilities across the country [5]. Health facility deliveries (also called institutional deliveries) and birth assistance from a skilled attendant (midwife, nurse or doctor who has received training in midwifery or obstetrics) have increased dramatically from less than 15% for both indicators in 2002 [6], rising to 32% of births at a health center and 34% with a skilled attendant in 2010 [7]. By 2015, these indicators had further improved with 48% of births occurring at a health facility and 51% of births assisted by a skilled provider [8]. These figures and other figures indicate that almost all skilled birth attendants are assisting women at health facilities: 99.5% of deliveries in health facilities are assisted by skilled providers compared to 13% of births that occur elsewhere and 11% of births where location was not reported [8].

Coverage of essential health interventions proven to improve maternal and neonatal health outcomes, particularly skilled birth attendance, remains unacceptably low among populations in the poorest quintile (22%) as compared to the richest (82%) and the rate of change in overall improvements for this indicator appears to be decreasing [8]. In rural areas, only 40% of birth occur at health facilities, compared to 76% in urban areas, and only [8]. Global evidence suggests that the "best intrapartum-care strategy is likely to be one in which women routinely choose to deliver in a health centre, with midwives as the main providers, but with other attendants working with them in a team" [9].

Improvements have occurred unequally with considerable barriers to much of the population maintained [10]. Skilled birth attendance in Afghanistan is strongly associated with wealth of households, literacy, and residing less than one hour from a health facility [11]. Studies indicate that distance from health facilities, lack of transport, and high cost of transportation to go to a health facility are commonly cited as barriers to accessing primary health services in Afghanistan [12, 13]. Although all public health services are supposed to be free of charge across the country, households bear costs even in the public sector including for transportation, food, and medicines. According to Afghanistan's National Health Accounts 2014, 73% of total health expenditure is comprised of household out-of-pocket expenses, and 7% of total household out-of-pocket expenditures is consumed by transportation related costs associated with health care [14].

The 'three delays model' represents the three main time-related factors that affect the outcome of an emergency presentation during pregnancy or child birth and are defined as: (i) delay in the decision to access care, (ii) delay in the identification of – and transport to – a medical facility, and (iii) delay in the receipt of adequate and appropriate treatment [15]. Women in Afghanistan experience all barriers, with the second delay being a particular challenge in rural areas. Additionally, Afghanistan is frequently classified as a 'fragile' state with high levels of ongoing conflict [16] and many women also lack power in the household to make decisions about health care for themselves and their children [17].

There are few studies which provide evidence on barriers to care-seeking for institutional delivery. The limited scope of available evidence combined with high concern for the low rates of skilled birth attendance and institutional delivery in the country merit additional investigation [18–20]. Some interventions, such as pay per performance of health facilities have shown minimal effect in Afghanistan, with inadequate attention to demand side factors as a possible reason. This study thus implemented a cross-sectional quantitative and qualitative study to assess the barriers associated with care-seeking among rural women who live in three disparate provinces in Afghanistan.

Methods

Design and setting

This study used a mixed methods approach – quantitative household questionnaire and qualitative data – to assess care-seeking behaviors and barriers to institutional delivery. The primary variables of interest were place of birth (facility or home) and reported barriers for facility-based birth. The household survey was organized in several sections or modules: respondent characteristics including socio-economic factors and childbearing history, maternal health seeking behavior, and service utilization. Given the nature of this study, including sensitivities around maternal in the country context, qualitative data is intended to complement and assist in explaining and interpreting quantitative findings.

The study was conducted from November to December 2016 in 12 districts across three provinces – Badghis, Bamyan, and Kandahar. Bamyan is a remote and rural mountainous province in the central Highlands region, Badghis and Kandahar are predominately rural with strong influence of anti-government groups, frequent conflict, and strict social norms. Badghis borders with Turkmenistan and has difficult and mountainous terrain, Bamyan is also very mountainous with remote settlements, while Kandahar is a southern region bordering Pakistan and is predominately flat and arid. The crude birth rate was 37 per 1000 population in rural areas; total fertility rate expressed per woman 16–49 years of age was 5.4 in rural areas compared to 4.8 in urban. The institutional delivery rates were 5.9% Badghis, 35.5% Kandahar and 46.2% Bamyan [8].

Sampling and inclusion criteria

The sample size, per province, was determined to account for later disaggregation between control and treatment districts, for a planned endline study. The sample size was based on a simple random sample and did not take into account clustering, for a total of target size of 2400 households from twelve districts. The primary sampling units selected were districts pre-defined on the basis of comparability between assigned treatment and control districts within the three provinces. The population assigned per district was based on population proportional to size sampling. Villages, the secondary sampling unit were selected randomly from lists identified through a combination of participatory mapping and data provided by Afghanistan's Central Statistics Organization. Eligible women respondents were selected randomly with approximately 20 households interviewed in each secondary sampling unit.

Respondents were selected through systematic random sampling using a 'random walk' protocol. A 'random walk' protocol was used instead of a household listing as there were no census data available [21]. Within urban areas, data collectors started at a central location, such as a mosque or school, stopping at every third house. Data collectors turned right at every corner to enable surveying of households off of the main roads. In rural areas, data collectors stopped at every third house. Within each household, eligible women who were married, aged 16–49 years and had had a still or live birth in the past two years were randomly selected from a household roster for quantitative interview. Women were purposively sampled for inclusion in the qualitative study based on eligibility per study group.

Data collection

For the quantitative study eight female data collectors were recruited from each of the three provinces for training on quantitative and qualitative data collection methods. A household questionnaire was used to collect data from the interviewees on key characteristics: demographics, socio-economic status, childbearing history, health transport and service costs, maternal health seeking behavior, service use, and reported barriers (for data collection instrument, see Additional file 1). For logistics reasons, namely that female data collectors were at specific rural sites and trained in both methods, quantitative and qualitative data were collected simultaneously.

Surveys were conducted using Electronic Tablet devices enabled with KoBo Toolbox questionnaire software and data were collected using the tablet and automatically input skip patterns.

For the qualitative component, two methods were used – focus group discussions (FGDs) and key informant interviews (KIIs) – using semi-structured data collection guides. These guides contained domains relevant to the study, namely maternal care-seeking around birth and associated barriers. For FGDs, the respondent categories included females of reproductive age and community leaders; for the KIIs, respondent categories included service providers, specifically community health workers, midwives, nurses, and doctors. Each FGD consisted of between 6 and 8 women and lasted two to three hours. Major themes included public health service use in general, specific health behaviours related to maternal and newborn health, the role of community health workers, and barriers to both general and maternal and newborn health service uptake. The location of each FGD was determined through consultation with community leaders to provide a safe space for female respondents. In some areas, the location was a local school or mosque. In others, it was an individual's house. The determination was based on local conditions including social norms, available space, and security. Recordings were transcribed and translated into English.

Data analysis

Quantitative data were reviewed, cleaned, and analyzed in STATA 13. As the primary purpose of this study was descriptive, no groupings or stratification occurred besides provincial level analyses. Cross tabulations were calculated to identify possible relationships between key variables and the likelihood of at least one child being born in a health centre.

Badghis province is well recognised to be one of the most disadvantaged and conservative provinces in Afghanistan [8]. Thus we also wished to assess if there were important differences between the proportion of women reporting barriers to institutional delivery in Badghis province compared to Kandahar and Bamyan provinces. We used univariable logistic regression in Stata version 15 to conduct these analyses.

Qualitative data from 9 FGDs and 16 KIIs (Table 1) was coded by theme and sub-theme and analyzed in Atlas.ti in combination with a manual review. Before coding the data, an a priori code list was developed and during coding emergent themes were added. The major themes were identified based on the overarching research questions of the analysis and harmonized between quantitative and qualitative data collection tools. Qualitative data were required to add nuance and contextualize quantitative data. As qualitative data were not collected in all areas of study, there was no effort to compare district-level observations across qualitative

Table 1 Sample by province and district for quantitative (including refusals and replacements) and qualitative (by type)

Province	District	Quantitative		Qualitative				
		Number of questionnaires administered (n)	Number of refusals/ replacements n (%)	Focus groups discussions		Key informant interviews		
				Females reproductive age	Community leaders	Community health workers	Doctors, Nurses	Midwives
Badghis	Qades	217	0	–	–	–	–	–
	Jowand	196	0 (0%)	1	–	–	1	1
	Abkamary	302	4 (1%)	–	1	1	1	–
	Moqur	100	0 (0%)	1	–	1	–	1
Bamyan	Punjab	312	0 (0%)	–	–	–	–	–
	Saighan	107	52 (49%)	1	–	1	–	1
	Waras	312	0 (0%)	–	1	1	–	–
	Kahmarad	109	2 (2%)	1	–	–	1	–
Kandahar	Arghandaab	159	5 (3%)	–	–	–	–	–
	Spin Boldak	258	28 (11%)	–	1	–	–	1
	Dand	228	1 (0%)	1	–	1	–	1
	Daman	179	5 (3%)	1	–	1	–	1
Total		2479	99 (4%)	6	3	6	3	6

and quantitative data. Rather, the qualitative data were used to triangulate findings from quantitative data and integrated into the analysis through summary of overall trends and observations.

Ethical approval

Informed verbal consent was obtained from all participants in the study, and marked at the beginning of each questionnaire. The study, final research protocol and data collection tools received full ethical approval from the Ministry of Public Health Institutional Review Board (IRB) in Afghanistan (#335540).

Results

Socio demographics of the study population

A total 2479 women who had given birth in the last two years were approached for interview across the three provinces. There were 99 refusals. Women who refused to participate were replaced using the random walk protocol to select the next available house. Of the 2479 women interviewed, approximately one-third were from each location: 840 (33.9%) were from Bamyan, 815 (32.9%) were from Badghis and 824 (33.2%) were from Kandahar (Table 1).

The majority of women interviewed were between 20 and 30 years old, and most had limited access to formal education. Literacy rates among respondents were low in all provinces, with around 20% of the respondents indicating they were literate and less than 20% reporting having attended formal schooling (Table 2). Across the study population in the three provinces, while access to formal education appeared to be low, literacy rates did not directly correspond to formal education rates.

On average, women had given birth to less than five children over their lifetime (mean $n = 4.5$). Birth rates were slightly higher in Kandahar compared to the other two provinces, with a wider range including three women who had birthed 15 or more children (Fig. 1). Bagdhis province showed a comparatively smaller range of births.

An average family size of 7.9 persons was reported, which is slightly larger than national averages from the 2013–2014 Afghanistan Living Conditions Survey (7.4) though in line with national estimates of average rural household size (8.2) as reported in the 2015 Afghanistan Demographic and Health Survey [3, 6].

Service use

Over 90% of respondents had visited a public health center at least one time in the past year. Almost half of respondents visited a public health facility between 1 and 5 times in the past year, with variation across the three provinces (Table 2). Of those who had visited a health center in the past year, the majority (60%) reported that a one-way trip was less than 30 km; however 28% responded that they did not know or provided no response, likely because they were not able to estimate distance to the nearest health facility.

Among women who had visited a public health facility in the past month, 86% ($n = 1013$) indicated that the health facility was less than two hours away (Table 2).

Over half of all women (52%) reported using mechanized transport (car or motorbike) to go to a health

Table 2 Literacy rates, number of health facility visits, time and method to nearest health facility

	Overall	Badghis	Bamyan	Kandahar
	100% (*n* = 2479)	33% (*n* = 815)	34% (*n* = 840)	33% (*n* = 824)
Mother's reported literacy				
Can read and write	20% (*n* = 508)	17% (*n* = 142)	23% (*n* = 192)	21% (*n* = 174)
Cannot read and write	79% (*n* = 1952)	82% (*n* = 670)	77% (*n* = 648)	80% (*n* = 634)
Don't know	0% (*n* = 6)	0% (*n* = 3)	0% (*n* = 0)	0% (*n* = 3)
Refused	1% (*n* = 13)	0% (n = 0)	0% (*n* = 0)	0% (*n* = 0)
Number of health facility visits (last 12 months)				
No visits	6% (*n* = 158)	10% (n = 81)	5% (*n* = 41)	4% (n = 36)
1–5 visits	46% (*n* = 1144)	68% (*n* = 551)	32% (*n* = 268)	40% (*n* = 325)
6–9 visits	29% (*n* = 719)	7% (*n* = 61)	50% (*n* = 421)	29% (*n* = 237)
10+ visits	12% (*n* = 290)	1% (n = 6)	13% (*n* = 105)	22% (*n* = 179)
Do not know/ no response	7% (*n* = 168)	14% (*n* = 118)	1% (n = 5)	5% (n = 47)
Time to public health facility				
Less than 30 mins	33% (*n* = 390)	52% (*n* = 77)	43% (*n* = 242)	16% (*n* = 71)
30 mins to 1 h	38% (*n* = 449)	28% (*n* = 42)	35% (*n* = 198)	46% (*n* = 209)
1–2 h	15% (*n* = 174)	10% (*n* = 15)	14% (*n* = 82)	17% (*n* = 77)
2 h to half a day	7% (*n* = 78)	2% (*n* = 3)	2% (*n* = 12)	14% (*n* = 82)
More than half a day	1% (*n* = 8)	0% (*n* = 0)	1% (n = 3)	1% (*n* = 5)
Don't know/ refused	6% (*n* = 68)	7% (*n* = 11)	5% (n = 30)	6% (*n* = 27)
Method of transport to health facility				
Mechanized[a]	52% (*n* = 580)	17% (*n* = 24)	54% (*n* = 289)	60% (*n* = 267)
Non-mechanized	11% (*n* = 124)	7% (*n* = 10)	0% (*n* = 1)	25% (*n* = 113)
Walking	37% (*n* = 417)	76% (*n* = 108)	46% (*n* = 243)	15% (*n* = 66)

[a] Private car (with or without payment), public bus/ mini-van, motorcycle

facility. More than one-third (37%) reported walking, and one in ten (11%) reported using a non-mechanized method (likely donkey) (Table 2). In study areas of Badghis province, there was noticeably less mechanized transport (17%), compared to more than 50% of respondents in Bamyan and Kandahar. More than three-quarters (76%) of respondents in Badghis indicated relying on walking to reach the nearest public health facility.

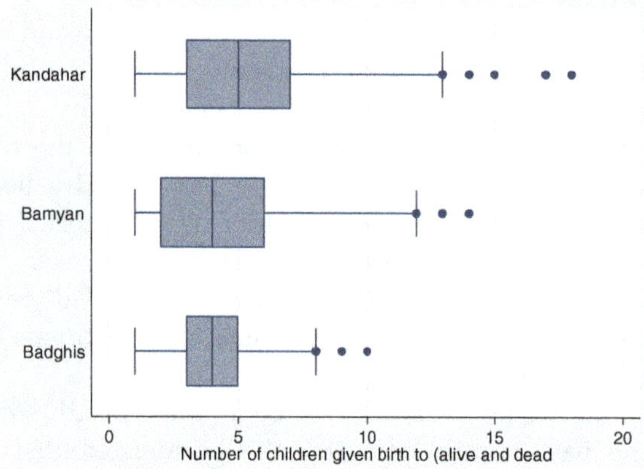

Fig. 1 Live and still births by province (mean, minimum and maximum)

On average, respondents in Kandahar and Badghis reported much lower transport and health service costs as compared to respondents in Bamyan. Interpreting the validity of cost estimates can be difficult, particularly when rural Afghan women, who are not generally in charge of payment and may lack numeracy skills, are asked for this information. This may help to explain high variation in cost estimates, ranging from 0 to 80,000 Afs. Figure 2 shows mean ranging from 163 Afs in Kandahar to a mean of 707 Afs in Bamyan. Figure 3 displays the variance in service costs reported by respondents who attended a public health centre between one and five times in the past year, with the widest variation occurring in Badghis.

Barriers to service use

In all provinces, the cost of health services and lack of transportation availability were among the top two most cited barriers to accessing institutional delivery among household questionnaire respondents in all provinces.

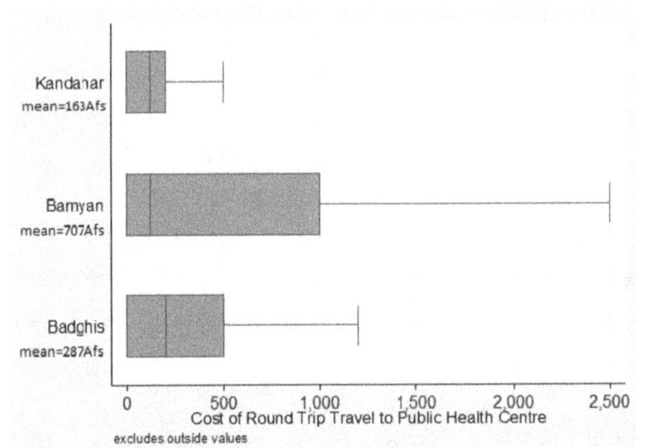

Fig. 2 Transport costs among respondents who travelled to a health facility between 1 and 5 times per year

Despite some consistent trends, a majority of respondents who identified specific barriers to institutional delivery varied greatly between provinces.

Among those respondents who had delivered none of their children in a health center, money to pay for services was the top reason for lack of attendance overall (56%, $n = 558$) and across the study locations in all three provinces (66% in Badghis, 52% in Bamyan, 39% in Kandahar). No transportation available was the second most widely cited reason (37%, $n = 368$ overall; 47% Bamyan, 43% Badghis, 12% Kandahar), followed by family restrictions ($n = 30\%$, $n = 302$). It is notable that family restrictions were comparatively higher in Badghis (46%, $n = 241$) and Kandahar (21%, $n = 47$), than in Bamyan (6%, $n = 14$) (Table 3). In addition, respondents in Badghis emphasised familial or cultural barriers as one of the top three barriers to institutional delivery, while respondents in other districts rarely mentioned this issue. Overall we found that the proportion of women reporting barriers to institutional delivery were 1.3–10.0 fold lower in Kandahar and Bamyan provinces than in Badghis province (Table 3).

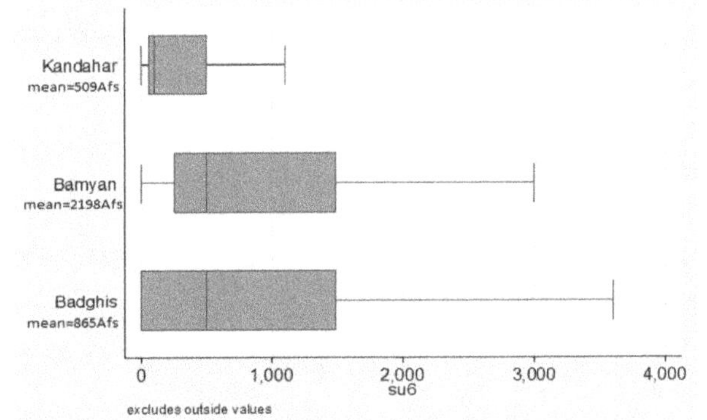

Fig. 3 Health service costs among respondents who had travelled to a health facility between 1 and 5 times per year

Qualitative data

A total of 9 FGDs and 16 KIIs were conducted by trained qualitative data collectors (Table 1). Although health care services are supposed to be free in Afghanistan, payment for services was a major and recurrent theme. Qualitative data from this study confirmed and provided more detail concerning barriers to health facilities and institutional delivery, in particular relating to cost. Some respondents referred to payment for midwives and doctors as 'sweets,' a term often used to imply traditional pressure to give gifts for service or after happy events, such as birth, or a subtler way of asking for a bribe. A community leader from Badghis reported: "A number of people give birth to children at home because they don't have money to pay 'sweets' to the midwives which is at least AFN 2,000 [about 29 USD) and this is a big amount for poor people. People who are good economically give birth to children in the clinic or hospital with midwives."

Another common theme was distance from health facilities and problems with transport availability, unsurprising as the sample is purposively selected to represent rural areas. One woman from Kandahar reported: "The problem is transportation. Vehicles break down on the way as the road is very bad." Problems are often confounded for rural woman, with many barriers present at once. For example, a woman from Badghis spoke of several barriers to institutional delivery: "The women face many problems during childbirth. The health centre is far and there is no ambulance to transfer the patient to the clinic, and they can't pay for a taxi because the rent is too high."

Discussion

This study contributes to understanding the barriers to institutional delivery in Afghanistan in rural locations of three provinces. Overall, barriers to institutional delivery are consistent with available evidence – though with some variation by location – indicating that distance, transport cost, and social factors act as inhibitors for women to access skilled care at health facilities.

Distance to the closest health facility is an important barrier to in-facility births in rural areas in Afghanistan and in other developing countries within the region and in other regions [22, 23]. A study in Afghanistan found: "small variations in distance were still associated with major differences in skilled birth attendant use" [8]. Distance to health facilities has improved overall in the last fifteen years, with new health facilities built, staffed, and equipped, so that now 88.2% of rural populations in Afghanistan are less than two hours from a health facility [3]. Still, in areas where geographic terrain is difficult, especially in the winter months – particularly Badghis and Bamyan – maldistribution of health facilities remains an issue for access.

Table 3 Barriers to institutional delivery among women who did not birth any children in a health centre among all respondents

	Province	Responses	Odds Ratio	95% CI	*P*-value
Money for health services	Badghis	62% (*n* = 508)	1.0		
	Bamyan	17% (*n* = 139)	0.110	0.092–0.145	< 0.001
	Kandahar	30% (n = 247)	0.750	0.209–0.316	< 0.001
	Overall	36% (*n* = 894)			
Money for transportation	Badghis	26% (*n* = 209)	1.0		
	Bamyan	6% (*n* = 54)	0.196	0.142–0.270	< 0.001
	Kandahar	27% (*n* = 223)	1.097	0.879–1.369	0.409
	Overall	20% (*n* = 486)			
No transportation available	Badghis	44% (*n* = 355)	1.0		
	Bamyan	16% (*n* = 137)	0.248	0.197–0.313	< 0.001
	Kandahar	13% (*n* = 107)	0.194	0.152–0.249	< 0.001
	Overall	24% (*n* = 599)			
Too far/no time	Badghis	28% (*n* = 229)	1.0		
	Bamyan	9% (*n* = 74)	0.249	0.188–0.332	< 0.001
	Kandahar	7% (*n* = 60)	0.205	0.151–0.279	< 0.001
	Overall	15% (*n* = 363)			
Not safe to travel	Badghis	13% (*n* = 102)	1.0		
	Bamyan	1% (*n* = 9)	0.075	0.037–0.150	< 0.001
	Kandahar	6% (*n* = 49)	0.446	0.312–0.637	< 0.001
	Overall	6% (*n* = 160)			
Family restrictions	Badghis	43% (*n* = 349)	1.0		
	Bamyan	2% (n = 15)	0.022	0.011–0.039	< 0.001
	Kandahar	12% (n = 102)	0.187	0.145–0.241	< 0.001
	Overall	19% (*n* = 466)			
No female staff	Badghis	13% (*n* = 103)	1.0		
	Bamyan	0% (n = 4)	0.032	0.011–0.088	< 0.001
	Kandahar	6% (*n* = 51)	0.436	0.305–0.622	< 0.001
	Overall	6% (n = 158)			
Poor quality care	Badghis	18% (*n* = 146)	1.0		
	Bamyan	2% (n = 16)	0.089	0.052–0.151	< 0.001
	Kandahar	6% (*n* = 53)	0.322	0.231–0.448	< 0.001
	Overall	9% (*n* = 215)			
Services not available/ did not know about services	Badghis	27% (*n* = 219)	1.0		
	Bamyan	4% (n = 34)	0.113	0.077–0.165	< 0.001
	Kandahar	10% (n = 81)	0.296	0.225–0.391	< 0.001
	Overall	13% (*n* = 334)			
Against religion	Badghis	3% (n = 28)	1.0		
	Bamyan	0% (n = 2)	0.066	0.015–0.278	< 0.001
	Kandahar	2% (n = 15)	0.520	0.276–0.982	0.044
	Overall	2% (*n* = 45)			
Did not think services were necessary	Badghis	20% (*n* = 159)	1.0		
	Bamyan	17% (n = 146)	0.846	0.658–1.087	0.192
	Kandahar	10% (*n* = 83)	0.424	0.316–0.569	< 0.001
	Overall	16% (*n* = 388)			

Associated with this finding of distance to health facilities being a barrier, transport was identified as a major obstacle for women in labour to reach a health facility. This relates to both availability of transport (mechanized and non-mechanized) and cost, particularly of mechanized transport. Potential solutions suggested by a recent systematic review include motorcycle ambulance programs, collaboration with taxi services, community education, subsidies, and vehicle maintenance [24].

Out-of-pocket spending on health in Afghanistan is high at 73% of total health expenditures [14], and especially affects rural population, who live far from facilities and generally have lower incomes. Studies in other low-income contexts demonstrated that economic status acts as a more crucial determinant than access (e.g. distance and other factors) for institutional deliveries, for example in India [25]. The wide variation in responses on costs of transport and services reported in this study make interpretation difficult as Afghan women, largely excluded from financial transactions, are less likely to be able to accurately report costs. However, women identified cost as a main barrier in the questionnaire, further supported by qualitative evidence.

One study based in Herat, the regional capital near Badghis, concluded social factors were felt to play an important role in decision-making to seek care and contributed to delays in seeking and obtaining care [18]. In this study, cultural barriers were also reported as more strongly influencing decisions around facility-based care.

This study has some limitations. First, the sample size does not account for any design effect introduced through cluster random sampling. Second, the sample within 12 districts was too small to draw nationally representative conclusions, though the sample – with almost 2500 women respondents – is larger than similar studies on maternal health conducted in Afghanistan. Variance at the community, district, and provincial levels also cannot be accurately represented with the sample size reported, though randomization did occur at village level to make the sample more representative. For each identified barrier, a chi-square test of independence was conducted to identify whether the rate of identification of this barrier was significantly different between provinces. Collecting data from female respondents, often excluded from financial transactions and with little educational exposure, likely reduces the accuracy of some data collected such as distance, time and cost of health services. Biases can occur in social desirability of responses, though this and other issues and techniques for quantitative and qualitative data collection were covered during the data collector training in efforts to minimize these biases.. The localised data collected in FGDs and KIIs is also not appropriate to be used in drawing representative conclusions about the study area as a whole. However, these data provide an additional level of insight into issues not available from quantitative information alone and are imperative to contextualizing findings and providing nuance to the evaluation of maternal and newborn service uptake, a complex and multidimensional process.

To further improve institutional deliveries in rural areas, schemes that provide conditional cash transfers which try to address multiple barriers of cost and distance have been examined in a number of settings. A systematic review of studies on conditional cash transfers aimed at improved maternal and newborn health outcomes, including studies from 8 countries, suggests that these programs have increased antenatal visits, skilled attendance at birth, delivery at a health facility, and tetanus toxoid vaccination for mothers and reduced the incidence of low birthweight [26]. Another study found that demand-side financing schemes can increase use of maternity services, though attention must be paid to supply-side components, implementation, and sustainability [27]. Findings from these studies will be tested during analysis of endline data which will be examined shortly.

Conclusion

There are major barriers a woman to have a safe delivery in Afghanistan. These include distance, cost, and social factors. Proven and promising approaches to overcome these barriers to institutional delivery in Afghanistan should be explored and studied. While the main issues are largely the same, the nuances/local conditions need to be explored to tailor programs appropriately given Afghanistan's varied ethnic, geographic, religious, and security makeup.

Abbreviations

FGD: Focus group discussion; KII: Key informant interview

Acknowledgements

The authors would like to acknowledge the dedicated work of the other members of the study implementation team Mohammad Attai, Emal Mujadidi, Ahmad Wahidi, Rabbani Wardak, and Sherin Varkey. The authors would also like to thank colleagues and collaborations from the Ministry of Public Health, UNICEF and other UN agencies.

Funding

Japan International Cooperation Agency (JICA).

Disclosure

All authors contributed in their individual capacities and the views that are expressed in this article do not necessarily reflect the views of their respective organization.

Authors' contributions

AHS provided technical inputs on study design, data collection, and prepared the manuscript. JB oversaw data collection, conducted data analyses, and drafted the full study report. AIF, FF, MN, SS, and KME provided oversight and technical support for the study. All authors provided substantive input in manuscript revisions and read and approved the final manuscript.

Competing interests

The authors declare that they have no competing interests.

Author details

[1]UNICEF Afghanistan, Kabul, Afghanistan. [2]ATR Consulting Afghanistan, Kabul, Afghanistan. [3]Afghanistan Ministry of Public Health, Kabul, Afghanistan. [4]United Nations Office Complex in Afghanistan (UNOCA), Jalalabad Road, Kabul, Afghanistan.

References

1. WHO, UNICEF, UNFPA, World Bank Group, and United Nations Population Division Maternal Mortality Estimation Inter-Agency Group. Maternal mortality in 1990-2015: Afghanistan http://www.who.int/gho/maternal_health/countries/afg.pdf?ua=1. Accessed 4 Apr 2018.
2. UN Inter-Agency Child Mortality Estimation Group (IGME). Levels and Trends of Child Mortality 2016. http://www.childmortality.org/. Accessed 4 Apr 2018.
3. Newbrander W, Ickx P, Feroz F, Stanekzai H. Afghanistan's basic package of health services: its development and effects on rebuilding the health system. Glob Public Health. 2014;9(Suppl 1):S6–S28.
4. Akseer N, Salehi AS, Hossain SMM, Mashal T, Rasooly MH, Bhatti Z, Rizvi A, Bhutta ZA. Achieving maternal and child health gains in Afghanistan: a countdown to 2015 country case study. Lancet Global Health. 2016;4(6): e395–413.
5. Central Statistics Organization. Afghanistan Living Conditions Survey 2013–14. National Risk and Vulnerability Assessment 2016. http://cso.gov.af/Content/files/ALCS/ALCS%20ENGLISH%20REPORT%202014.pdf. Accessed 22 Jan 2018.
6. Transitional Islamic State of Afghanistan Central Statistics Office 2003. Afghanistan Progress of Provinces Multiple Indicator Cluster Survey. https://mics-surveys-prod.s3.amazonaws.com/MICS2/South%20Asia/Afghanistan/2003/Final/Afghanistan%202003%20MICS_English.pdf. Accessed 22 Jan 2018.
7. Afghanistan Central Statistics Organisation, UNICEF. Afghanistan Multiple Indicator Cluster Survey 2010-2011: Final Report. Kabul: Central Statistics Organisation (CSO) and UNICEF; 2012. http://cso.gov.af/Content/files/AMICS-Jun24-2012-FINAL.pdf. Accessed 22 Jan 2018
8. Afghanistan Central Statistics Organization, Afghan Ministry of Public Health and The DHS Programme. Afghanistan Demographic and Health Survey 2015. Kabul: 2017. https://dhsprogram.com/pubs/pdf/FR323/FR323.pdf. Accessed 22 Jan 2018.
9. Campbell OMR, Graham WJ. The lancet maternal survival series steering group. Strategies for reducing maternal mortality: getting on with what works. Lancet. 2006;368:1284–99.
10. Akseer N, Bhatti Z, Rizvi A, Salehi AS, Mashal T, Bhutta ZA. Coverage and inequalities in maternal and child health interventions in Afghanistan. BMC Public Health. 2016;16(Suppl 2):797.
11. Mayhew, et al. Determinants of skilled birth attendant utilization in Afghanistan: a cross-sectional study. Am J Public Health. 2008;98(10): 1849 56.
12. Newbrander W, Natiq K, Shahim S, Hamid N, Skena NB. Barriers to appropriate care for mothers and infants during the perinatal period in rural Afghanistan: a qualitative assessment. Glob Public Health. 2014;9(Suppl 1): S93–S109.
13. Singh L, Sharma A, Kumar M, Shinwari S. Public health care in Afghanistan: an investigation in suboptimal utilization of facilities. Health. 2012;4:794–801.
14. Afghanistan Ministry of Public Health. Afghanistan National Health Accounts 2014.
15. Thaddeus S, Maine D. Too far to walk: maternal mortality in context. Soc Sci Med. 1994;38(8):1091–110.
16. Fund for Peace. 2017 Fragile States Index. http://fundforpeace.org/fsi/. Accessed 22 Jan 2018.
17. Mashal T, Takano T, Nakamura K, Kizuki M, Hemat S, Watanabe M, Seino K. Factors associated with the health and nutritional status of children under 5 years of age in Afghanistan: family behaviour related to women and past experience of war-related hardships. BMC Public Health. 2008;8:301.
18. Hirose A, Borchert M, Niksear H, Alkozai AS, Cox J, Gardiner J, Osmani KR, Filippi V. Difficulties leaving home: a cross-sectional study of delays in seeking emergency obstetric care in Herat, Afghanistan. Soc Sci Med. 2011; 73(7):1003–13.
19. Azimi DA, Najafizada SAM, Khaing IK, Hamajima N. Factors influencing non-institutional deliveries in Afghanistan: secondary analysis of the Afghanistan mortality survey 2010. Nagoya J Med Sci. 2015;77(1–2):133–43.
20. Hadi A, Rahman T, Khuram D, Alam A. Raising institutional delivery in war-torn communities: experience of BRAC in Afghanistan. Asia Pacific Family Medicine. 2007.
21. United Nations. Designing Household Survey Samples: Practical Guidelines. New York: 2005. https://unstats.un.org/unsd/demographic/sources/surveys/Handbook23June05.pdf. Accessed 22 Jan 2018.
22. Bohren MA, Hunter EC, Munthe-Kaas HM, Souza JP, Vogel JP, Gülmezoglu. Facilitators and barriers to facility-based delivery in low- and middle-income countries: a qualitative evidence synthesis. Reprod Health. 2014;11:71.
23. Moyer CA, Mustafa A. Drivers and deterrents of facility delivery in sub-Saharan Africa: a systematic review. Reprod Health. 2013;10:40.
24. Wilson A, et al. A systematic review and thematic synthesis of qualitative studies on maternal emergency transport in low- and middle-income countries. Int J Gynecol Obstet. 2013;122(3:192–201.
25. Kesterton AJ, Cleland J, Sloggett A, Ronsman C. Institutional delivery in rural India: the relative importance of accessibility and economic status. BMC Pregnancy and Childbirth. 2010;10:30.
26. Glassman A, et al. Impact of conditional cash transfers on maternal and newborn health. J Health Popul Nutr. 2013;31(4 Suppl 2):S48–66.
27. Murray SF, Hunter BM, Bisht R, Ensor T, Bick D. Effects of demand-side financing on utilisation, experiences and outcomes of maternity care in low- and middle-income countries: a systematic review. BMC Pregnancy and Childbirth. 2014;14:30.

12

Systematic review of community participation interventions to improve maternal health outcomes in rural South Asia

Binod Bindu Sharma[1,2*], Lisa Jones[3,4], Deborah Joanne Loxton[5,6], Debbie Booth[2] and Roger Smith[7,8,9]

Abstract

Background: This is a systematic review on the effectiveness of community interventions in improving maternal health care outcomes in South Asia.

Methods: We searched electronic databases to June 2017. Randomised or cluster randomised studies in communities within rural/remote areas of Nepal, Bangladesh, India and Pakistan were included. Data were analysed as risk ratios (RR) or odds ratios (OR), and effects were adjusted for clustering. Meta-analyses were performed using random-effects and evidence quality was assessed.

Results: Eleven randomised trials were included from 5440 citations. Meta-analysis of all community interventions combined compared with control showed a small improvement in the number of women attending at least one antenatal care visit (RR 1.19, 95% CI 1.06 to 1.33). Two community mobilisation sub groups: home care using both male and female mobilisers, and education by community mobilisers, improved the number of women attending at least one antenatal visit. There was no difference in the number of women attending at least one antenatal visit for any other subgroup. There was no difference in the number of women attending 3 or more antenatal visits for all community interventions combined, or any community subgroup. Likewise, there was no difference in attendance at birth between all community interventions combined and control. Health care facility births were modestly increased in women's education groups (adjusted RR (1.15, 95% CI 1.11 to 1.20; 2 studies)). Risk of maternal deaths after 2 years (RR 0.63, 95% CI 0.24 to 1.64; 5 studies), and 3 years (RR 1.11, 95% CI 0.52 to 2.36; 2 studies), were no different between women's education groups and control. Community level mobilisation rather than health care messages at district level improved the numbers of women giving birth at health care facilities (RR1.09 (95%CI 1.06 to 1.13; 1 study)). Maternal health care knowledge scores improved in two community-based interventions, one involving education of male community members.

Conclusion: Women's education interventions may improve the number of women seeking birth at a health care facility, but the evidence is of low quality. No impact on maternal mortality was observed Future research should explore the effectiveness of including male mobilisers.

Keywords: Community, Networks, Rural, Pregnancy, Antenatal care, Delivery, Pregnancy complications, Maternal death

* Correspondence: BinodBindu.Sharma@uon.edu.au
[1]Mothers and Babies Research Centre, Hunter Medical Research Institute, Lookout Rd, New Lambton Heights, NSW 2305, Australia
[2]The University of Newcastle, Callaghan, Australia
Full list of author information is available at the end of the article

Background

More than 800 women worldwide die each day from pregnancy and childbirth-related complications [1] with 99% of these occurring in low and lower middle-income countries [2–5]. South Asian and sub-Saharan African countries bear the highest burden of maternal death [6]. The widest level of disparity in maternal mortality is between low/lower middle, and high-income countries. The lifetime risk of maternal death in high income countries is one in 3700, compared with one in 160 live births in low income countries [7]. It has been estimated that 16% to 33% of all maternal mortality may be avoided by preventing complications through the provision of skilled personnel at birth [8].

Quality care throughout pregnancy and childbirth is associated with good maternal and infant outcomes [9]. Antenatal care uptake in rural settings is dependent on social and cultural factors [10]. Increased access to antenatal care, provision of skilled birth attendants and pregnancy care awareness programs at the local level contribute to safer pregnancies and childbirth [11]. In rural families, money, food and other logistics have all been seen to have an important influence on maternal health outcomes [12]. For instance, in Nepal, pregnancy and childbirth are considered to be the domain of women [13]. Although mothers-in-law commonly make decisions on pregnancy-related issues [14], permission must be sought from the male head of the household for any costs associated with seeking pregnancy care. As it is very uncommon for men to take an interest in pregnancy-related care issues, the resulting lack of communication limits women's access to pregnancy care [15]. Gender disparity and discrimination is common in South Asian countries like Nepal and is particularly prevalent in rural settings [16].

Health care interventions are often limited to a rigid and structured operational framework rather than being designed to meet the socio-cultural and economic realities of the communities they serve [17]. National programs and strategies often fail to consider the hardship imposed by distance and lack of infrastructure that is peculiar to people living within rural settings [18]. Poor social status among women in South Asian countries is a great contributor to lack of family planning and a rising population growth. This "feminisation of poverty" in the region is a fundamental anomaly that has impaired societal development [19]. Engaging local people to educate and mobilise the community has the capacity to provide multidimensional benefits [20] such as: helping to modify practices [21], encouraging a sense of community [22], and emboldening the identification of local methods to address problems [23].

Changing people's attitudes is required, but the best method for doing this is unclear. This systematic review aimed to compare the overall effect of different approaches to community participation in maternal health care education compared with health service or control/standard care interventions, on important maternal health outcomes. Furthermore, this systematic review aimed to examine which interventions promote husband, family and community awareness and involvement in maternal health care and result in better maternal health care-seeking and utilisation of maternal health services for improved maternal health outcomes in rural South Asian countries.

The overall objective of this systematic review was to compare the effectiveness of interventions to promote family and community participation in maternal health care against standard health care and health service led programs on the outcomes: indicators of maternal health care knowledge improvement, maternal health care utilisation (antenatal care, facility birth, skilled birth attendant use), and maternal mortality in rural-remote regions of the South Asian countries, Bangladesh, India, Nepal, and Pakistan.

Methods

Search strategy and selection criteria

Database searches were initially conducted in November 2015 and updated in June 2017. No restriction was placed on language or year of publication (refer Medline search strategy, Additional file 1). Hand searches were conducted on the reference lists of included studies.

This systematic review and meta-analysis were conducted according to a prospectively registered protocol (PROSPERO CRD42016033201) dated 14 January, 2016 and reported as per the Preferred Reporting in Systematic Reviews and Meta analyses (PRISMA) Guidelines [24].

We included cluster randomised trials or randomised trials evaluating different community health promotion interventions compared against each other, or against control or health service-based interventions, involving women, men, family and community members living within rural areas of Nepal, Bangladesh, India and Pakistan. We excluded studies of urban populations, and middle to high-income countries. Primary outcomes included: indicators of improved knowledge among women of childbearing age, their husbands/partners, family and community members, skilled provider attendance at birth (formal provider, traditional birth assistant), delivery at a health care facility and maternal mortality. The secondary outcome was male involvement in supporting access to maternal health care provision defined as; the supportive role played by men particularly husband, father-in-law and others with decision making capacity to access care during pregnancy, childbirth and postnatal period [25]. Traditional birth assistant (TBA) is defined as; *"a person normally a female, who assists mothers during childbirth and who initially learns her skills delivering babies by herself or by working with another more experienced TBA"* [26].

Two authors (BBS, LJ) independently extracted data from the full-text articles using the Covidence program [27]. Any differences in opinion were resolved by consensus. Data were cross-checked for accuracy by both authors. Reviewers (BBS, LJ) independently assessed the risk of bias (low, high, or unclear) (refer Additional file 2) of all included trials using the Cochrane 'Risk of bias' tool and evidence quality was assessed using GRADE [28, 29]. Any disagreements were resolved by discussion until consensus was reached. Data were analysed using Review Manager Version 5.3. Meta-analyses were performed using fixed-effects modelling, random-effects modelling was substituted in situations where heterogeneity (I^2) was greater than 20%. Publication bias was assessed by visual inspection of funnel plots and incorporated in GRADE quality assessment [30]. Results for dichotomous data were presented as risk ratios (RR) with 95% confidence intervals (CI) [30. Continuous data were reported using mean difference (MD) or standardised mean difference (SMD) where appropriate [30]. All trials randomised the intervention at village or district level. To avoid unit of analysis error caused by clustering, the intra-cluster coefficient (ICC) was used to calculate the effective sample size of both intervention and control arms which was then used to adjust the standard error for all analyses [30]. Where not provided in the study, ICC estimates were imputed from other sources [31]. Data were entered into the analysis as inverse ratios (logOR or logRR) and adjusted standard errors. Sensitivity analyses were conducted including only trials of moderate quality or above [30].

In order to consider a study as overall having low risk of bias we defined that it had to have none of the domains considered as high risk of bias and at least four (not counting 'Other biases') considered as low risk of bias, and two of these must include 'random sequence generation' and 'incomplete outcome data' as the domains most likely to influence overall measurements of effect.

Results

We identified 5440 citations in our search strategy, removed 525 duplicates and screened title and abstracts of 4915 (refer to Fig. 1 'Study selection'), resulting in 115 articles which we assessed in full text against the inclusion and exclusion criteria. Of the 45 articles remaining, we excluded nine studies that did not report any of the stated review outcomes, 15 contained insufficient information to make a judgement on whether they should be included or excluded, and six related to registered trial protocols awaiting publication of results. Of the 15 remaining publications there were only 11 independent studies as four studies had appeared in more than one publication.

Pregnant women and women of reproductive age (15 to 49 years or < 50 years) were most commonly targeted (9 studies), in addition to their in-laws (1 study), community members of any age (2 studies), and both women and men of reproductive age (1 study) (Tables 1 and 2). All studies were from rural and remote areas of low or lower middle income South Asian countries sharing a similar burden of maternal morbidity and mortality, including India (3 studies), Nepal (2 studies), Bangladesh (4 studies) and Pakistan (2 studies). Population sample sizes ranged from 1058 to 29,889 pregnant women, communities (health units, rural unions) or live births.

Eleven studies randomly allocated communities to community interventions; 10 studies compared a community intervention to a standard health care or control group (Table 1), and one (Acharya) compared different types of community intervention combinations at village or district level (Table 2). Two studies (Baqui, Midhet) assessed a community intervention against standard care or control group and provided data for comparisons between different community interventions. Four studies (Acharya, Baqui, Bhutta, Sharma) involved the use of community members to mobilise their community to take part in maternal health education and take practical steps to improve maternal health care within the community. Baqui compared the use of both male and female community mobilisers with the use of female mobilisers only. Darmstadt used community health workers to deliver a community education intervention. Six studies (list studies) involved the participation of community women in maternal health education groups. The intervention periods occurred over approximately 2 years.

In addition to examining the results for each outcome, all community interventions were compared against:

a) standard care or control (10 studies) (Table 1), and;
b) other community interventions (3 studies) (Table 2);

We identified the following post-hoc Community intervention subgroups:

1) Use of community mobilisers to deliver maternal health education;
    a. Home care by male and female mobilisers.
    b. Community care by female mobilisers.
2) Community education by health care workers.
3) Women's maternal health care education groups.
4) Women's and men's maternal health care education groups.

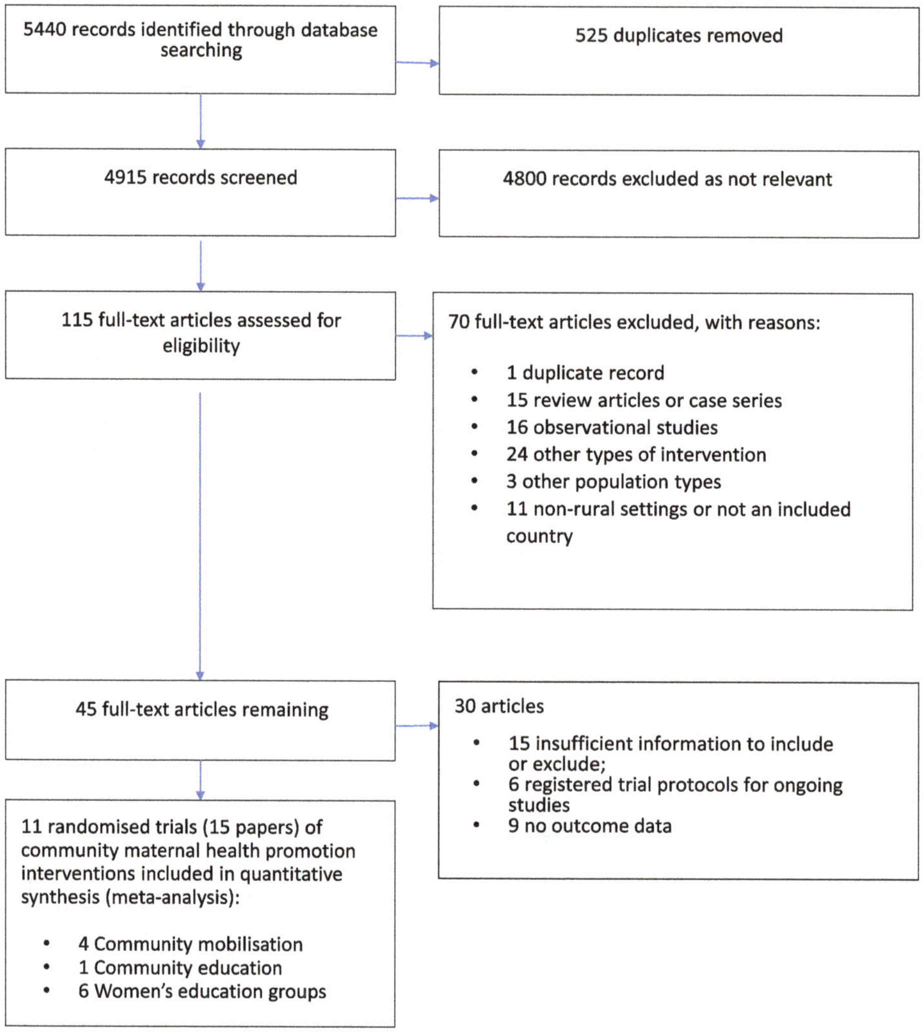

Fig. 1 Study selection

As the design of cluster randomised studies is likely to have made it difficult to provide blinded participation and assessment, we rated all studies not blinded or not reporting blinding, as unclear risk performance and detection bias. The main domains of interest for these study designs were random sequence generation, allocation concealment, incomplete outcome data and subjective reporting.

Overall, six studies were assessed as low risk of bias, two (Tripathy 2010, 2016) as unclear risk, and three (Azad, Baqui, Midhet) as high risk. Azad, Baqui and Midhet reported > 10% losses of population outcome data to the final analysis over the study follow-up period. Although population outcome data losses at follow-up were < 10%, Tripathy 2010 excluded twice as many women and live births in the control group (169 women, 171 births from a total of 9260 births; 1.8% losses) compared with that of the intervention group (83 women, 84 births from a total of 9770 births; 0.9%) due to deaths, stillbirths and migration. Similarly, Tripathy 2016 excluded a greater percentage of population outcome data from the final analysis in the intervention group (6238 women from 82,702; 7.6%) compared with the control group (28 women from 73,817; 0.04%).

The individual results of all included studies are shown in Tables 1 and 2.

Two studies (Darmstadt, Sharma) reported improved mean knowledge scores among women of childbearing age, their partners, and family and community members. There was a small improvement in knowledge of maternal danger signs RR 1.40 (95% CI 1.12, 1.75) in receiving community education intervention by community health workers compared with a control group, whilst Sharma demonstrated improvement in maternal health care knowledge among community members receiving health care messages in a community singing intervention compared with control. Post-intervention, knowledge doubled in the intervention group from a mean of 11.60/36

Table 1 Characteristics of studies. Community interventions versus health services, standard care or control

Study/Year published Country Duration of intervention	Design	Population	n	Risk of Bias [a]	Intervention	Control	Outcome	OR	RR
Azad [42] Bangladesh 2005 to 2007	Cluster RCT 18 clusters	Women aged 15 to 49 years having given birth during the study period	29,889	1. Low 2. Unclear 3. Unclear 4. Low 5.High 6.Low 7.Low Overall: High	Women's education groups plus health system improvement	Control (health system improvement)	Antenatal care		
							any	0.78 [0.51, 1.19]*	0.91 [0.76, 1.09]**
							≥ 4 visits	0.15 [0.06, 0.40]*	0·79 [0.46, 1.37]***
							Skilled birth attendant formal provider	0.45 [0.19, 1.11]*	0.90 [0.72, 1.14]**
							Delivery at a health care facility	0.75 [0.62, 0.89]***	0.97 [0.77, 1.24]**
							Maternal deaths		
							2 years	–	1.80 [1.2, 3.17]*
							3 years (N = number of live births for all outcomes above)	–	1.67 [1.00, 2.79]*
							MMR (over 3 years) (live births per 100,000)	388.9 vs. 189.10	2.02 [1.11, 3.68]** 1.74 [0.97, 3.13]#
Baqui [49] Bangladesh 2003 to 2006	Cluster RCT 24 clusters	All married women of reproductive age (15–49 years)	5110	1.Low 2.Low 3.Unclear 4.Low 5.High 6.Low 7.Low Overall: High	Community mobilisation: home care by female mobilisers visiting every 8 months	control	Antenatal care Any (N = number of live births)	1.70 [1.07, 2.68]*	1.13 [0.93, 1.36]*
					Community mobilisation: Community care by male mobilisers visiting every 10 months and female mobilisers visiting every 4 months	control	Antenatal care		
							Any (N = number of live births)	2.67 [1.70, 4.21]*	1.47 [1.21, 1.70]*
					Community mobilisation: Both community and home care	control	Antenatal care		
							Any (N = number of live births)	2.13 [1.33, 3.39]*	1.37 [1.15, 1.63]*
Bhutta [50] Pakistan 2006 to 2008	Cluster RCT 16 clusters	Pregnant women and women of reproductive age (15–49 years)	4474	1.Low 2.Unclear 3.Unclear 4.Low 5.Low 6.Low 7.Low Overall: Low	Community mobilisation	Healthcare workers (standard healthcare)	Antenatal care		
							Any	1.64 [1.03, 2.62]*	1.20 [1.01, 1.42]*
							≥ 4 visits	1.51 [0.79, 2.88]*	1.44 [0.75, 2.77]*
							Delivery at a health care facility (any) (N = number of women for all outcomes)	1.53 [1.36, 1.72]***	1.24 [1.17, 1.32]***

Table 1 Characteristics of studies. Community interventions versus health services, standard care or control *(Continued)*

Study/Year published Country Duration of intervention	Design	Population	n	Risk of Bias [a]	Intervention	Control	Outcome	OR		RR	
Darmstadt [51] Bangladesh 2004 to 2006	Cluster randomised trial 12 clusters	All married women of reproductive age (15–49 years)	3491	1.Low 2.Unclear 3.Unclear 4.Low 5.Low 6.Low 7.Low Overall: Low	Community education by community health care workers	Control	Antenatal care				
							Any	2.29 [1.34, 3.91]*		1.40 [1.12, 1.75]*	
							Skilled birth attendant	Not reported		Not reported	
							Delivery at health care facility (N = number of women for all outcomes)	1.20 [0.62, 2.29]***		1.19 [0.63, 2.27]***	
							Maternal danger sign knowledge score:	Mean score Intervention		Mean score Control	
								Pre	Post	Pre	Post
							a. Antenatal [0–10]	1.0	2.9	1.1	2.2
							b. Labor/ delivery [0–11]	1.1	2.4	1.2	1.9
							c. Postpartum [0–9]	1.0	2.5	1.0	2.5
Fottrell [52] Bangladesh 2005 to 2007	Cluster randomised trial 18 Clusters	Ever-married women of reproductive age (15–49 years) who were permanent residents including in-laws and adolescent girls	17,940	1.Low 2.Unclear 3.Unclear 4.Low 5.Low 6.Low 7.Unclear Overall: Low	Women's education groups plus health system improvement	Control (health system improvement)	Antenatal care				
							≥ 4 visits	1.37 [0.99–1.88]**		1.28 [0.13, 12.11]*	
							Skilled birth attendant	0.54 [0.38, 0.78]**		0.92 [0.71, 1.20]*	
							Delivery at health care facility (any) (N = number of births for above outcomes)	1.05 [0.88, 1.25]**		0.94 [0.55, 1.59]***	
							Maternal deaths 2 years (N = number of live births)	–		0.59 [0.30, 1.18]*	
							MMR (over 2 years) (per 100,000 live births)	153.4 vs. 276.10		0.74 [0.34, 1.64]**	
Midhet** [53] Pakistan 1998–2002	Cluster randomised trial 24 clusters	Women and men of reproductive age (all ever-married women under 50 years of age)	2564	1.Low 2.Unclear 3.Unclear 4.Low 5.High 6.Unclear 7.Low Overall: High	Women's and men's education groups	Control	Antenatal care				
							Any	2.83 [1.60, 5.00]**		1.35 [0.81, 2.25]*	
							Delivery at health care facility (any) (N = number of pregnant women for all outcomes)	1.3 [0.6, 2.7]**		1.28 [0.84, 1.96]***	
					Women's education	Control	Antenatal care				

Table 1 Characteristics of studies. Community interventions versus health services, standard care or control *(Continued)*

Study/Year published Country Duration of intervention	Design	Population	n	Risk of Bias [a]	Intervention	Control	Outcome	OR	RR
					groups		Any	2.45 [1.40, 4.30]**	1.32 [0.79, 2.20]*
							Delivery at a health care facility (N = number of pregnant women for all outcomes)	1.3 [0.7, 2.5]**	1.32 [0.86, 2.02]***
					Both interventions combined (women's education groups and women's and men's education groups)	Control	Antenatal care		
							Any	1.38 [0.82, 1.34]*	1.33 [0.84, 2.10]*
							Delivery at health care facility (any) (N = number of pregnant women for all outcomes)	1.46 [0.99, 2.15]***	1.43 [0.99, 2.07]***
Osrin [54] Nepal 1998–2000	Randomised trial 24 Clusters	Women (aged 15–49 years) and key members of the community in improving perinatal health outcomes	4241	1.Low 2.Unclear 3.Unclear 4.Low 5.Low 6.Low 7.Low Overall: Low	Women's education groups	Control	Antenatal care		
							Any	2.82 [1.41, 5.62]**	1.32 [1.08, 1.60]*
							(N = number of pregnancies) Skilled birth attendant		
							Any	2.50 [1.51, 4.16]*	2.26 [1.43, 3.57]*
							formal health provider (doctor or nurse)	3.13 [1.62, 6.03]**	2.96 [1.50, 5.84]*
							Traditional birth assistant (N = number of deliveries)	1.70 [0.93, 3.11]**	1.71 [0.89, 3.31]*
							Delivery at health care facility	3.54 [1.56, 8.05]**	3.38 [2.57, 4.45]***
							Maternal deaths 2 years		0.18 [0.14, 0.24]*
							MMR (over 3 years) (per 100,000 live births)	69 vs 341	0.22 [0.05, 0.90]**
Sharma 2018 [34] Nepal	Pre and post-test randomised	All community members (all ages eligible)	1572	1.Low 2.Unclear 3.Unclear 4.Low 5.Low 6.Low 7.Unclear Overall: Low	Community mobilisation: Community singing to deliver healthcare messages	Control	1. Mean change in knowledge scores (se):		
							a. Importance of antenatal examination (out of 7)	2·12 [0·06] vs 4.89 [0.06]	
							b. Importance	3·71 [0·07]	0.12 [−0.22,

Table 1 Characteristics of studies. Community interventions versus health services, standard care or control *(Continued)*

Study/Year published Country Duration of intervention	Design	Population	n	Risk of Bias [a]	Intervention	Control	Outcome	OR	RR
							of supplementary diet and rest during pregnancy (out of 9)	vs 6·84 [0·06]	0.46]
							c. Importance of delivery care (out of 12)	2·95 [0·08] vs 5·09 [0·07]	
							d. Importance of childbirth planning (out of 8)	2·81 [0·08] vs 5·50 [0·06]	−0.71[−1.3, −0.11]
							e. Overall knowledge (out of 36)	11·60 [0·24] vs 22·33 [0·18]	−1.02 [−2, −0.03]
Tripathy 2010 [55] India 2005 to 2008	Cluster RCT 18 clusters	Women of reproductive age (15–49 years)	17,335	1.Low 2.Unclear 3.Unclear 4.Low 5.Unclear 6.Low 7.Unclear Overall: Unclear	Women's education groups plus health system improvement	Control (health system improvement)	Antenatal care		
							Any	0.97 [0.48, 1.97]**	1.11 [0.99, 1.23]*
								1·60 (0·65–3·92)#	
							> 3 visits	0.68 [0.37, 1.24]**	0.70 [0.57, 0.87] *
							Skilled birth attendant		
							Any	0.52 [0.37, 0.74]**	0.70 [0.57, 0.87]*
							Formal provider	0.59 [0.37, 0.94]*	0.67 [0.46, 1.00]*
							Traditional birth assistant	0.82 [0.43, 1.56]*	0.88 [0.68, 1.13]*
							Delivery at health care facility(any) (*N* = number of pregnant women for all outcomes)	0.64 [0.39, 1.04]**	0.71 [0.66, 0.75]***
							Maternal deaths		
							2 years		0.82 [0.51, 1.33]*
							3 years		0.77 [0.53, 1.13]*
							MMR (over 3 years) (per 100,000 live births)	517.5 vs 680.3	0.70 [0.46, 1.07]**
Tripathy 2016 [56] India 2009 to 2012	Randomised Controlled Trial 30 clusters	Women of reproductive age (15–49 years)	7100	1.Low 2.Unclear 3.Unclear 4.Low 5.Unclear 6.Low 7.Low	Women's education groups plus health system improvement	Control (health system improvement)	Antenatal Care		
							Any	0.82 [0.35, 1.92]**	0.90 [0.75, 1.07]*
								0·63 [0·35–1·16]#	1.17 [0.78, 1.77]*

Table 1 Characteristics of studies. Community interventions versus health services, standard care or control *(Continued)*

Study/Year published Country Duration of intervention	Design	Population	n	Risk of Bias [a]	Intervention	Control	Outcome	OR	RR
				Overall: Unclear			> = 3 visits (N = number of births)	1.08 [0.58, 2.01]*	1.16 [1.12, 1.20]**
							Delivery at health care facility	1.23 [0.58, 2.60]**	0.63 [0.25, 1.42]**
							Maternal deaths 2 years (N = number of live births for all of the above outcomes)	–	0.63 [0.26, 1.55]*
							MMR (over 2 years) (per 100,000 live births)	222 vs. 349 0.63 [0.25, 1.42]***	

[a]Risk of Bias tool (Cochrane)
*Adjusted estimate using outcome specific ICC
**Adjusted estimate reported by authors – adjusted for clustering and stratification
***Unadjusted estimate reported by authors
#Adjusted estimate reported by authors – adjusted for clustering, stratification and baseline covariates

to 22.33/36, an increase of 10.69 points [$P < 0.001$], with only a modest change in the control population [17.48/36 to 18.26/36].

For the meta-analyses, all community interventions combined increased attendance of at least one antenatal visit compared with control by an average of 19% (RR 1.19, 95% CI 1.06 to 1.33; participants = 75,737; studies = 8; I^2 = 58%) (Fig. 2). Intervention sub groups: use of community mobilisers, community care using female mobilisers, home care using both male and female mobilisers, and community education by health workers, had a similar effect (Fig. 2). However, there was no difference in effect in the number of women seeking at least one antenatal visit for community care using female mobilisers, women's education groups, and women's and men's education groups. There was no difference in the number of women attending three or more antenatal visits from any community interventions, or any intervention subgroups, compared with control (Fig. 3). Likewise, there was no difference in attendance by a person of any skill level, formal provider (doctor or nurse) or traditional birth attendant between community intervention and control groups (Fig. 4). Deliveries in health facilities were increased in women's education groups for meta-analyses of studies reporting adjusted RR 1.15 (95% CI 1.11 to 1.20; participants = 36,989; studies = 2; I^2 = 48%) but not in meta-analyses of studies reporting adjusted OR 1.19 (95% CI 0.71 to 1.99; participants = 49,590; studies = 4; I^2 = 76%) (Fig. 5). Estimates of RR and OR are more likely to be similar when the number of events is rare, which may explain the difference between OR and RR for antenatal care attendance as the number of events are comparatively much higher. For this reason, we have based our discussion and conclusions on RR in preference to OR. There was no difference in risk of maternal deaths at two (RR 0.63, 95% CI 0.24 to 1.64; participants = 61,487; studies = 5; 94%), and 3 years (RR 1.11, 95% CI 0.52 to 2.36; participants = 48,921; studies = 2; I^2 = 82%), between women's education groups and health service, standard care or control (Fig. 6).

No studies reported on the secondary outcome, indicators of male involvement (fathers-in-law and male partners) in maternal health care.

In addition to the varying results and evidence quality in the interventions and intervention subgroups described above, further investigation of potential contributors to heterogeneity by population (country), and outcome measurement (follow-up period 2 years vs. 3 years) subgroups showed no reduction in heterogeneity for any combination of community mobilisation interventions versus standard healthcare or control. There were insufficient data to explore the effect of these on the remaining comparisons.

Discussion

Overall, meta-analysis of all community interventions combined showed modest benefits of in terms of improving attendance of at least one antenatal care visit

Table 2 Community participation interventions versus combined health service and community interventions or other types of community-based interventions

Study/Year published Country Duration of intervention	Design	Population	n	Risk of Bias [a]	Community and Health Service Intervention	Health Service Intervention	Outcome	OR	RR
Acharya 2015 [57] India 2005 to 2011	RCT	Women becoming pregnant or giving birth during the study period (average age 27 years) and their families		1. Low 2. Unclear 3. Unclear 4. Low 5. Low 6. Low 7. Unclear Overall: Low	Community mobilisation at community level (L2)	Community mobilisation at community level combined with health care messages at district level (L1 and L2)	Antenatal care		
							Any	1.21 [0.86, 1.70]*	1.04 [0.97, 1.10]*
							Skilled birth attendant	0.90 [0.56, 1.43]*	0.91 [0.61, 1.35]*
							Delivery at a health facility (*N* = number of women for all outcomes)	1.10 [1.03, 1.17]**	1.04 [1.02, 1.07]**
					Community mobilisation at community level (L2)	Healthcare messages at district level (L1)	Antenatal care:		
							Any		1.07 [0.98, 1.17]*
							Skilled birth attendant		0.83 [0.64, 1.07]*
							Delivery at a health facility		1.09 [1.06, 1.13]**
							(*N* = number of women for all outcomes)		
					Community mobilisation at community level (L2) involving 'Sure Start' community field workers working directly with ASHAs and strengthening village health and sanitation committees, and health care messages at district level (L1)	Healthcare messages at district level (L1)	Antenatal care:		
							Any		0.76 [0.19, 3.08]*
							Skilled birth attendant		0.83 [0.64, 1.07]*
							Delivery at a health facility (any)		1.05 [1.02, 1.08]**
							(*N* = number of women for all outcomes)		
Baqui [49] Bangladesh 2003 to	Cluster RCT 24 clusters	All married women of reproductive age		1.Low 2.Low 3.High	Community mobilisation: home care with female mobilisers visiting every	Community mobilisation: Community care	Antenatal care:		
							Any		0.76

Table 2 Community participation interventions versus combined health service and community interventions or other types of community-based interventions *(Continued)*

Study/Year published Country Duration of intervention	Design	Population	n	Risk of Bias [a]	Community and Health Service Intervention	Health Service Intervention	Outcome	OR	RR
2006		(15–49 years)		4.High 5.High 6.Low 7.Low Overall: High	8 months	with Male mobilisers visiting every 10 months and Female mobilisers visiting every 4 months	(N = number of live births, % = cluster averages)		[0.19, 3.08]* 0.94 [0.89, 1.00]**
Midhet** [53] Pakistan 1998–2002	Cluster randomised trial 32 clusters	Women and men of reproductive age (all ever-married women under 50 years of age)		1.Low 2.Unclear 3.Unclear 4.Unclear 5.High 6.Unclear 7.Low Overall: High	Women's and men's education groups	Women's education groups	Antenatal care		
							Any	1.42 [0.99, 2.05]*	1.05 [0.89, 1.24]*
							Delivery at a health facility (N = number of pregnant women for all outcomes)	1.01 [0.65, 1.56]**	1.01 [0.67, 1.53]**

[a]Risk of Bias tool (Cochrane)
*Adjusted estimate using outcome specific ICC (Page 1)
**Adjusted estimate reported by authors – adjusted for clustering and stratification
***Unadjusted estimate reported by authors
[#]Adjusted estimate reported by authors – adjusted for clustering, stratification and baseline covariates

but not the recommended four antenatal visits recommended by the World Health Organisation. Meta-analysis showed no difference in assistance of birth attendants at birth between all community interventions combined, or any community intervention subgroup and control. Women's education group interventions rather than health service or control, and community level mobilisation rather than health care messages at a district level, increased the numbers of women delivering at a health care facility. There was no difference in maternal mortality for meta-analyses between community intervention groups, intervention subgroups and health service, standard care or control. A community-based health promotion intervention [32], including men, women and community members from rural Nepal, showed an improvement in overall knowledge scores for antenatal care and skilled birth attendance.

There were several limitations to the findings of this review. Evidence quality varied across the outcomes for the three main comparisons (refer Additional file 2 GRADE tables). There was moderate to considerable heterogeneity for all outcomes. As the majority of studies were primarily designed to evaluate neonatal rather than maternal outcomes, there were no outcome specific ICC available to calculate adjusted estimates of effect for some maternal outcomes, meaning that some study data for some outcomes, such as institutional delivery, could not be included in the analysis. Studies reported different maternal health knowledge outcome categories which could not be combined in a meta-analysis.

Our review demonstrated improved maternal health outcomes where male community mobilisers were involved in home-based community interventions. Previous evidence suggests that the need to prioritise male involvement in maternal health care education in addition to measures that aim to improve women's education and their status in the family [33]. Involvement of the male family members in maternal health care education is of particular importance in low socioeconomic and uneducated community environments [34]. Intervention strategies involving men and community leaders in maternal health care programs in Bolivia resulted in improved maternal health outcomes in a low resource environment [35]. A study carried out in Maharashtra, India concluded that the maternal mortality ratio was three times higher among women with uneducated husbands compared to

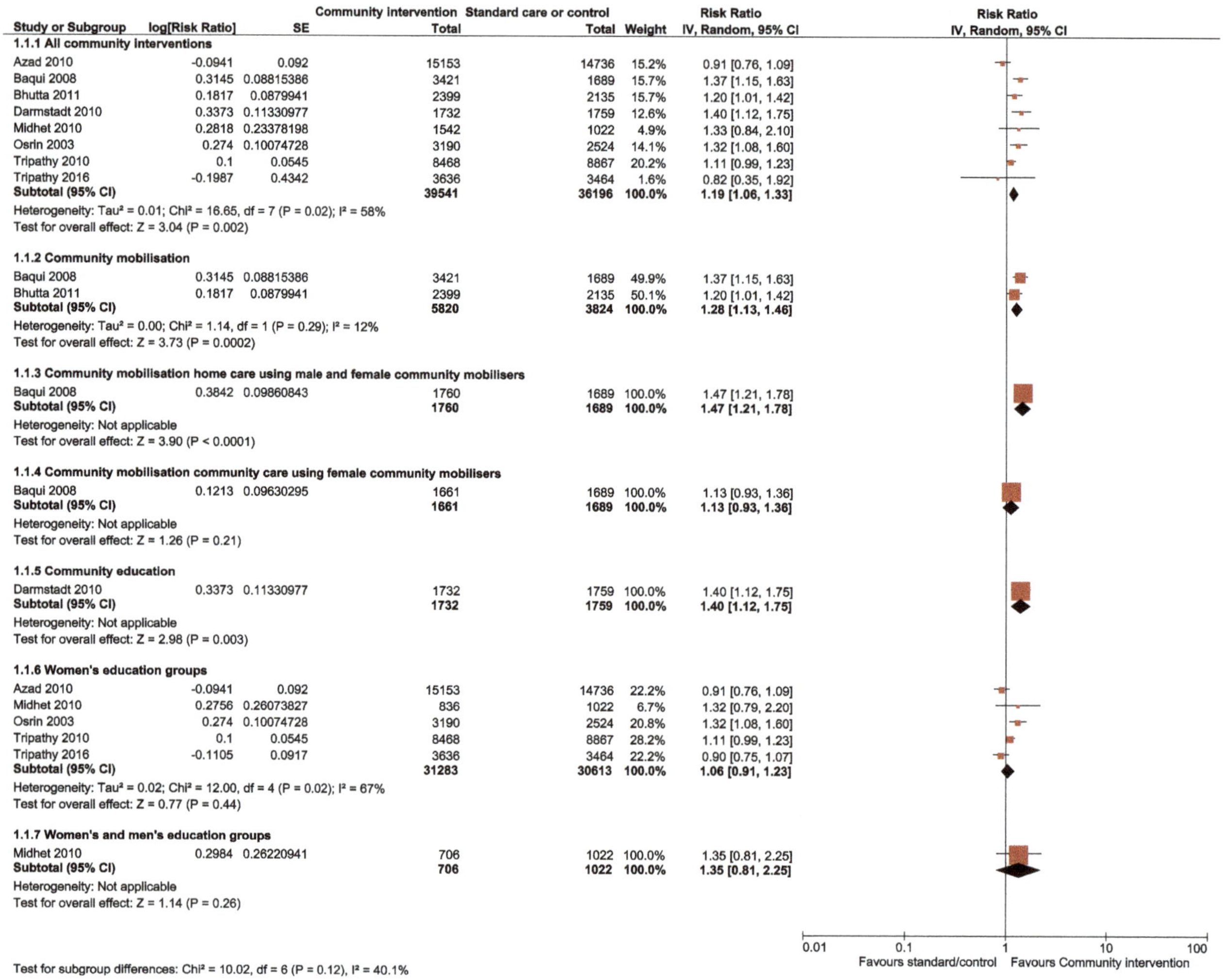

Fig. 2 Forest plot of comparison: 4 Community interventions vs. standard health care, control or no intervention (all adjusted RR), outcome: Antenatal Care (any) adjusted RR

the group of women with college-educated husbands [36]. The involvement of husbands in the utilization of maternal care needs to be included as equally important as the improvement of women's education and their status in the family [33]. Although the involvement of male (fathers-in-law and husbands) members in maternal health care is critical, [37] only one study reported this outcome.

Previous research has concluded that women from deprived communities with poor access to health care and low levels of education have an increased risk of mortality [38]. All community interventions, and use of community mobilisers were more effective than health service, standard care or control, while women's education groups, female mobilisers, women's and men's (couples) education were not. The selection of suitable interventions is critical. This could be one of the reasons that, although worldwide maternal mortality seems to be decreasing, there has not been a similar change for women in rural/remote areas of lower and lower-middle income countries in South Asia [39]. A study carried out in Tamil Nadu, India showed improved maternal health care knowledge among both males and females following education via mobile phone text messaging. Ninety eight percent of participants surveyed responded that text messaging was an effective means of health education [40]. Although this study was carried out in a rural setting, the high level of literacy in Tamil Nadu may have influenced this result. This evidence may therefore not apply to all rural environments of South Asian countries, as use of mobile phone demands many prerequisites such as: ability to read and write, buying a mobile phone, and accessibility to mobile networks in remote locations.

Our meta-analysis found that there was no difference in the risk of maternal death in communities allocated to women's education groups compared to standard care or control. In a systematic review of women's participatory

Study or Subgroup	log[Risk Ratio]	SE	Experimental Total	Control Total	Weight	Risk Ratio IV, Random, 95% CI
1.2.1 All community interventions						
Azad 2010	-0.2309	0.2784	15153	14736	23.1%	0.79 [0.46, 1.37]
Bhutta 2011	0.3669	0.3333	2399	2135	16.1%	1.44 [0.75, 2.77]
Fottrell 2013	0.2448	1.14776391	9106	8834	1.4%	1.28 [0.13, 12.11]
Tripathy 2010	-0.3575	0.3122	2457	2235	18.3%	0.70 [0.38, 1.29]
Tripathy 2016	0.1611	0.2084	1640	1612	41.2%	1.17 [0.78, 1.77]
Subtotal (95% CI)			**30755**	**29552**	**100.0%**	**1.01 [0.78, 1.31]**
Heterogeneity: Tau² = 0.00; Chi² = 3.85, df = 4 (P = 0.43); I² = 0%						
Test for overall effect: Z = 0.07 (P = 0.94)						
1.2.2 Community mobilisation						
Bhutta 2011	0.3669	0.3333	2399	2135	100.0%	1.44 [0.75, 2.77]
Subtotal (95% CI)			**2399**	**2135**	**100.0%**	**1.44 [0.75, 2.77]**
Heterogeneity: Not applicable						
Test for overall effect: Z = 1.10 (P = 0.27)						
1.2.4 Women's education groups						
Azad 2010	-0.2309	0.2784	15153	14736	34.7%	0.79 [0.46, 1.37]
Fottrell 2013	0.2448	1.14776391	9106	8834	2.0%	1.28 [0.13, 12.11]
Tripathy 2010	-0.3575	0.3122	2457	2235	27.6%	0.70 [0.38, 1.29]
Tripathy 2016	-0.3575	0.2747	1640	1612	35.6%	0.70 [0.41, 1.20]
Subtotal (95% CI)			**28356**	**27417**	**100.0%**	**0.74 [0.54, 1.02]**
Heterogeneity: Tau² = 0.00; Chi² = 0.36, df = 3 (P = 0.95); I² = 0%						
Test for overall effect: Z = 1.84 (P = 0.07)						

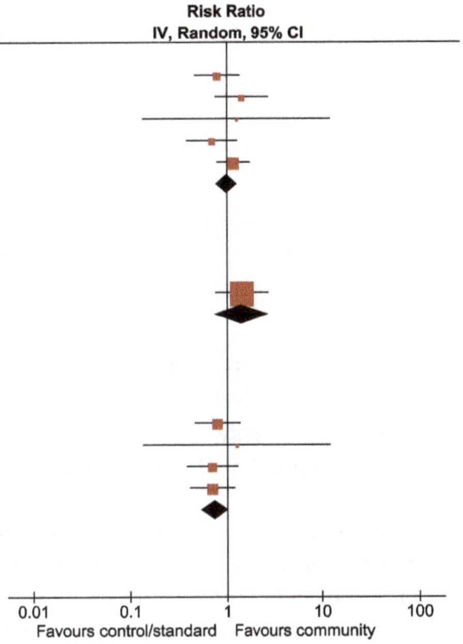

Test for subgroup differences: Chi² = 4.06, df = 2 (P = 0.13), I² = 50.8%

Fig. 3 Forest plot of comparison: 1 Community interventions vs. standard health care, control or no intervention (all adjusted RR), outcome: Antenatal Care (≥ 3 visits)

groups in Nepal, Malawi, India and Bangladesh, also no difference in overall maternal mortality was found [41]. After having further divided the women's group according to the percentage of pregnant women attending, Prost [41] found that maternal mortality was halved only in those groups having > 30% pregnant women (OR 0.51, 95CI 0.29–0.89). Similarly, in our analysis, the only study showing increased risk of mortality, Azad [42], at 3 %, had the lowest proportion of pregnant women attending women's education groups out of all the studies in the meta-analysis. It is possible that women's education interventions may need to include a larger proportion of pregnant women in order to be more successful in reducing maternal mortality.

Another systematic review assessing the impact of community interventions on maternal health in resource poor economies, revealed that community-based programs integrated with multiple interventions greatly improved maternal health outcomes [43]. A review of randomised trials aiming to improve antenatal care practice

Study or Subgroup	log[Risk Ratio]	SE	Community interventions Total	Standard care/control Total	Weight	Risk Ratio IV, Random, 95% CI
1.3.1 Skilled birth attendant (any)						
Osrin 2003	0.8171	0.2329	3190	2524	48.4%	2.26 [1.43, 3.57]
Tripathy 2010	-0.3536	0.1079	9468	8865	51.6%	0.70 [0.57, 0.87]
Subtotal (95% CI)			**12658**	**11389**	**100.0%**	**1.24 [0.39, 3.90]**
Heterogeneity: Tau² = 0.65; Chi² = 20.80, df = 1 (P < 0.00001); I² = 95%						
Test for overall effect: Z = 0.37 (P = 0.72)						
1.3.6 Skilled birth attendant (formal provider)						
Azad 2010	-0.1057	0.1208	15153	14736	30.1%	0.90 [0.71, 1.14]
Fottrell 2013	-0.0808	0.13308067	9106	8834	29.3%	0.92 [0.71, 1.20]
Osrin 2003	1.0855	0.3463	2945	3270	15.9%	2.96 [1.50, 5.84]
Tripathy 2010	-0.3931	0.2001	9468	8835	24.7%	0.67 [0.46, 1.00]
Subtotal (95% CI)			**36672**	**35675**	**100.0%**	**1.02 [0.70, 1.48]**
Heterogeneity: Tau² = 0.10; Chi² = 13.82, df = 3 (P = 0.003); I² = 78%						
Test for overall effect: Z = 0.11 (P = 0.92)						
1.3.7 Skilled birth attendant (traditional birth attendant)						
Osrin 2003	0.5382	0.3365	2945	3270	39.3%	1.71 [0.89, 3.31]
Tripathy 2010	-0.1332	0.13033649	8084	7034	60.7%	0.88 [0.68, 1.13]
Subtotal (95% CI)			**11029**	**10304**	**100.0%**	**1.14 [0.60, 2.17]**
Heterogeneity: Tau² = 0.16; Chi² = 3.46, df = 1 (P = 0.06); I² = 71%						
Test for overall effect: Z = 0.40 (P = 0.69)						

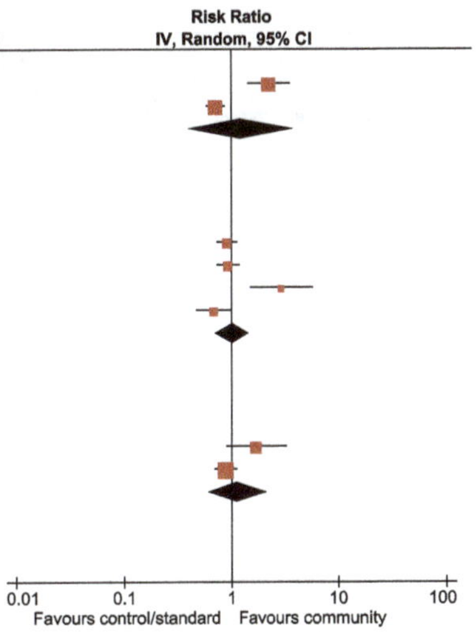

Test for subgroup differences: Chi² = 0.16, df = 2 (P = 0.92), I² = 0%

Fig. 4 Forest plot of comparison: 1 Community interventions vs. standard health care, control or no intervention (all adjusted RR), outcome: Skilled birth attendant

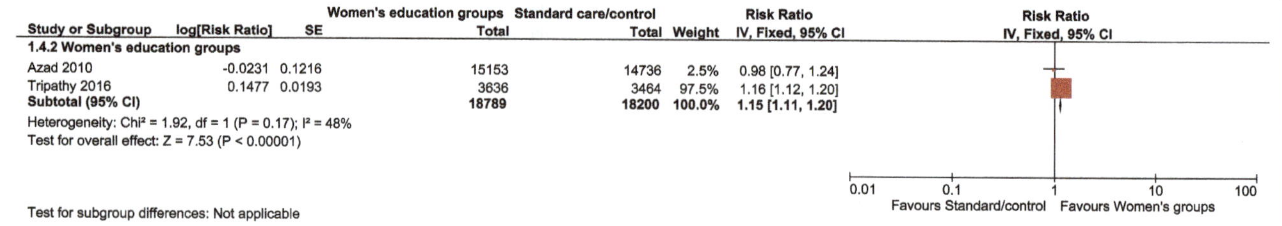

Fig. 5 Forest plot of comparison: 1 Community interventions vs. standard health care, control or no intervention (all adjusted RR), outcome: Delivery at a health facility (all adjusted RR)

demonstrated a reduction in maternal mortality (OR 0.62, 95% CI 0.39–0.98) [44]. The effectiveness of these community level interventions on maternal outcomes challenges the viewpoint that these programs are not worth the cost.

Women's education group interventions did not improve the use of skilled care at birth. It is possible that the involvement of men who control finances and family decisions and improving infrastructure may have improved this outcome. For pregnant women to obtain necessary antenatal visits and skilled care during childbirth, it is necessary to discuss and plan pregnancy care with the men who are responsible for decision-making within the family [45]. Antenatal care is essential to help prevent pregnancy complications and minimize maternal mortality.

Our meta-analysis showed that the numbers of women attending at least one antenatal visit were greater among women receiving any type of community intervention and intervention sub groups. This finding is supported by a study conducted in Nepal that demonstrated improvement in maternal health care outcomes in rural communities using a female facilitator in organizing monthly meetings with women's groups [46].

Increased access to antenatal care, provision of skilled birth attendants and pregnancy care awareness programs at local level contributes to safer pregnancies and childbirth [11]. Previous studies have concluded that delivery in a health care facility offers much needed emotional support to pregnant women [47]. Presence of skilled professionals, lifesaving drugs and equipment help to reduce the risk of complications and death of mother and baby [48]. However, our meta-analysis demonstrated unexpected outcomes of community intervention. For example, none of the interventions were effective in increasing the number of women receiving any level of trained or skilled assistance at birth.

Conclusion

A range of community interventions are likely to be successful in improving antenatal care attendance. Pregnant women receiving women's education group interventions were more likely to deliver at a health care facility. However, women's education groups were less likely to seek antenatal care or have a formal provider attend at birth. The contributing factors to this are unclear, but it has been previously suggested [41] that the varying

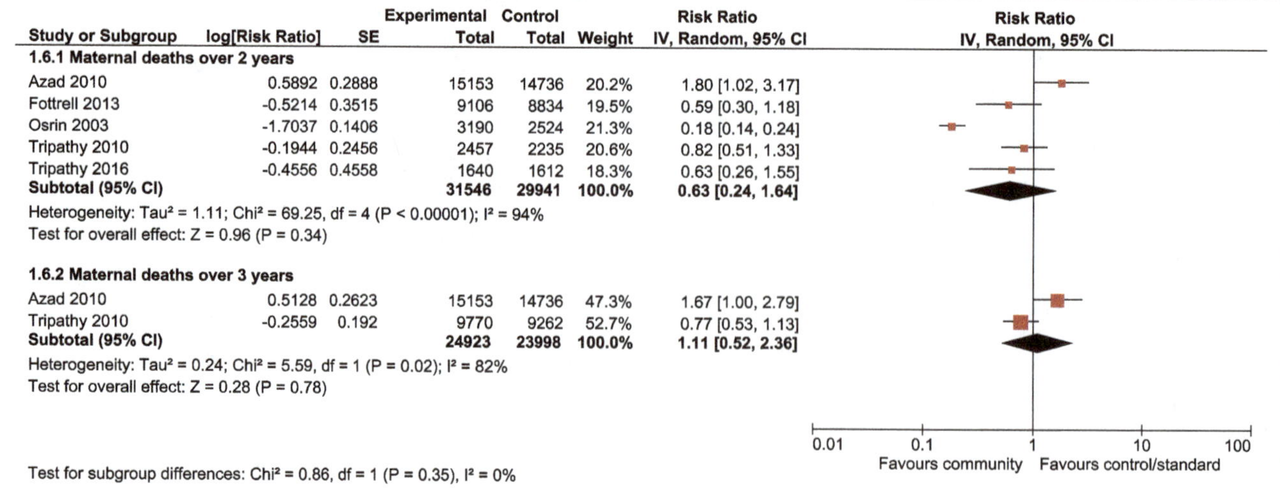

Fig. 6 Forest plot of comparison: 1 Community interventions vs. standard health care, control or no intervention (all adjusted RR), outcome: Maternal deaths (N = number of live births) STATA one-way ICC

proportion of pregnant women attending women's education interventions among the included studies may have been an important factor. Moderate quality evidence from a single study suggests including male alongside female mobilisers in community mobilisation home care programs [34] may improve the success of women's groups on maternal health care outcomes. Further research is needed on the impact of male involvement in community interventions to supplement women's involvement in community mobilisation, which up until now has been the primary focus, and the impact of couple's education in preference to women only. National health guidelines should include evidence from current systematic reviews of randomised trials, when planning interventions to promote community education on maternal health care.

Abbreviations

CI: Confidence interval; GRADE: Grading of Recommendations Assessment, Development and Evaluation.; ICC: Interclass correlation coefficient; MD: Mean difference; OR: Odds ratio; PRISMA: Preferred Reporting in Systematic Reviews and Meta analyses; RCT: Randomised controlled trial; RR: Risk ratio; SD: Standard deviation; SMD: Standardised mean difference; TBA: Traditional Birth Attendant

Acknowledgements

The authors would like to thank the University of Newcastle, Hunter Medical Research Institute HMRI) and staff and students of the Mothers and Babies Research Centre and Priority Research Centre for Generational Health and Ageing for their support during the study. We thank all the authors who provided additional information. Our thanks also go to HMRI Clinical Research Design and Stats Support Unit (CReDITSS)s for their generous support.

Funding

BBS received a 50:50 PhD scholarship from the University of Newcastle, Australia.

Authors contributions

BBS and LJ wrote and registered the protocol. DL and RS commented on the protocol and provided guidance for the searches. BBS, LJ, and DB finalised the search strategies and DB conducted the database searches for related articles. BBS and LJ screened the search results, assessed the eligibility of all relevant studies for inclusion and extracted data BBS and LJ contacted the authors of respective studies for additional information, LJ conducted the quality assessment and analysed data, both were checked by DB. BBS, LJ, and DB contributed to the final manuscript. RS and DL edited and commented on the draft and provided overall supervision for the systematic review. All authors contributed intellectually to the work. All authors read and approved the final manuscript.

Competing interests

The authors declare that they have no competing interests.

Author details

[1]Mothers and Babies Research Centre, Hunter Medical Research Institute, Lookout Rd, New Lambton Heights, NSW 2305, Australia. [2]The University of Newcastle, Callaghan, Australia. [3]Department of Neonatology, John Hunter Hospital, Lookout Rd, New Lambton Heights, NSW 2305, Australia. [4]Department of Obstetrics and Gynaecology, Sydney Medical School, University of Sydney, Camperdown, Australia. [5]Priority Research Centre for Generational Health and Ageing, The University of Newcastle, Callaghan, Australia. [6]Hunter Medical Research Institute, Lot 1 Kookaburra Circuit, New Lambton Heights, NSW 2305, Australia. [7]Mothers and Babies Research Centre, Hunter Medical Research Institute, Lot 1 Kookaburra Circuit, New Lambton Heights, NSW 2305, Australia. [8]Department of Endocrinology, John Hunter Hospital, Lookout Rd, New Lambton Heights, NSW 2305, Australia. [9]Priority Research Centre for Reproductive Science, The University of Newcastle, Callaghan, Australia.

References

1. Griffin S. Partners in health engage at UNCA: promoting global health through advocacy, education, and fundraising. J Undergrad Neurosci. 2016; IV:1–9.
2. Nour NM. An introduction to maternal mortality. Glastonbury: Rev Obstet Gynecol. 2008;1:77.
3. Pathmanathan I, Liljestrand J. Investing in maternal health: learning from Malaysia and Sri Lanka. Washington, DC: World Bank Publications; 2003.
4. Koblinsky MA. Reducing maternal mortality: learning from Bolivia, China, Egypt, Honduras, Indonesia, Jamaica, and Zimbabwe: World Bank Publications; 2003.
5. Pillai G. Reducing deaths from pregnancy and childbirth. Asia Links. 1993;9: 11–3.
6. Ronsmans C, Graham WJ. Lancet Maternal Survival Series Steering Group. Maternal mortality: who, when, where, and why. Lancet. 2006;368:1189–200.
7. WHO, UNICEF. UNFPA, The World Bank, United Nations Population Division. Trends in maternal mortality: 1990 to 2013. Estimates by WHO, UNICEF. In: UNFPA, The World Bank and the United Nations Population Division. Geneva: World Health Organization; 2014.
8. Graham WJ, Bell JS, Bullough CH. Can skilled attendance at delivery reduce maternal mortality in developing countries. Safe Mother Strat: A Rev Evid. 2001;17:97–130.
9. Paudel DP, Nilgar B, Bhandankar M. Antenatal care service utilization and contributing factors: a community based study in rural Belgaum, Karnataka, India. IOSR J Dent Med Sci. 2013;9:25–31.
10. Simkhada B, Teijlingen ER, Porter M, Simkhada P. Factors affecting the utilization of antenatal care in developing countries: systematic review of the literature. J Adv Nurs. 2008;61:244–60.
11. Baral OP, Vashisth K. Goal, strategies and programme of safe motherhood in Nepal. Acad Voices Multidiscipl J. 2014;3:19–23.
12. Shiffman J. Can poor countries surmount high maternal mortality? Stud Fam Plan. 2000;31:274–89.
13. Brunson J. Confronting maternal mortality, controlling birth in Nepal: the gendered politics of receiving biomedical care at birth. Soc Sci Med. 2010; 71:1719–27.
14. Simkhada B, Porter M, van Teijlingen E. My mother-in-law tells me what to do. Midwives. 2011;14:34–6.
15. Nwakwuo GC, Oshonwoh FE. Assessment of the level of male involvement in safe motherhood in Southern Nigeria. J Community Health. 2013;38:349–56.
16. Fikree FF, Pasha O. Role of gender in health disparity: the South Asian context. BMJ. 2004;328:823.
17. Stone L. Cultural influences in community participation in health. Soc Sci Med. 1992;35:409–17.
18. Soto EJ, La Vincente S, Clark A, Firth S, Morgan A, Dettrick Z, et al. Investment case for improving maternal and child health: results from four countries. BMC Public Health. 2013;13:601.
19. Bhutta ZA, Gupta I, de'Silva H, Manandhar D, Awasthi S, Hossain SM, et al. Maternal and child health: is South Asia ready for change? BMJ 2004;328: 816–819.

20. Jinadasa WMPK. The study of the potentials of folk-media performance as a form of effective communication in community mobilization. Proc Annual Res Symp. 2006;56
21. Ghosh SK, Patil RR, Tiwari S, Dash AP. A community-based health education programme for bio-environmental control of malaria through folk theatre (Kalajatha) in rural India. Malar J. 2006;5:123.
22. Jinadasa WMPK. Community development programmes and folk-media: a communication model for Sri Lankan rural society. Glob Media J. 2011;2:1–16.
23. Leong CML, Pan SL, Ractham P, Kaewkitipong L. ICT-enabled community empowerment in crisis response: Social media in Thailand flooding 2011. J Assoc Inf Syst. 2015;16:1.
24. Liberati A, Altman DG, Tetzlaff J, Mulrow C, Gøtzsche PC, Ioannidis JP, et al. The PRISMA statement for reporting systematic reviews and meta-analyses of studies that evaluate health care interventions: explanation and elaboration. PLoS Med. 2009;6:e1000100.
25. Kululanga LI, Sundby J, Chirwa E. Striving to promote male involvement in maternal health care in rural and urban settings in Malawi-a qualitative study. Reprod Health. 2011;8:36.
26. Leedam E. Traditional birth attendants. Int J Gynecol Obstet. 1985;23:249–74.
27. Covidence systematic review software. http:///covidence.org [Accessed 20 Nov 2017].
28. Schünemann H, Brożek J, Guyatt G, Oxman A. GRADE handbook for grading quality of evidence and strength of recommendations. 2017. The GRADE Working Group, 2013.
29. Review Manager (RevMan). Copenhagen, The Cochrane Collaboration; 2014.
30. Higgins J, Green S, editors. Cochrane handbook for systematic reviews of interventions Chichester. West Sussex: Wlley-Blackwell; 2011.
31. Pagel C, Prost A, Lewycka S, Das S, Colbourn T, Mahapatra R, et al. Intracluster correlation coefficients and coefficients of variation for perinatal outcomes from five cluster-randomised controlled trials in low and middle-income countries: results and methodological. Trials. 2011;12:151.
32. Sharma BB, Loxton DJ, Murray H, Angeli GL, Oldmeadow C, Chiu S, Smith R. Singing Health Messages is Effective in Transmitting Knowledge Regarding Antenatal Care in Nepal. Am J Obstet Gynecol. Under review.
33. Halim N, Bohara AK, Ruan X. Healthy mothers, healthy children: does maternal demand for antenatal care matter for child health in Nepal? Health Policy Plan. 2011;26:242–56.
34. Bhalerao VR, Galwankar M, Kowli SS, Kumar R, Chaturvedi RM. Contribution of the education of the prospective fathers to the success of maternal health care programme. J Postgrad Med. 1984;30:10–2.
35. Morrison J, Tamang S, Mesko N, Osrin D, Shrestha B, Manandhar M, et al. Women's health groups to improve perinatal care in rural Nepal. BMC Pregnancy Childbirth. 2005;5(6):1–12.
36. Ganatra BR, Coyaji KJ, Rao VN. Too far, too little, too late: a community-based case-control study of maternal mortality in rural west Maharashtra, India. Bull World Health Organ. 1998;76:591–8.
37. Chattopadhyay A. Men in maternal care: evidence from India. J Biosoc Sci. 2012;44:129–53.
38. Bhandari A, Gordon M, Shakya G. Reducing maternal mortality in Nepal. BJOG. 2011;118:26–30.
39. Dhakal S. Maternal mortality falls in Nepal but inequalities exist. Lancet. 2007;370:1301.
40. Datta SS, Ranganathan P, Sivakumar KS. A study to assess the feasibility of text messaging service in delivering maternal and child healthcare messages in a rural area of Tamil nadu, India. Austral Med J. 2014;7:175–80.
41. Prost A, Colbourn T, Seward N, Azad K, Coomarasamy A, Copas A, et al. Women's groups practising participatory learning and action to improve maternal and newborn health in low-resource settings: a systematic review and meta-analysis. Lancet. 2013;381:1736–46.
42. Azad K, Barnett S, Banerjee B, Shaha S, Khan K, Rego AR, et al. Effect of scaling up women's groups on birth outcomes in three rural districts in Bangladesh: a cluster-randomised controlled trial. Lancet. 2010;375:1193–202.
43. Nyamtema AS, Urassa DP, van Roosmalen J. Maternal health interventions in resource limited countries: a systematic review of packages, impacts and factors for change. BMC Pregnancy Childbirth. 2011;11:30.
44. Kidney E, Winter HR, Khan KS, Gülmezoglu AM, Meads CA, Deeks JJ, et al. Systematic review of effect of community-level interventions to reduce maternal mortality. BMC Pregnancy Childbirth. 2009;9:2.
45. Li J. Gender inequality, family planning, and maternal and child care in a rural Chinese county. Soc Sci Med. 2004;59:695–708.
46. Manandhar DS, Osrin D, Shrestha BP, Mesko N, Morrison J, Tumbahangphe KM, et al. Effect of a participatory intervention with women's groups on birth outcomes in Nepal: cluster-randomised controlled trial. Lancet. 2004; 364:970–9.
47. Tumblin A, Simkin P. Pregnant women's perceptions of their nurse's role during labor and delivery. Birth. 2001;28:52–6.
48. Kesterton AJ, Cleland J, Sloggett A, Ronsmans C. Institutional delivery in rural India: the relative importance of accessibility and economic status. BMC Pregnancy Childbirth. 2010;10:30.
49. Baqui AH, Williams E, El-Arifeen S, Applegate JA, Mannan I, Begum N, et al. Effect of community-based newborn care on cause-specific neonatal mortality in Sylhet district, Bangladesh: findings of a cluster-randomized controlled trial. J Perinatol. 2016;36:71–6.
50. Bhutta ZA, Soofi S, Cousens S, Mohammad S, Memon ZA, Ali I, et al. Improvement of perinatal and newborn care in rural Pakistan through community-based strategies: a cluster-randomised effectiveness trial. Lancet. 2011;377:403–12.
51. Darmstadt GL, Choi Y, Arifeen SE, Bari S, Rahman SM, Mannan I, et al. Evaluation of a cluster-randomized controlled trial of a package of community-based maternal and newborn interventions in Mirzapur, Bangladesh. PLoS One. 2010;5:e9696.
52. Fottrell E, Azad K, Kuddus A, Younes L, Shaha S, Nahar T, Aumon BH, Hossen M, Beard J, Hossain T, et al. The effect of increased coverage of participatory women's groups on neonatal mortality in Bangladesh: A cluster randomized trial. JAMA Pediatr. 2013;167:816–25.
53. Midhet F, Becker S. Impact of community-based interventions on maternal and neonatal health indicators: results from a community randomized trial in rural Balochistan, Pakistan. Reprod Health. 2010;7:10.
54. Osrin D, Mesko N, Shrestha BP, Shrestha D, Tamang S, Thapa S, Tumbahangphe KM, Shrestha JR, Manandhar MK, Manandhar DS, et al. Implementing a community-based participatory intervention to improve essential newborn care in rural Nepal. Trans R Soc Trop Med Hyg. 2003; 97:18–21.
55. Tripathy P, Nair N, Barnett S, Mahapatra R, Borghi J, Rath S, et al. Effect of a participatory intervention with women's groups on birth outcomes and maternal depression in Jharkhand and Orissa, India: a cluster-randomised controlled trial. Lancet. 2010;375:1182–92.
56. Tripathy P, Nair N, Sinha R, Rath S, Gope RK, Rath S, Roy SS, Bajpai A, Singh V, Nath V. Effect of participatory women's groups facilitated by Accredited Social Health Activists on birth outcomes in rural eastern India: a cluster-randomised controlled trial. Lancet Glob Health. 2016;4:e119–e28.
57. Acharya A, Lalwani T, Dutta R, Knoll Rajaratnam J, Ruducha J, Varkey LC, et al. Evaluating a large-scale community-based intervention to improve pregnancy and newborn health among the rural poor in India. Am J Public Health. 2015;105:144–52.

13

Effects of a community-based data for decision-making intervention on maternal and newborn health care practices in Ethiopia

Ali Mehryar Karim[1*], Nebreed Fesseha Zemichael[1], Tesfaye Shigute[1], Dessalew Emaway Altaye[1], Selamawit Dagnew[1], Firew Solomon[1], Mulu Hailu[1], Gizachew Tadele[1], Bantalem Yihun[1], Nebiyu Getachew[2] and Wuleta Betemariam[1]

Abstract

Background: Community participation and community health volunteer programs are an essential part of the health system so that health services are responsive and accountable to community needs. Information systems are necessary for community health volunteer programs to be effective, yet effectiveness evaluations of such information systems implemented at scale are rare. In October 2010, a network of female volunteers with little or no literacy, the Women's Development Army (WDA), was added to extend Ethiopia's Health Extension Program services to every household in the community. Between July 2013 and January 2015, a health management information system for the WDA's Community-Based Data for Decision-Making (CBDDM) strategy was implemented in 115 rural districts to improve the demand for and utilization of maternal and newborn health services. Using the CBDDM strategy, Health Extension Workers (HEWs) fostered the WDA and community leaders to inform, lead, own, plan, and monitor the maternal and newborn health interventions in their *kebeles* (communities). This paper examines the effectiveness of the CBDDM strategy.

Methods: Using data from cross-sectional surveys in 2010–11 and 2014–15 from 177 kebeles, we estimated self-reported maternal and newborn care practices from women with children aged 0 to 11 months (2124 at baseline and 2113 at follow-up), and a CBDDM implementation strength score in each kebele. Using kebele-level random-effects models, we assessed dose-response relationships between changes over time in implementation strength score and changes in maternal and newborn care practices between the two surveys.

Results: Kebeles with relatively high increases in CBDDM implementation strength score had larger improvements in the coverage of neonatal tetanus-protected childbirths, institutional deliveries, clean cord care for newborns, thermal care for newborns, and immediate initiation of breastfeeding. However, there was no evidence of any effect of the intervention on postnatal care within 2 days of childbirth.

Conclusions: This study shows the extent to which an information system for community health volunteers with low literacy was implemented at scale, and evidence of effectiveness at scale in improving maternal and newborn health care behaviors and practices.

Keywords: Community-based information system, Community engagement, Community health workers, Women's development army of Ethiopia, Health extension program of Ethiopia

* Correspondence: mehryar.karim62@gmail.com
[1]The Last Ten Kilometers Project (L10K) 2020, JSI Research & Training Institute, Inc, Bole Sub-City, Kebele 03/05, Hs # 2111, Addis Ababa, Ethiopia
Full list of author information is available at the end of the article

Background

The World Health Organization envisions community engagement as a critical component of health care delivery systems [1–3]. Community engagement and community-based health programs are expected to ensure that health services are responsive to individual and community needs, adaptive to local cultural practices that influence health care behavior, accountable to the community, and desirable [2, 4–7]. Consequently, community engagement strategies and voluntary community health worker programs are increasingly being used to improve access and utilization of health care services in many settings [4, 5, 8]. For the community engagement and voluntary community health worker programs to achieve their objectives, community-led monitoring and evaluation of health service delivery, including a community-based health information system, are essential [9–11].

Community-led monitoring and evaluation, including community-based health information use, has many forms. Broadly, a community-based health information system is defined as community members actively collaborating with representatives from the health system to gather, analyze, interpret and use data to improve the efficiency of the delivery of health services to the community [9–13]. There are several examples of implementing health information systems for community-based programs to improve uptake of health services [8, 13–24]. These community-based information systems can be categorized into two types: (a) as a part of the health management information system of a national program, where salaried community health workers collect and use data to deliver and ensure quality of services, and the data are then aggregated and used at higher levels of the health system for program monitoring and planning purposes; and (b) a strictly community-level health information system in which health workers in the formal health system facilitate community health volunteers and community representatives to collect data and use it to plan and improve uptake of health services. For example, the Community Health Information System of the Health Extension Program of Ethiopia is part of the national health management information system [14], and the community-based health information systems of orphan and vulnerable children programs of Kenya, Tanzania, and Zambia are part of health management information systems of donor-funded programs implemented at scale [20–22]. There are several examples of strictly community-based health information systems or community-based program monitoring and evaluation systems where the information systems are implemented and used within the local community to improve the uptake of health services [18, 23–25]. Although there is evidence that the strictly community-based health information systems in Honduras, Kenya, and Nigeria were effective in improving health care utilization [13, 18, 23], and that in Uganda, community-based monitoring and evaluation improved health outcomes [24], these community-based health information systems were pilot studies, or they were implemented on a small scale.

A recent systematic literature review indicates that there is a need for more quantitative studies to assess the effectiveness of community engagement in maternal and newborn health services [8]. However, despite calls for effectiveness evaluations of large-scale programs [26], there are no examples of effectiveness in strictly community-based health information systems implemented at scale. We designed, tested and implemented Community-Based Data for Decision-Making (CBDDM) — a strictly community-based health information system for community health volunteers with little or no literacy — in 115 rural agrarian districts in the Amhara, Oromia, Southern Nations, Nationalities, and Peoples' (SNNP), and Tigray regions of Ethiopia, covering about 17 million people, which is about 19% of the total population.

This paper is the second in a series of four, investigating innovations designed to support the flagship Health Extension Program of Ethiopia to improve the maternal and newborn health of the country. The other three papers consider the Women's Development Army (WDA) strategy [27], the use of a Participatory Community Quality Improvement strategy [28]; and the Family Conversation strategy [29]. This study analyzes the effects of CBDDM on maternal and newborn health care practices in 83 districts covering a population of about 12 million people, a sub-set of 115 districts implementing CBDDM at the time.

Methods

Study settings

In Ethiopia, the rural district health system includes one primary hospital per district with 4–5 primary health care units—each primary health care unit comprises one health center with five satellite health posts to serve about 25,000 people. Health centers, staffed with health officers, nurses, midwives and laboratory technicians, provide preventive and clinical services. Health posts, each serving a *kebele* (community), are staffed by two female Health Extension Workers (HEWs) supported by a network of WDA volunteers in the community with little or no literacy, provide 18 packages of mainly promotive, preventive and selected curative services as part of the country's flagship Health Extension Program. Since 2004, the Health Extension Program has established about 16,000 health posts and deployed about 38,000 HEWs [30–32]. The WDA is also known as the Health Development Army.

One of the initial tasks of the HEWs was to train and graduate "model households", households that practiced proper household hygiene and sanitation and utilized basic service provisions (such as childhood vaccination and family planning) [33]. Building on the graduated model households, the Federal Ministry of Health introduced the concept of the WDA in 2010. The WDA strategy fostered community engagement to ensure that health care services were responsive to individual and community needs by engaging women volunteers from model families to disseminate health information and to facilitate uptake of high-impact interventions. Under the guidance of HEWs, the WDA network members were organized into groups, with one WDA team leader for every six WDA volunteers, each of whom was responsible for five or six households. Thus, each WDA team leader was responsible for linking 30 households in her neighborhood to use the services provided by the Health Extension Program. To date, the Health Extension Program has established a network of about 3 million WDA members [32, 34], which has led to improved maternal and newborn health care behaviors and practices [27].

The intervention

To support the Health Extension Program to implement high-impact maternal, newborn, and child health services, the Last 10 Kilometers (L10K) Project has implemented innovative, community-based strategies (see Additional files 1–3 of the first paper in this supplement) [27]. In partnership with 12 local civil society organizations, L10K has enhanced the interactions between frontline health workers and communities to achieve more accessible, efficient, and equitable maternal, newborn, and child health services [35]. Between 2013 and 2015, the L10K Platform strategy was implemented in 115 districts, covering about 3070 kebeles. The platform strategy included CBDDM; Family Conversation, a forum conducted at the household of the pregnant women with her family members during the antenatal period to reinforce birth preparedness; and Birth Notification to ensure early postnatal care. The current study was limited to the 2150 kebeles from the 83 districts in which L10K implemented only its platform strategy.

CBDDM fostered the kebeles to generate and use data to improve maternal and newborn health practices. The strategy identified underserved households and linked them with HEWs and kebele command post leaders (kebele administrators) to address the barriers in access to maternal and newborn health services. Accordingly, HEWs were trained to support WDA team leaders to map the 30 households in their catchment areas, to keep each under surveillance, and to ensure maternal and newborn health services along the continuum of care: through pre-pregnancy, pregnancy, childbirth, postnatal care — including newborn care, to childhood immunization (Fig. 1). The surveillance system used images so that it could be maintained and updated by individuals with little or no education. HEWs collected data from WDA team leaders' surveillance and drew on the kebele leaders to identify and address barriers to access maternal and newborn health services.

HEWs were required to visit households routinely to update the information in the Family Folders, the central piece of the Community Health Information System of the Health Extension Program [14]. Each household within a kebele has a Family Folder, which is kept at the

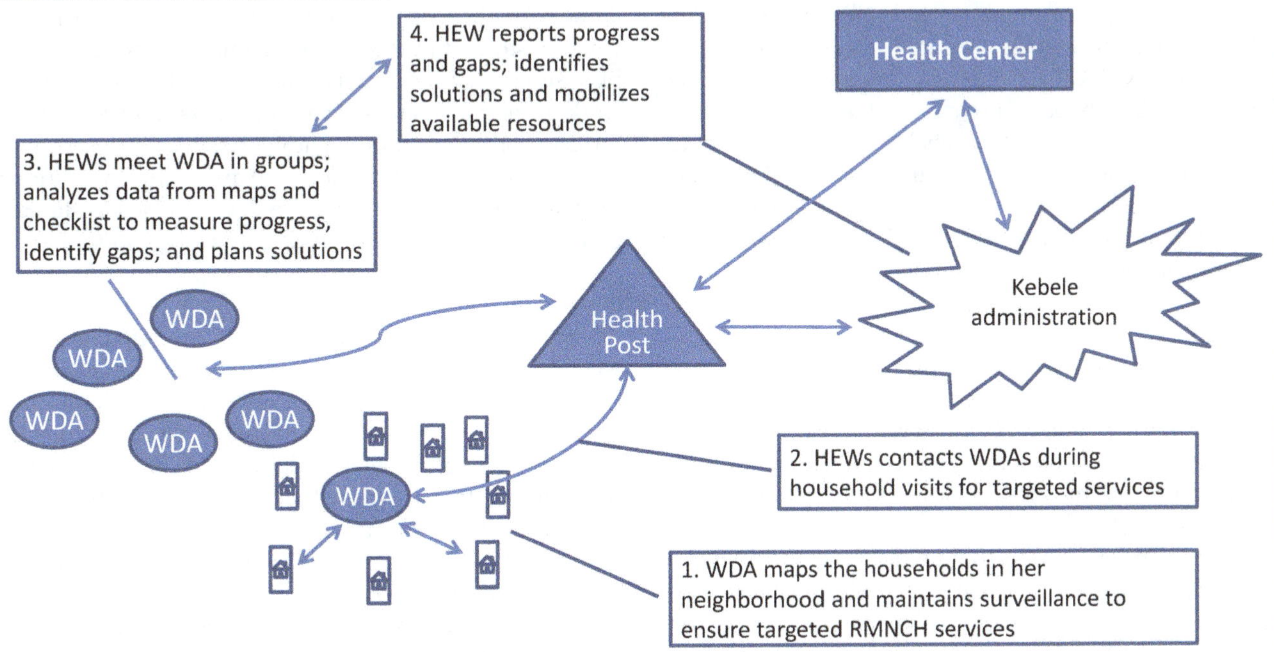

Fig. 1 Activities involved in Community-Based Data for Decision-Making

health post. It holds information on the family members, water supply and sanitation characteristics, and maternal and child care management records [14]. The CBDDM strategy gave an effective tool to HEWs to organize their household visits and to interact with the WDA to update the Family Folders. Although the policy to implement the Community Health Information System began in 2008, the actual implementation was initiated in October 2010 [14]; thus, the Community Health Information System was being rolled out at the same time as the CBDDM strategy was beginning to be scaled-up in the L10K areas. In the L10K areas the CBDDM was an important supplement of the Community Health Information System, which helped HEWs to personify and visualize the locations of their clients, whose records they maintained in the Family Folders.

Before the CBDDM strategy was implemented, it was prototyped in selected districts, among which were 14 of the 83 districts included in this study. Nonetheless, during the study period there were no additional inputs in the prototyping areas. We anticipated that there would be natural variability in the implementation intensity of the CBDDM strategy across the 2150 kebeles in the 83 study districts.

Study design

Using before-and-after cross-sectional household and health post surveys conducted in 2010–11 and 2014–15, we applied an internal comparison group design to examine dose-response relationships between improvements in CBDDM implementation strength in 177 kebeles during the observation period and improvements in maternal and newborn health care behaviors and practices during the same period. We measured the CBDDM implementation strength through interviews with HEWs and CBDDM activity records we obtained during the health post survey. Women with children aged 0 to 11 months in the kebeles reported care practices for their most recent pregnancy and childbirth. The hypothesis was that kebeles with a higher CBDDM implementation strength would have better improvements in maternal and newborn health care practices.

Sample size

We used data from the before and after household and health post surveys conducted in December 2010–January 2011 and December 2014–February 2015 to evaluate the larger L10K program. The survey design for the evaluation of the broader L10K program including sample size estimation parameters for the surveys are provided in Additional files 1–3 of the first paper in this supplement [27]. For the current study, the data were first restricted to the 195 kebeles included in the surveys where only L10K Platform activities were taking place, and which were visited for data collection during both the surveys. However, data from 18 kebeles were dropped, due to missing values of some of the kebele-level variables, leaving 177 kebeles in the study. The final sample size of women with children aged 0 to 11 months was 2124 in 2010–11 and 2113 in 2014–15.

Data collection and study participants

The household survey applied a two-stage cluster sampling method: at the first stage, kebeles were selected as primary sampling units with the probability of selection being proportionate to the population. At the second stage, the sampling strategy described by Lemeshow and Robinson (1985) was used to select the household with the target respondents [36]. The first household was selected randomly from the middle of the kebele, and from there every fifth household was visited, moving away from the middle. If the household visited had women with children aged 0 to 11 months, the women were interviewed, after seeking their consent. If a respondent was under 18 years old, then consent was sought from her husband, parents, or guardian. A quota of 12 women was interviewed from each kebele to obtain information on their socio-demographic background and the maternal and newborn health care behavior and practices associated with their most recent pregnancy and childbirth. The health posts within the sampled kebeles were visited, the HEWs based there were interviewed and the health post records were reviewed to obtain information on CBDDM implementation strength.

The data collection from households was carried out by health professionals working for regional health bureaus at zonal or woreda levels. They were recruited in consultation with the regional health bureaus. The supervisors were mostly from L10K's implementing partners. To avoid bias, supervisors and interviewers did not conduct survey work in their own areas. The supervisors were responsible for data collection from the health posts.

Ethical clearance was obtained from the Institutional Review Boards of the respective Regional Health Bureaus and that of the JSI Research & Training Institute, Inc.

Dependent variables

The maternal and newborn health care practices that were expected to improve due to the intervention were the coverage of four or more antenatal care visits to a health facility (ANC 4+), neonatal tetanus-protected childbirth (defined below), delivery at health facilities, receiving postnatal care within 48 h of childbirth (PNC in 48 h), clean umbilical cord care for home births, thermal care of the newborn, and initiation of breastfeeding within 30 min of childbirth.

If the mother reported receiving at least two tetanus toxoid injections during her lifetime, the last of which had occurred less than 3 years previously; if she received at least three tetanus toxoid injections during her lifetime, the last of which had occurred in the previous 5 years; if she received at least four tetanus toxoid injections during her lifetime, the last of which occurred in the previous 10 years; or if she had received at least five tetanus toxoid injections during her lifetime, her last birth was considered to be protected from neonatal tetanus. Clean cord care was defined as the umbilical cord being cut with a sterile instrument, the cord tied with sterile thread, and either nothing or only chlorhexidine applied to the cut end of the umbilical cord. Thermal care was defined as the newborn being dried and wrapped immediately after birth, delayed bathing of the newborn by 6 hours or more, and maintaining skin-to-skin contact with the baby. The analysis of clean cord care and thermal care was restricted among home deliveries.

Independent variables

The independent variable of interest for this study was the CBDDM implementation strength. During the follow-up survey, each kebele was assigned a CBDDM implementation strength score based on four items obtained during the health post survey: (a) the proportion of WDA team leaders in the kebele who had a surveillance map of their neighborhood; (b) the proportion of WDA team leaders who had either reported surveillance data to the HEW, or from whom the HEW had collected it, during the last 3 months; (c) whether or not the HEW had updated health post records of surveillance data; and (d) whether the kebele leaders had used surveillance data to monitor the utilization of maternal and newborn health services during the last 3 months. The first three items were measured from WDA activity records maintained by HEWs, while for the fourth item, HEWs were asked if there had been any meeting of kebele leaders (kebele command post meeting) at which maternal and newborn health issues were discussed. If the response was yes, then they were asked whether CBDDM data were used during that meeting. After verifying the responses from meeting minutes, they were recorded.

The first two item scores were probabilities ranging between 0 and 1, while the last two items score were binary responses, where kebeles received a score of 1 for yes and null for no. Each of these was standardized (with mean 0 and variance 1), and then all four were added together to obtain a scale. Cronbach's alpha, which reflects the internal reliability of the four items in constructing the scale, was 0.75.

The kebeles were ranked according to the score of the scale from the follow-up survey and then divided into three terciles. Due to ties, the three terciles were not equal. There were 68 kebeles in the lowest and middle terciles, and 41 kebeles in the highest tercile. The lowest, middle and highest CBDDM implementation strength score terciles were scored 1, 2, and 3 and named low, medium and high CBDDM implementation strength, respectively. At baseline, the CBDDM implementation strength score was assumed to be zero. Higher scores indicated better CBDDM implementation strength.

The independent variables that were considered as controls for the multivariate analysis were the individual, household, and contextual characteristics of the sample. The individual-level characteristics were age, education, marital status, parity and religion of the respondents; the household-level characteristics were household wealth and distance of the respondents' household from the nearest health facility; and the contextual characteristics were the HEW-to-population ratio of the kebele, administrative regions, and program stratum. The program stratum was an indicator variable indicating areas in which CBDDM was prototyped prior to the study period.

A single wealth index score was constructed for each household for both survey periods using principal component analysis of household possessions (electricity, watch, radio, television, mobile phone, telephone, refrigerator, table, chair, bed, electric stove, and kerosene lamp) and household characteristics (type of latrine and water source). Households from both the surveys were ranked according to wealth score and then divided into five quintiles [37].

Statistical analysis

First, we assessed the difference in the characteristics of the respondents between the two survey periods using Pearson's chi-square statistics adjusted for cluster survey design effects. Then we analyzed the distribution properties of the four items of the CBDDM implementation strength score using box plots. We assessed whether the background characteristics of the respondents were systematically associated with the CBDDM implementation strength score during the follow-up survey using Pearson's chi-squared statistics adjusted for cluster survey design effects.

We estimated the changes in the outcomes of interest between the two surveys and their 95% confidence intervals using post-estimation procedures following logistic regression models. The survey period was the only predictor in the logit models, and the models accounted for cluster survey design effects, using the Taylor series linearization technique for estimating variances [38].

We estimated the dose-response associations between changes in the CBDDM implementation strength score and the changes in maternal and newborn health care practices using kebele-level random effect models. We used Stata's '*xtlogit*' command for this purpose [38]. The models accounted for cluster survey design [39], secular change over time, and the individual, household and contextual characteristics of the respondents. We accounted for the secular change of the maternal and newborn health care indicator between the two survey periods by including the survey period as an indicator variable. The CBDDM implementation strength score entered the models as a linear term to identify dose-response association or the trend effect. To assess the contribution of the independent variables to the model, we grouped them into individual, household, and contextual factors. First, we estimated the model with all three groups of independent variables. Then we assessed the statistical significance of each of the three groups one by one using a likelihood ratio test. If a particular group was not statistically significant at $p < 0.05$, we dropped it [40]. We assessed the goodness of fit of the models using global Wald's statistic and the likelihood ratio test of the kebele-level random effects.

If the linear term for the CBDDM implementation strength score was statistically significant ($p < 0.05$) in the final model, then we tested it for departure from linearity (i.e. not a trend effect). We used the likelihood ratio test to compare the final model with the score as a linear term (restricted model) with the unrestricted model where the score was a categorical variable. If the two models were not statistically significantly different ($p > 0.05$) then we considered the linear term for CBDDM implementation score as adequate, and we concluded that there was a dose-response relationship, or trend effect [41].

Lastly, if we found a trend effect in the CBDDM implementation score, we did a counterfactual analysis to quantify the average treatment effects (ATEs) of CBDDM for maternal and newborn health care practices. We used Stata's post-estimation 'margins' command for the purpose [38]. The regression models were simulated to predict two values for each maternal and newborn health care practice. The first value was the predicted (adjusted) maternal and newborn health care practice when the CBDDM implementation strength score did not change from the baseline value (zero); and the second value was the adjusted maternal and newborn health care practice holding the CBDDM implementation strength score at its mean value during the follow-up survey. The difference between the second and first values estimated the effect of CBDDM on the maternal and newborn health care practice – the ATE.

Table 1 Sample characteristics by survey period

Characteristic		2010–11		2014–15		*p*-value
		%	*n*	%	*n*	
Women's age (years)	15–19	8	168	10	202	0.150
	20–34	77	1629	74	1566	
	35–49	15	327	16	341	
Education	None	73	1559	57	1204	< 0.001
	Primary	16	330	23	487	
	Secondary or higher	11	234	20	417	
Marital status	Single	5	105	4	75	0.034
	In union	95	2019	97	2034	
Number of children	1	21	448	29	609	< 0.001
	2	17	356	18	372	
	3	17	361	14	300	
	4+	45	959	39	827	
Religion	Orthodox	63	1342	62	1302	0.468
	Protestant	19	396	20	431	
	Muslim	17	358	17	355	
	Traditional/other	1	27	1	21	
Distance to any health facility	< 30 min.	64	1365	55	1163	0.002
	30 min - < 1 h	26	545	30	636	
	1 - < 2 h	10	214	15	309	
Wealth quintile	Lowest	28	604	13	256	< 0.001
	Fourth	21	447	18	380	
	Middle	20	426	19	407	
	Second	17	369	23	475	
	Highest	13	279	27	572	
Region	Tigray	13	284	14	286	0.317
	Amhara	38	808	38	791	
	Oromia	28	589	28	583	
	SNNP	21	443	21	449	
Population to HEW ratio	2500 or less	50	1059	47	996	0.407
	2501 – 3500	25	521	25	519	
	3501 – 5000	17	349	15	309	
	> 5000	9	195	14	285	
Program stratum	CBDDM only	76	1606	76	1607	0.427
	Prior program areas	24	518	24	506	
No. of respondents		100	2124	100	2113	

CBDDM Community-Based Data for Decision-Making, *HEW* Health Extension Worker, *WDA* Women's Development Army

Results

We found statistically significant ($p < 0.05$) evidence of change over time between the 2010–11 and 2014–15 surveys for the following background characteristics: education, marital status, parity, household distance from the nearest health facility, and household wealth (Table 1). Compared with the 2010–11 survey, respondents from the 2014–15 survey were more likely to be educated, had fewer children and were wealthier. The increase in wealth between the two surveys was mainly due to the comparatively higher proportion of households with electricity, mobile phones, household furniture, and piped water as the source of drinking water. Contrary to expectations, the respondents from the follow-up survey (2014–15) were more likely to be living

Table 2 Kebele-level measures of CBDDM implementation strength score and the items, 2014–15

CBDDM Implementation Strength Score Items	CBDDM Implementation Strength			Total
	Low	Medium	High	
% of WDA team leaders on average to have CBDDM map (Mapped)	82	98	99	92
% of WDA team leaders on average who reported CBDDM data in the previous month (Reported)	11	57	95	48
% of kebele command post leaders who used CBDDM data for monitoring maternal and newborn health services in the last 3 months (Used)	9	50	100	46
% of kebeles that have updated CBDDM registers (Updates data)	39	67	97	63
Number of kebeles	68	68	41	177

CBDDM Community-Based Data for Decision-Making, *WDA* Women's Development Army

further away from health facilities than those in the baseline survey (2010–11). The difference in the marital status of respondents between the survey periods was small.

The CBDDM implementation strength score during 2010–11 was assumed to be null. During 2014–15, on average 92% of the WDA team leaders had mapped their neighborhood for surveillance, while 48% of them had reported surveillance data to the HEWs. In 63% of the kebeles HEWs were maintaining CBDDM activity registers and 46% of the kebeles were using CBDDM data to monitor access to maternal and newborn health services (Table 2). Figure 2 provides the distribution properties of the CBDDM activity measures according to the CBDDM implementation strength score categories.

Table 3 compares sample characteristics of the respondents according to the CBDDM implementation strength score during the 2014–15 survey. Distance of the respondents' households from the nearest health facility was systematically associated ($p < 0.05$) with CBDDM implementation strength. Respondents in kebeles with relatively high CBDDM implementation strength scores were more likely to live nearer to health facilities. Parity was also associated ($p < 0.05$) with CBDDM implementation strength, but the association did not have any systematic pattern. Although the proportion of respondents in the prior CBDDM program area kebeles appeared to be relatively high in the kebeles with higher CBDDM implementation strength score, this effect was not statistically significant (because the unit of analysis was the kebele, which had a small sample size).

There was no evidence of change ($p > 0.05$) in PNC coverage, while the proportion of women who practiced clean cord care of their newborn among home deliveries declined ($p < 0.05$) between 2010 and 11 and 2014–15 (Table 4). We found some evidence of improvement for all other maternal and newborn health care practices during the observation period ($p < 0.05$).

We used random-effects logit models to assess the linear effects of CBDDM implementation strength on maternal and newborn care practices (Table 5). All the three groups of the respondents' characteristics were statistically significant ($p < .05$) in all the final models. The kebele-level random effects and the goodness of fit were also statistically

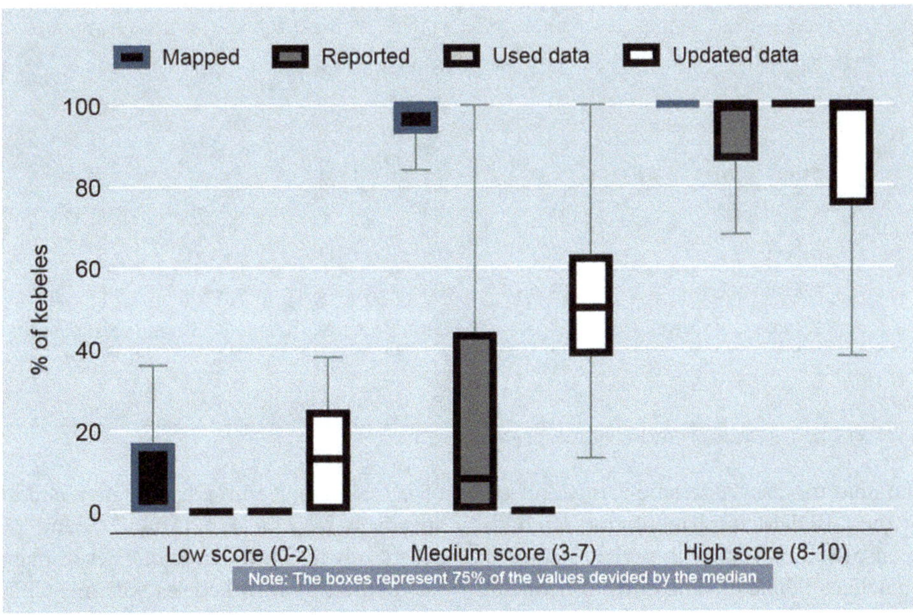

Fig. 2 CBDDM activities by CBDDM implementation strength score during 2014–15

Table 3 Sample characteristics by CBDDM implementation strength score at follow-up survey

Characteristic		CBDDM Implementation Strength						p-value
		Low		Medium		High		
		%	N	%	N	%	N	
Women's age (years)	15–19	11	93	9	69	8	40	0.506
	20–34	72	593	76	620	74	356	
	35–49	17	137	15	122	17	82	
Education	None	61	500	57	463	51	244	0.203
	Primary	22	178	23	190	25	121	
	Secondary or higher	18	146	20	159	24	113	
Marital status	Single	3	29	4	28	4	18	0.971
	In union	97	795	97	783	96	460	
Number of children	1	31	257	24	194	33	160	0.032
	2	16	133	21	167	15	74	
	3	13	110	15	119	15	72	
	4+	39	324	41	332	36	173	
Religion	Orthodox	57	465	62	506	70	333	0.179
	Protestant	24	201	15	124	22	107	
	Muslim	18	144	21	174	8	37	
	Traditional/other	2	13	1	7	0	1	
Distance to any health facility	< 30 min.	46	378	59	480	65	309	< 0.001
	30 min - < 1 h	33	275	28	230	28	132	
	1 - < 2 h	21	170	13	102	8	37	
Wealth quintile	Lowest	13	107	14	114	11	55	0.533
	Fourth	18	152	19	156	15	72	
	Middle	21	169	16	133	22	106	
	Second	24	200	22	176	21	99	
	Highest	24	194	29	233	30	146	
Region	Tigray	12	97	14	114	16	74	0.512
	Amhara	31	252	39	314	47	227	
	Oromia	35	287	26	207	19	89	
	SNNP	23	186	22	176	18	88	
Population to HEW ratio	2500 or less	44	365	48	392	50	241	0.533
	2501 – 3500	20	167	21	169	39	184	
	3501 – 5000	13	107	20	162	8	39	
	> 5000	22	183	11	89	3	14	
Program stratum	CBDDM only	81	669	76	618	67	320	0.251
	Prior program areas	19	154	24	193	33	158	
No. of respondents		100	823	100	811	100	478	
No. of communities			68		68		41	

CBDDM Community-Based Data for Decision-Making, *HEW* Health Extension Worker

significant for all the final models. Assessment of trend effects indicated that the CBDDM implementation strength score had dose-response relationships with several maternal and newborn care practices (Table 5). The odds of neonatal tetanus-protected childbirth, institutional deliveries, clean cord care and thermal care of the newborn, and initiation of breastfeeding immediately after childbirth increased respectively by 23%, 47%, 21%, 29% and 27% when we compared kebeles with low CBDDM implementation strength (at follow-up) with kebeles with no CBDDM implementation strength (at baseline); or when we compared kebeles with medium CBDDM implementation strength with

Table 4 Maternal and newborn health care practices during 2010–11 and 2014–15 surveys

Maternal and Newborn Health Care Practice	2010–11	2014–15	Change		
	(%)	(%)	%-points	(95% CI)	*p*-value
ANC 4+	28	52	24	(20, 28)	< 0.001
Neonatal tetanus protected birth	57	63	6	(2, 10)	0.004
Institutional delivery	9	53	43	(39, 48)	< 0.001
PNC in 48 h	10	11	1	(−2, 4)	0.426
Clean cord care among home deliveries	44	38	−6	(−12, 0)	0.036
Thermal care	26	57	30	(26, 35)	< 0.001
Immediate initiation of breastfeeding	53	76	23	(20, 27)	< 0.001

ANC 4+ received four or more antenatal care visits, *PNC* postnatal care

kebeles with low CBDDM implementation strength; or when we compared kebeles with high CBDDM implementation strength with kebeles with medium CBDDM implementation strength. However, we found no evidence that CBDDM implementation strength was associated with utilization of four or more antenatal care services and early postnatal care, which we defined as a visit within 2 days of delivery.

The ATEs of CBDDM on maternal and newborn care practices ranged between 8 and 15 percentage-points (Table 6). For example, 15 percentage-points of the institutional delivery rate at follow-up were attributable to the CBDDM strategy.

Discussion

We sought to assess the effectiveness of a community-based health information system, designed for a low-literacy community health volunteer program and implemented at scale, to improve maternal and newborn care behaviors and practices. We found strong evidence of a dose-response relationship between the implementation strength of CBDDM and better care practices, indicating that the strategy was effective. The findings were consistent with an earlier analysis of the effects of CBDDM on the utilization of maternal and newborn health care services, using program monitoring data and service statistics [42]. Engaging communities to collect and use data to plan and improve the uptake of maternal and newborn care services has been effective in other developing country settings [18, 23, 24].

The HEWs were mainly responsible for supporting the WDA to implement the CBDDM strategy. They used the strategy to provide targeted maternal and newborn health services and to maintain the Community Health Information System. Thus, the observed effects of CBDDM on maternal newborn care practices may partly reflect the efforts of HEWs, including the influence of the Community Health Information System. The effects of CBDDM are likely to be mediated by HEWs, including through their use of the Community Health Information System. Nonetheless, we concluded that the CBDDM strategy most likely improved the efficiency of the Health Extension Program.

With only 3.2 skilled health workers (doctors, nurses, and midwives) per 10,000 people, in 2012 [43], Ethiopia was far from the World Health Organization's recommended minimum of 23 skilled health workers per 10,000 people required to provide the health coverage needed to achieve the health-related Millennium Development Goals (MDGs) [44]. As it was committed to reach the health-related MDGs, the Federal Ministry of Health addressed the shortfall of skilled health workers by establishing the Health Extension Program in 2003 and task shifting some of the basic maternal, newborn and child health services from skilled health workers to HEWs, with a more basic level of training [31, 32, 45]. The Health Extension Program contributed towards achieving the MDG target for child survival [46]. Thus, the Health Extension Program is expected to play a key role in achieving the health-related targets of the Sustainable Development Goals set for 2030. Realizing that CBDDM is a useful tool for the WDA to carry out its responsibilities, mainly

Table 5 Linear effects of CBDDM implementation strength score and test of trend

Maternal and Newborn Health Care Practice	Linear Effects of CBDDM			Test for Trend	
	OR	(95% CI)	*p*-value	*p*-value[a]	Dose-Response Relationship
ANC 4+	1.12	(0.99, 1.26)	0.067	ND	No
Neonatal tetanus protected birth	1.23	(1.09, 1.38)	< 0.001	0.056	Yes
Institutional delivery	1.47	(1.25, 1.73)	< 0.001	0.748	Yes
PNC in 48 h	1.07	(0.91, 1.27)	0.418	ND	No
Clean cord care among home deliveries	1.21	(1.01, 1.44)	0.039	0.827	Yes
Thermal care	1.29	(1.08, 1.55)	0.006	0.136	Yes
Immediate initiation of breastfeeding	1.27	(1.10, 1.46)	0.001	0.596	Yes

CBDDM Community-Based Data for Decision-Making, *OR* odds ratio, *ND* not done, *ANC 4+* received four or more antenatal care visits, *PNC* postnatal care. [a]Null hypothesis: Not a trend effect

Table 6 Average treatment effects (ATEs) of CBDDM from simulation of models that concluded dose-response relationships

Maternal and Newborn Health Care Practice	ATE of CBDDM		
	%-points	(95% CI)	*p*-value
Neonatal tetanus protected birth	9	(4, 14)	0.001
Institutional delivery	15	(9, 20)	< 0.001
Clean cord care among home deliveries	7	(1, 14)	0.030
Thermal care	10	(3, 17)	0.003
Immediate initiation of breastfeeding	8	(3, 13)	0.002

ATE average treatment effect, *CBDDM* Community-Based Data for Decision-Making

facilitating the uptake of high-impact interventions by underserved households, the Health Extension Program has adopted it within its national WDA program to improve its efficiency.

The recent and impressive increase in institutional deliveries in Ethiopia —from 10% in 2011 to 28% in 2016 [47]— is likely due to national government strategies, including mobilizing communities to encourage pregnant mothers to give birth in health facilities, creating effective supportive and referral linkages between communities and health facilities, staffing health centers with midwives to ensure the continuous availability of basic emergency obstetric care services and the provision of ambulances to districts to mitigate transportation barriers [48]. The current study indicates that the CBDDM strategy augmented this national effort.

The practice of clean cord care among home deliveries declined during the observation period. During 2010–11 almost all women were delivering at home. As more and more women give birth at health facilities, over time, it is likely that those who deliver at home will be less aware of the best maternal and newborn health care behaviors and practices. However, in kebeles where the CBDDM implementation strength was relatively low, the decline in clean cord care was also relatively low.

Interestingly, we found no evidence that CBDDM affected early postnatal care. Further investigations will be required to identify the barriers and to address them.

There are several limitations to this study. First, the household selection for data collection can be criticized because the interviewers may have avoided hard-to-reach areas and non-responders were not revisited [36]. The increase in the average distance of the respondents' household from the nearest health facility between the two survey periods most likely indicates that the interviewers during the 2014–15 survey made greater efforts to interview households from hard-to-reach areas than those during the 2010 11 survey. The possible bias that the change in the households' distance to the nearest health facility could introduce was minimized by controlling for distance to any health facility in our analysis and by using multi-level analysis. Second, the outcomes considered are associated with the most recent birth among women with surviving children aged 0 to 11 months old, excluding women whose children died before the women had the opportunity for an interview. It is likely that such cases would have relatively poor practices; their exclusion would, therefore, result in overestimating care practices. Nevertheless, there are few such women and also, since the sampling method was consistent between the surveys, the sampling strategy to interview women with living children does not affect the internal validity of this study. Third, the CBDDM effects could be biased due to unmeasured confounders. The respondents living in kebeles with relatively high CBDDM implementation strength were nearer to health facilities. Although we controlled for distance of the respondents' household from the nearest health facility, there could be other unmeasured confounders. For example, the effects to CBDDM could be overestimated if the CBDDM implementation strength was higher in kebeles where there have been improvements in other unmeasured developmental factors that also influenced maternal and newborn care practices. Lastly, there could be reverse causality; kebeles with better household practices selecting more motivated WDA team leaders who implemented the CBDDM strategy better.

Conclusion

The CBDDM strategy demonstrated that data can be obtained and used by community members who have no or little education and used at the community level to support Ethiopia's Health Extension Program —thus underscoring the importance of a local information system to engage communities effectively to improve the performance of health systems. Potentially, the strategy could be adapted to community-based maternal and newborn health care systems elsewhere that have similar settings. Nonetheless, further research will be required to understand why the strategy fell short in improving the coverage of early postnatal care.

Abbreviations

ANC 4+: Four or more antenatal care visits at a health facility; ATE: Average treatment effect; CBDDM: Community-Based Data for Decision-Making; CI: Confidence interval; HEW: Health Extension Worker; L10K: The Last Ten Kilometers; MDG: Millennium Development Goal; PNC: Postnatal care; SDG: Sustainable Development Goal; SNNP: Southern Nations, Nationalities and Peoples; WDA: Women's Development Army

Acknowledgements
We thank the Health Extension Workers and Women's Development Army members for their contribution towards implementing the intervention. We are also thankful to the women respondents who voluntarily participated in this study. The support from the Regional Health Bureaus of Amhara, Oromia, SNNP and Tigray regions, and the L10K implementing partners, i.e., Amhara Development Association, Bench Maji Development Association, Ethiopian Kale Hiwot Church, Fayyaa Integrated Development Organization, Illu Women and Children Integrated Development Association, Kaffa Development Association, Oromia Development Association, Relief Society of Tigray, Sheka Peoples' Development Association, Siltie Development Association, Southern Region's Women's Association, and Women's Association of Tigray were critical for the data collection.

Funding
Funding for the study and for publication was provided by the Bill & Melinda Gates Foundation.

Authors' contributions
Conceived and designed the experiment: AK. Performed the experiment: NF TS DE SD FS MH GT BY NG. Analyzed the data: AK. Contributed materials/ analysis tools: AK, DE, GT, BY, NG. Wrote the paper: AK WB. All authors read and approved the final version of the manuscript.

Competing interests
All authors declared that they do not have any competing interest.

Author details
[1]The Last Ten Kilometers Project (L10K) 2020, JSI Research & Training Institute, Inc, Bole Sub-City, Kebele 03/05, Hs # 2111, Addis Ababa, Ethiopia. [2]Ethiopia Performance Monitoring and Evaluation Service (EPMES), Social Impact, Bole Sub-City, Woreda 13, House # 478, Addis Ababa, Ethiopia.

References
1. Tunçalp Ö, Were WM, MacLennan C, Oladapo OT, Gülmezoglu AM, Bahl R, et al. Quality of care for pregnant women and newborns - the WHO vision. BJOG. 2015;122(8):1045–9.
2. Pathé S, Habib B, Joses S, Kirigia M, Nyoni J, Bessaoud K, et al. The Ouagadougou declaration on primary health care and health systems in Africa: achieving better health for Africa in the new millennium. Afr Health Monit. 2010;12:10–21. http://www.aho.afro.who.int/en/ahm/issue/12/reports/ouagadougou-declaration-primary-health-care-and-health-systems-africa-achieving. (Accessed: 27 Oct 2017
3. World Health Organization (WHO). Rio political declaration on social determinants of health. Rio de Janeiro: WHO; 2011. http://www.who.int/sdhconference/declaration/en/. Accessed: 15 Apr 2018
4. Liu A, Sullivan S, Khan M, Sachs S, Singh P. Community health workers in global health: scale and scalability. Mt Sinai J Med. 2011;78(2):173–81.
5. Singh P, Sachs JD. 1 million community health workers in sub-Saharan Africa by 2015. Lancet. 2013;382(9889):363–5.
6. Campbell C, Jovchelovitch S. Health, community and development: towards social psychology of participation. J Community Appl Psychol. 2000;10(4):255–70.
7. Jewkes R, Murkott A. Community representatives: representing the "community"? Soc Sci Med. 1998;46(7):843–58.
8. Marston C, Renedo A, McGowan CR, Portela A. Effects of community participation on improving uptake of skilled care for maternal and newborn health: a systematic review. PLoS One. 2013;8(2):1–9.
9. Global Fund. Community systems strengthening framework. Geneva: Global Fund; 2014. https://www.theglobalfund.org/media/6428/core_css_framework_en.pdf?u=636637834640000000. Accessed: 6 Aug 2018
10. Marsh D. Population-based health information systems. In: Lippeveld T, editor. Design and implementation of health information systems. Geneva: WHO; 2000. p. 146–73. http://apps.who.int/iris/bitstream/10665/42289/1/9241561998.pdf. Accessed 15 Apr 2018.
11. Azim T, Tilahun B, Mullen S. Use of community health data for shared accountability: guidance. Measure Evaluation: Chapel Hill; 2018. https://www.measureevaluation.org/our-work/data-demand-and-use/useofcommunityhealthdata. Accessed 15 Apr 2018
12. de la Torre C, Unfried K. Monitoring and evaluation at the community level: a strategic review of MEASURE evaluation, phase III accomplishments and contributions. MEASURE Evaluation: Chapel Hill; 2014. http://www.cpc.unc.edu/measure/publications/sr-14-114. Accessed 15 Apr 2018
13. Rosales A. A community based health information system in rural Honduras: CRS/COCEPRADII experience. Washington DC: American Public Health Association; 2003. https://apha.confex.com/apha/131am/techprogram/paper_53322.htm. Accessed 15 Apr 2018
14. Chewicha K, Azim T. Community health information system for family centered health care: scale-up in southern nations nationalities and People's region. Ethiop Minist Heal Q Heal Bull. 2013;5(1):49–53. https://www.measureevaluation.org/resources/publications/ja-13-161. Accessed 15 Apr 2018
15. Damtew ZA, Moges AS. From multiple register to family folder: the transition of data collection and reporting tools for health extension Workers in Ethiopia. J Health Inform Dev Ctries. 2013;7(2):99–112.
16. MEASURE Evaluation. Community-based health information systems in the global context: A review of the literature. Chapel Hill: MEASURE Evaluation; 2016. Report No.: WP-16-161. https://www.measureevaluation.org/resources/publications/wp-16-161. Accessed 15 Apr 2018.
17. Odhiambo-otieno GW, Management H, Health P. Implementing a community-based health management information system in Bungoma district, Kenya. Heal Policy Dev. 2005;3(2):170–7.
18. Sabitu K, Iliyasu Z, Hassan SS, Mande AT. Evaluation of a community level nutrition information system for action in a rural community of Zaria, Northern Nigeria. Ann Afr Med. 2004;3(3):120–5.
19. Jeremie N, Kaseje D, Olayo R, Akinyi C. Utilization of community-based health information systems in decision making and health action in Nyalenda, Kisumu County, Kenya. Univers J Med Sci. 2014;2(4):37–42.
20. MEASURE Evaluation. Case study series: community-based information systems: Tanzania. MEASURE Evaluation: Chapel Hill; 2014. https://www.measureevaluation.org/resources/publications/sr-14-105b. Accessed 15 Apr 2018
21. MEASURE Evaluation. Case study series: community-based information systems: Kenya. Chapel Hill: MEASURE Evaluation; 2014. https://www.measureevaluation.org/resources/publications/sr-14-105a. Accessed 15 April 2018
22. MEASURE Evaluation. Case study series: community-based information systems: Zambia. MEASURE Evaluation: Chapel Hill; 2014. https://www.measureevaluation.org/resources/publications/sr-14-105c. Accessed 15 Apr 2018
23. Kaseje D, Olayo R, Musita C, Oindo C, Wafula C, Muga R. Evidence-based dialogue with communities for district health systems' performance improvement. Glob Public Health. 2010;5(6):596–610.
24. Björkman M, Svensson J. Power to the people: evidence from a randomized field experiment on community-based monitoring in Uganda. Q J Econ. 2009;124(2):735–69.
25. Akinyi C, Nzanzu J, Kaseje D. Effectiveness of community health workers in promotion of maternal health services in Butere district, rural western Kenya. Univers J Med Sci. 2015;3(1):11–8.
26. Editorial. Evaluation: the top priority for global health. Lancet. 2010; 375(9714):526.
27. Damtew ZA, Karim AM, Willey B, Tesfaye C, Fesseha Zemichael N, Yeshanew B, et al. Correlates of the Women's Development Army strategy implementation strength with household reproductive, maternal, newborn and child healthcare practices: a cross-sectional study in four regions of Ethiopia. BMC Pregnancy Childbirth. 2018;18(Suppl 1) https://doi.org/10.1186/s12884-018-1975-y.
28. Wereta T, Betemariam W, Karim AM, Fesseha Zemichael N, Dagnew S, Wanboru A, et al. Effects of a participatory community quality improvement strategy on improving household and provider health care behaviors and practices: a propensity score analysis. BMC Pregnancy Childbirth. 2018; 18(Suppl 1) https://doi.org/10.1186/s12884-018-1977-9.

29. Emaway Altaye D, Karim AM, Betemariam W, Fesseha Zemichael N, Shigute T, Scheelbeek P. Effects of family conversation on health care practices in Ethiopia: a propensity score matched analysis. BMC Pregnancy Childbirth. 2018; 18(Suppl 1) https://doi.org/10.1186/s12884-018-1978-8.
30. Federal Ministry of Health, Ethiopia. Health Sector Transformation Plan. Addis Ababa: FMOH; 2015. http://www.globalfinancingfacility.org/sites/gff_new/files/documents/HSTP Ethiopia.pdf. Accessed 17 Oct 2017
31. Wakabi W. Extension workers drive Ethiopia's primary health care. Lancet. 2008;372(9642):880.
32. Admasu K, Balcha T, Getahun H. Model villages: a platform for community-based primary health care. Lancet. 2016;4(2):e78–9.
33. Karim AM, Admassu K, Schellenberg J, Alemu H, Getachew N, Ameha A, et al. Effect of Ethiopia's health extension program on maternal and newborn health care practices in 101 rural districts: a dose-response study. PLoS One. 2013;8(6):e65160.
34. Federal Ministry of Health, Ethiopia. The Health Development Army: Its origins, development and current status, The Health Documentation Initiative. Addis Ababa: FMOH; 2016.
35. Darmstadt GL, Marchant T, Claeson M, Brown W, Morris S, Donnay F, et al. A strategy for reducing maternal and newborn deaths by 2015 and beyond. BMC Pregnancy Childbirth. 2013;13:216.
36. Lemeshow S, Robinson D. Surveys to measure programme coverage and impact: a review of the methodology used by the expanded programme on immunization. World Heal Stat Q. 1985;38:115–32.
37. Filmer D, Pritchett L. Estimating wealth effects without expenditure data– or tears: an application to educational enrollment in states of India. Demography. 2001;38(1):115–32.
38. StataCorp. Stata base reference manual, Release 14. College Station, TX: StataCorp LP; 2015.
39. Angeles G, Guilkey DK, Mroz T. The impact of community-level variables on individual-level outcomes: theoretical results and applications. Sociol Methods Res. 2005;34(1):76–121.
40. Hosmer D, Lemeshow S. Applied logistic regression. 2nd ed. New York: Wiley; 1989.
41. Clayton D, Hill M. Statistical models for epidemiology. Oxford: Oxford University Press; 1993.
42. Karim A. Effectiveness evaluation of a large-scale community-based program: lessons from Ethiopia. Ann Glob Heal. 2015;81:192.
43. Feysia B, Herbst CH, Lemma W, Soucat A, Zhao F, Kedir N, et al. The health workforce in Ethiopia: addressing the remaining challenges. Washington DC: The World Bank; 2012.
44. World Health Organization. Working together for health: the world health report 2006. Geneva: WHO; 2006. http://www.who.int/whr/2006/en/. Accessed 15 Apr 2018
45. Bhutta Z, Lassi Z, Pariyo G, Huicho L. Global experience of community health workers for delivery of health related millennium development goals: a systematic review, country case studies, and recommendations for integration into national health systems. Community Dent Health. 2010; http://www.who.int/workforcealliance/knowledge/publications/alliance/Global_CHW_web.pdf. Accessed 17 Oct 2017
46. Ethiopia Public Health Institute, Federal Ministry of Health, Countdown to 2015, UNICEF. Countdown to a healthier Ethiopia: building on successes to accelerate newborn survival. Addis Ababa: UNICEF; 2015. http://countdown2030.org/documents/EthiopiaBrief.pdf. Accessed 15 Apr 2018
47. Central Statistical Agency, Ethiopia. Ethiopia Demographic and Health Survey 2016 Key indicators. Addis Ababa, Ethiopia and Rockville, Maryland, USA: CSA; 2016.
48. Admasu K, Balcha T, Ghebreyesus TA. Pro-poor pathway towards universal health coverage: lessons from Ethiopia. J Glob Health. 2016;6(1):1–4.

14

Cancer related maternal mortality and delay in diagnosis and treatment

Jorine de Haan[1,2*], Christianne A. R. Lok[3], Joke S. Schutte[4], Lia van Zuylen[5] and Christianne J. M. de Groot[1]

Abstract

Background: Cancer during pregnancy is relatively rare but may lead to maternal mortality. We aimed to assess the incidence of cancer related maternal mortality and the neonatal outcome in these patients. Also, doctor- and patient-related delay in cancer diagnosis and therapy among patients with cancer related maternal mortality is assessed.

Methods: Maternal mortality was defined as death during pregnancy or within 1 year after delivery. Data of the Dutch Maternal Mortality Committee was used to calculate the cancer related maternal mortality rate and to assess neonatal outcome in the Netherlands. Delay was scored by ten medical specialist based on case descriptions.

Results: Cancer related maternal mortality rate was 1.23 per 100,000 live births. Delay in either diagnosis or treatment occurred in 65%. Delay in diagnosis was more frequent then delay in treatment, and was mainly caused by health care providers. Only 77% of pregnancies were ongoing, and 65% ended preterm of which 85% was induced.

Conclusions: Avoiding delay in diagnosis and therapy in case of pregnancy related cancer could potentially improve maternal and neonatal outcome. It is therefore essential to increase awareness among health care providers about the occurrence and recurrence of cancer in pregnancy and the possibilities of diagnostic and therapeutic interventions in these women.

Keywords: Cancer, Pregnancy, Delay, Preterm delivery, Mortality

Background

In western countries, maternal mortality, defined as death occurring during pregnancy or within the first year after delivery, is a relatively small but still serious problem. Most women die of pregnancy related problems, but approximately 25% of the maternal deaths are non- pregnancy related. Pregnancies complicated by cancer are a potential threat for both maternal and fetal wellbeing. Incidence of cancer during pregnancy has been estimated to be one in 1000 pregnancies, but due to increasing maternal age and the increasing incidence of risk factors for cancer, e.g. obesity, this incidence is rising [1, 2]. Schutte et al. reported no cancer related maternal deaths between 1983 and 1992 and three between 1993 and 2005 [3].

If standard therapy is started without delay, prognosis of pregnant patients is comparable to non-pregnant patients when corrected for maternal age and stage. Cancer related symptoms can mimic those of physiological pregnancy changes [4]. They may be interpreted by both patient and health care providers as pregnancy related, delaying an accurate diagnosis [5, 6]. This delay can lead to a more advanced stage of disease, causing a higher mortality rate [7].

In the management of pregnant patients with cancer, the unborn child is an important second patient that needs to be taken care of. Treatment regimens must be carefully evaluated in order to ensure fetal safety. Recent

* Correspondence: j.dehaan11@vumc.nl
[1]Department of Obstetrics and Gynaecology, VU University Medical Center, De Boelelaan 1118, 1081, HZ, Amsterdam, The Netherlands
[2]Department of Oncology, KU Leuven, Herestraat 49, 3000 Leuven, Belgium
Full list of author information is available at the end of the article

studies have shown that several cancer treatments seem to be feasible during pregnancy without increasing the change of congenital malformations [8, 9]. Chemo- and radiotherapy during pregnancy does not seem to affect the neuropsychological development up to 3 years. Unfortunately, substandard and/or delayed treatment and iatrogenic preterm birth is still a major problem in this specific patient group [10]. In fact, preterm delivery is a high risk factor for developmental problems later in life [8].

In advanced stages of disease, treatment is often more extensive and maternal condition deteriorated. Minimizing delay in diagnosis will not prevent all maternal deaths, but the outcome for both mother and neonate is likely to be improved. However, literature on current cancer related maternal mortality is scarce. Therefore, in the present study the incidence of cancer related maternal mortality in the Netherlands will be calculated and the occurrence of doctor- and patient-related delay in diagnosis and therapy will be evaluated. Finally, the neonatal outcome of the children of the mothers that died of cancer during pregnancy will be analysed.

Methods

This study is a nationwide observational cohort study using the non-public database of the Dutch Maternal Mortality Committee (MMC) after written permission of the board of the committee. The methods of the MMC and definitions of maternal mortality used have been described previously [3]. Briefly, the MMC discusses reported cases, collects missing data and evaluates the avoidability of maternal mortality. Maternal mortality is defined as death occurring during pregnancy or within the first year after delivery. Their database is cross-checked with the Central Bureau of Statistics of the Netherlands (CBS). Missing cases are anonymously added to the database.

Selection criteria and data collection

Patients registered between 2001 and 2012 by the MMC who died during pregnancy or within 1 year postpartum were screened. We selected the patients that died because of (recurrent) cancer. Patients with cancer related symptoms during pregnancy but diagnosed after delivery were included. If patients died from cancer but only showed symptoms after delivery, they were not eligible. Missing data in the reports of the MMC were completed by review of the medical files. Ten medical specialists from different disciplines, including medical oncologists, gynaecological oncologists and obstetricians, were provided detailed case descriptions, with information on diagnosis and therapy. They scored anonymously whether delay had occurred and whether this was doctor- and/or patient-related delay. Delay was defined as an extension of the period between symptoms/presentation and diagnosis, and diagnosis and treatment, compared to optimal care based on expert opinions. For the patients with recurrent disease during pregnancy, delay was assessed from the moment of the new onset of symptoms caused by recurrent disease. Delay due to other primary health care providers like midwifes were considered to be doctor-related delay.

Statistical analysis

Because of the observational nature of this study, statistical analysis was restricted to descriptive statistics and the evaluation of inter-observer agreement with a kappa score. Because our data was scored by a fixed number of observers using a numeric scorings system the Fleiss kappa score was used.

Results

Incidence and maternal mortality rate

Between 2001 and 2012, 32 cancer related maternal deaths were reported to the MMC. Four of these cases were excluded: two patients were treated with chemotherapeutic agents for other indications than malignant disease, one patient had a benign brain tumour and one patient became symptomatic after delivery. Two additional anonymous cases were reported by the CBS, which were included but could only be used to calculate the incidence of cancer related maternal mortality. The 26 remaining cases were available for analysis of delay. With an average number of 188,604 live births per year (range 202,603 in 2001 to 175,959 in 2012) in the Netherlands, the Dutch cancer related MMR between 2001 and 2012 was 1.23 per 100,000 live births [11].

Patient characteristics

Brain tumours, gastro-intestinal tumours and melanomas were the most common types of cancer causing maternal mortality. Patient characteristics are shown in Table 1. The median maternal age at diagnosis was 34 years (range 27–45 years). Of the 26 patients, 73% was diagnosed during pregnancy; one patient (4%) was diagnosed in the first trimester, ten patients (39%) in the second trimester and eight patients (31%) in the third trimester. Seven patients (27%) were diagnosed after delivery, but experienced cancer related symptoms during pregnancy. Median survival after diagnosis was 101 days with a range of 3–352 days. Stage IV disease was present at diagnosis in 90% of the patients; the other 10% had stage III disease. Four patients had recurrent disease during pregnancy and were diagnosed with advanced stage disease at recurrence while pregnant; one melanoma and three astrocytomas.

Standard curative therapy was applied in nine cases. Four patients received adjusted treatment because of

Table 1 Patient characteristics

Patient	Tumour	Parity	GA a.d. (wks)	Stage/grade a.d. (TNM/FIGO)	Survival after diagnosis (days)	One-year survival in general (%)	Patient/ doctor delay in diagnosis	Patient/doctor delay in treatment	Obstetrical outcome
1	Adrenal carcinoma	G5P3	Pp	IV	133	Unknown	Inconclusive	No	GA 36 weeks; induction for suspicion of HELLP syndrome, but were metastasis.
2	Astrocytoma	G1P0	Pp	II	92	84	Yes, both	Yes, doctor	GA 38 weeks; induction for HELLP syndrome
3	Breast cancer	G2P1	Pp	IV	9	72	Yes, doctor	No	GA 37 weeks; SVD
4	Breast cancer	G9P6	12	IV	310	72	NA	No	GA 32 weeks; emergency CS when patient was found in coma.
5	Breast cancer	G3P2	Pp	IV	126	72	Yes, patient	Yes, patient	GA 39 weeks; induction for excessive skeletal pains
6	Cervical carcinoma	G2P1	25	IV	352	44–54	No	No	GA 34 weeks; maternal deterioration
7	Cholangio-carcinoma	G3P0	28	IV	81	13	Yes, doctor	No	GA 28 weeks; CS for fetal distress
8	Esophagus carcinoma	G5P4	28	IV	78	20	No	No	GA 36 weeks; induction for therapy planning
9	Esophagus carcinoma	G1P0	17	Unknown	110	29	NA	Yes, doctor	IUFD at GA 22 weeks
10	Gastric carcinoma	G3P1	23	IV	78	17	No	No	GA 29 weeks; CS for maternal deterioration and breech position
11	Gastric carcinoma	G2P1	18	IV	171	17	Yes, doctor	No	GA 18 weeks; immature delivery after surgery.
12	Glioblastoma multiforme	G14P10	16	IV	87	38	No	No	IUFD at GA 27 weeks
13	Glioblastoma multiforme	G2P1	28	IV	270	38	Yes, doctor	Yes, patient	GA 34 weeks; CS for twin and maternal deterioration
14	Glioblastoma multiforme	G4P3	16	IV	15	38	Yes, doctor	No	Died while pregnant (GA 18 weeks)
15	Lung carcinoma	G2P1	36	IV	149	22	Yes, both	NA	GA 36 weeks; induction for therapy planning
16	Melanoma	G1P0	26	IV	15	32	No	NA	Died while pregnant (GA 29 weeks)
17	Melanoma	G2P1	21	IIIC	154	82	No	Yes, doctor	Term; SVD
18	Melanoma	G4P2	Pp	IV	47	32	Yes, doctor	No	GA 40 weeks; SVD
19	Melanoma	G1P0	16	IV	167	32	No	Yes, patient	GA 32 weeks; fetal distress
20	Non-Hodgkin lymphoma	G3P2	Pp	IVB	20	67	Yes, doctor	No	Term; SVD
21	Ovarian carcinoma	G2P1	34	IIIB	176	77	Yes, patient	No	GA 35 weeks; induction for therapy planning
22	Pancreatic carcinoma	G1P0	24	IV	37	10	No	No	GA 28 weeks; SVD
23	Pilocytic astrocytoma	G2P1	17	I	3	89	No	No	Died during pregnancy (GA 17 weeks)
24	Rectum carcinoma	G2P1	37	IV	134	46–70	Yes, doctor	No	GA 37 weeks; induction after diagnosis.
25	Satellite tumour CNS	G1P0	21	III	130	61	No	Yes, doctor	GA 34 weeks; CS for maternal deterioration
26	Unknown primary tumour	G1P0	Pp	IV	82	–	Yes, NA	No	GA 26 weeks; CS for HELLP. Neonatal death after 4 days.

Pp postpartum, *G* gravidity, *P* parity, *a.d.* at diagnosis, *NA* not assessable, *GA* gestational age, *HELLP* hemolysis, elevated liver enzymes, and low platelet count, *CS* caesarean section, *SVD* spontaneous vaginal delivery, *IUFD* intra-uterine fetal death, *CNS* central nervous system pregnancy or complications. In six cases, the patient decided to postpone treatment until a higher gestational age (GA). Four of these patients were still induced preterm. Palliative care was the only option for six patients. For one patient, data on therapeutic decision-making was not available.

Obstetrical outcome

Obstetrical outcome was available for all 26 patients with detailed case information (Fig. 1). Five pregnancies were complicated by intra-uterine fetal death: 1) at a GA of 17 weeks, when mother died of an astrocytoma, 2) at a GA of 18 weeks, when mother died of a glioblastoma multiforme, 3) at a GA of 22 weeks after suboptimal intubation during surgery, 4) at a GA of 27 weeks, when mother was admitted with a status epilepticus due to progressive glioblastoma multiforme, and 5) at a GA of 29 weeks, when the mother died suddenly at home due to metastatic melanoma. One patient experienced an immature delivery at a GA of 18 weeks after a bilateral laparotomic oophorectomy.

Of the 20 ongoing pregnancies ending in a live birth, one was a twin pregnancy resulting in 21 live newborns. However, one of the children died 4 days after caesarean section at a GA of 26 weeks due to complications of extreme preterm delivery. Caesarean section was performed because of presumed HELLP syndrome. After delivery, the complaints progressed and stage IV cancer of unknown origin with liver metastases was diagnosed.

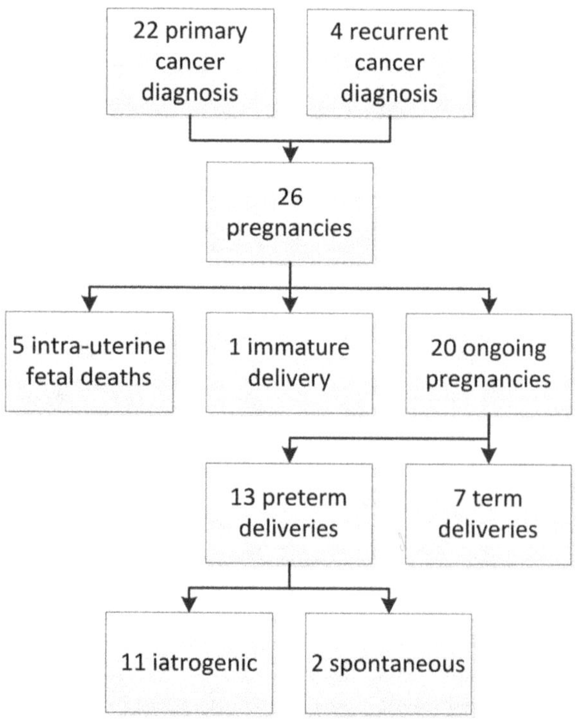

Fig. 1 Obstetrical outcome for all 26 pregnancies

Median GA at delivery of all 20 ongoing pregnancies was 35 weeks (range 26–40 weeks). Thirteen (65%) of these ended preterm, of which 11 deliveries (85%) were vaginally induced (n = 3) or terminated by caesarean section (n = 8). Reasons for iatrogenic preterm delivery were maternal deterioration (n = 4), therapy planning (n = 4) or obstetrical complications (n = 3).

Doctor-related and patient-related delay

Ten medical specialists dealing with pregnant cancer patients from six different medical centres independently scored all 26 case descriptions on delay in diagnosis and treatment. The score was considered conclusive if six or more specialists shared the same opinion.

See Table 2 for an overview of the types of delay. In 65% of patients (n = 17) delay was found to be present, 50% (n = 13) or all patients were found to have delay in diagnosis and 27% (n = 7) in starting therapy. Three patients were considered to have both types of delay. Regarding the other nine cases, six showed no signs of delay, two had not enough information available for adequate evaluation and one score was inconclusive. Even in patients with recurrent disease, delay in diagnosis occurred in 50%. In one of these patients with recurrent astrocytoma, delay was caused by doctors in a non-academic centre where symptoms like increasing blood pressure, headache and general seizure were interpreted as eclampsia, for which delivery was induced. In the other patients with delay in diagnosis with recurrent melanoma, progressive back pain and pain on her ribcage at a GA of 35 weeks, was treated with pain medication until 2 weeks after delivery. Diagnostic investigations showed wide spread melanoma metastasis including bones and lungs.

Inter-observer agreement on the presence of delay in diagnosis was found to be substantial, with a Fleiss Kappa

Table 2 Delay in diagnosis and treatment

Type of delay	No.	%
Overall delay	17	65
Delay in diagnosis	13	50
- Doctor-related[a]	8	62
- Patient-related[a]	2	15
- Doctor- and patient related[a]	2	15
- Not assessable[a]	1	4
Delay in therapy	7	27
- Doctor-related[a]	4	15
- Patient-related[a]	3	12

[a]Of all patients with delay

score of 0.71. The agreement for the delay in therapy was less, with a score of 0.33, which is a fair agreement.

In the cases where delay in diagnosis was caused, the origin was evaluated to assess whether the delay was caused by the involved health care provider or by the patient. In eight of 13 patients with delay in diagnosis, doctor-related delay was considered to have influenced the time between presentation of symptoms and diagnosis. In two additional cases, both the health care provider and the patient caused delay. For the ten patients with doctor-related delay, delay was caused by the midwife ($n = 5$), general practitioner ($n = 2$) and by doctors from a non-academic centres ($n = 2$) and in two patients, multiple non-academic health care workers caused delay. In nine cases, symptoms were described as pregnancy related complaints, and in one patient, a wrong diagnosis was made based on additional diagnostic tests. In one patient, delay was caused by a long period between referral to a hospital and actual diagnostic evaluation. Patient-related delay in diagnosis was present in only two cases, and in one case enough information was not available to evaluate the cause of delay.

Doctor-related delay in therapy was found in four of the seven cases. In the other three cases, patients refused the advised treatment during pregnancy and wished to delay until after delivery.

Discussion

This is, to our knowledge, the second study to evaluate specific cancer related MMR and the first to report on delay in either diagnosis or treatment and obstetrical outcome in this specific population. The cancer related MMR in the Netherlands between 2001 and 2012 was 1.23 per 100,000 live births, with the highest incidence of cause related death due to brain tumours, gastrointestinal tumours and melanomas. Delay in diagnosis was more frequent than delayed treatment, and was mainly caused by health care providers. Of the 77% ongoing pregnancies, 65% delivered preterm, often after induction of labour for oncological reasons. One neonatal death occurred.

The only other article published on cancer related maternal mortality, in 1990 by Sachs et al. [12], reported on their population-based study in the USA between 1954 and 1985 and found a cancer related MMR of 1.44. They defined maternal mortality as death during pregnancy or within 90 days after delivery. Because this is different from the current WHO definition used in our study, comparing these results to this present study is not feasible [12].

The outcome for pregnant patients with cancer is not different from non-pregnant patients when corrected for stage and age at diagnosis [7]. Previous literature has reported that patients with cancer during pregnancy present with a more advanced stage of disease due to delay in diagnosis [5, 6]. Since stage of disease at diagnosis is strongly correlated to prognosis, this delay may contribute to a worse maternal outcome and should be avoided where possible. For some tumours, the effect of delay on the prognosis is less, since lower stage of disease still has a poor prognosis. However, even in these cases, prognosis is better when diagnosed in an earlier stage.

Delay in therapy until after delivery may postpone adequate therapy for the mother, thereby contributing to a worse maternal prognosis. If preterm induction of labour is aimed for to start therapy postpartum, the prognosis of the unborn child is influenced as well. A recent study [8] showed that there was no difference between neuropsychological development between children exposed to chemotherapy in utero and healthy controls. In fact, preterm birth had a bigger impact on neuropsychological outcome in both groups with an increase of 2.6 IQ points per week gestation at birth [8]. In our study population, delay in diagnosis may have contributed to a more advanced stage of disease requiring systemic therapy in order to improve survival. In 27% of the cases, therapy was delayed until spontaneous delivery or until a certain GA was reached and pregnancy could be terminated. Raising awareness on cancer in pregnancy and the possibilities in diagnostic and therapeutic treatment modalities among health care providers may help in reducing the morbidity and mortality of these patients and their children.

One of the main limitations of our study include that reporting fatalities to the Dutch MMC is on a voluntary basis. Even though the committee is well known among gynaecologists, it is possible that a year after pregnancy, the relation between death and pregnancy by other medical professionals may be overlooked. Cross checking with the CBS database revealed only two more cases, but the actual number of cancer related (late) mortalities might be higher than reported. Furthermore, there are some difficulties in studying delay, as the extent of delay for one tumour will not have the same consequences as delay for another, more aggressive, tumour and if curative therapeutic options are not available, delay will not change the fatal outcome. However, the various medical specialists reached an overall agreement on the occurrence of delay, which makes our findings more reproducible. Our study population is small, because of the low incidence of cancer related maternal mortality.

We cannot exclude that treatment in a multidisciplinary team may influenced outcome. Practitioners with experience in oncologic treatment in pregnancy will probably hesitate less to start treatment, but they are often dependent on referral from first-line healthcare workers and they cannot change the stage of cancer. This emphasizes that awareness in all practitioners is essential.

Conclusions

In conclusion, cancer related maternal mortality is rare but contributes to high neonatal morbidity and mortality rates, mainly due to iatrogenic preterm delivery. Delay in diagnosis and treatment occurs frequently in this group and is mainly caused by health care providers. This can only be resolved by increased awareness among health-care professionals.

Abbreviations

CBS: Central Bureau of Statistics; GA: Gestational age; MMC: Maternal Mortality Committee; MMR: Maternal mortality rate

Acknowledgements

The authors thank all the medical specialists and outpatient department managers who helped collecting all data necessary for completing the database and scoring the case reports. No funding was received.

Funding

No funding was obtained for this project.

Authors' contributions

JH contributed to the article with the design of the protocol, planning of the project, data collection, analysis of hospital files, interpretation of data, statistical analysis and writing the article. CL contributed to the article with the design of the protocol, support in planning the project, supervising data collection, analysis and interpretation of collected data, and critical revision of the article. JS contributed to the article with the data collection of maternal deaths during many years as member of the MMC, scoring of all cases and revision of the article. LZ contributed to the article with the scoring of all cases and revision of the article. CG contributed to the article with the design of the protocol, supervision of planning the project and of analysis of data and final revision of the article. All authors read and approved the final manuscript.

Competing interests

The authors declare that they have no competing interests.

Author details

[1]Department of Obstetrics and Gynaecology, VU University Medical Center, De Boelelaan 1118, 1081, HZ, Amsterdam, The Netherlands. [2]Department of Oncology, KU Leuven, Herestraat 49, 3000 Leuven, Belgium. [3]Department of Gynaecologic Oncology, Center for Gynaecologic Oncology Amsterdam, Amsterdam, The Netherlands. [4]Department of Obstetrics and Gynaecology, Isala Clinics, Zwolle, the Netherlands. [5]Department of Medical Oncology, Erasmus MC Cancer Institute, Rotterdam, the Netherlands.

References

1. Lee YY, Roberts CL, Dobbins T, Stavrou E, Black K, Morris J, et al. Incidence and outcomes of pregnancy-associated cancer in Australia, 1994–2008: a population-based linkage study. BJOG An Int J Obstet Gynaecol. 2012;119:1572–82.
2. Parazzini F, Franchi M, Tavani A, Negri E, Peccatori FA. Frequency of pregnancy related cancer: a population based linkage study in Lombardy, Italy. Int J Gynecol Cancer. 2017;27:613–9.
3. Schutte JM, Steegers EAP, Schuitemaker NWE, Santema JG, de Boer K, Pel M, et al. Rise in maternal mortality in the Netherlands. Br J Obstet Gynaecol. 2010;117:399–406.
4. de Haan J, Vandecaveye V, Han SN, Van de Vijver KK, Amant F. Difficulties with diagnosis of malignancies in pregnancy. Best Pract. Res. Clin. Obstet. Gynaecol. 2016;33:19–32.
5. Andersson TM, Johansson ALV, Fredriksson I, Lambe M. Cancer during pregnancy and the postpartum period: a population-based study. Cancer. 2015;121:2072–7.
6. Voulgaris E, Pentheroudakis G, Pavlidis N. Cancer and pregnancy: a comprehensive review. Surg Oncol. 2011;20:e175–85.
7. Stensheim H, Møller B, Van Dijk T, Fosså SD. Cause-specific survival for women diagnosed with cancer during pregnancy or lactation: a registry-based cohort study. J Clin Oncol. 2009;27:45–51.
8. Amant F, Vandenbroucke T, Verheecke M, Fumagalli M, Halaska MJ, Boere I, et al. Pediatric outcome after maternal cancer diagnosed during pregnancy. N Engl J Med. 2015;373:1824–34.
9. Amant F, Han SN, Gziri MM, Vandenbroucke T, Verheecke M, Van Calsteren K. Management of cancer in pregnancy. Best Pract Res Clin Obstet Gynaecol. 2015;29:741–53.
10. Han SN, Kesic VI, Van Calsteren K, Petkovic S, Amant F. Cancer in pregnancy: a survey of current clinical practice. Eur J Obstet Gynecol Reprod Biol. 2013; 167:18–23.
11. Central Bureau of Statistics of the Netherlands. Geboorte naar diverse kenmerkingen. [cited 2015 Nov 1]. Available from: http://statline.cbs.nl/StatWeb/publication/?VW=T&DM=SLNL&PA=37422ned&D1=0,4-5,7,9,11,13,17,26,35,40-41&D2=0,10,20,30,40,(l-4)-l&HD=090218-0953&HDR=G1&STB=T.
12. Sachs BP, Penzias AS, Brown DA, Driscoll SG, Jewett JF. Cancer-related maternal mortality in Massachusetts, 1954–1985. Gynecol Oncol. 1990;36:395–400.

15

The relationship of prenatal maternal depression or anxiety to maternal caregiving behavior and infant behavior self-regulation during infant heel lance

Fay F. Warnock[1,2*], Kenneth D. Craig[3], Roger Bakeman[4], Thaila Castral[5] and Jila Mirlashari[6]

Abstract

Background: Sensitive and responsive maternal caregiving behavior strengthens infant self-regulatory capacities (HL), but this regulatory role may be diminished in some mothers with second-trimester prenatal exposure to depression and/ or anxiety (MDA). This study examined maternal and infant behavior during infant heel lance (HL) when mothers had or did not have MDA. Ethological methods and micro-analytic approaches capable of distinguishing and comparing time-based patterning in maternal and infant behavior were used to clarify biological mechanisms, such as MDA, that may underlie observed behavior. Aims were to examine group differences in caregiving behavior between mothers with and without MDA 5 min Pre-HL and 5 min Post-H, and relationships between MDA, maternal caregiving behavior and infant pain behavior self-regulation, concurrently.

Methods: At second trimester, mothers were assessed for symptoms of mild-severe depression or anxiety. Mothers whose scores exceeded predetermined cut-off scores on one or more of the mental health measures were allocated to the MDA-exposure group, those below to the non-MDA-exposure group. Reliable observers, blinded to MDA status and study phases, coded video records of the caregiving behavior of each study mother for the full duration of the 5 min Pre-HL and 5 min Post-HL study phases. Group differences and associations between mean measures of maternal mental health scores, time-based measures of maternal behavior, and time-based measures of infant pain behavior regulation (previously coded) were concurrently analyzed using comparative and correlational statistics.

Results: MDA-exposed mothers spent significantly more time not embracing, engaging or responding to infant cues than maternal controls Pre-HL and Post-HL. MDA was associated with atypical maternal caregiving behavior, which in turn was related to atypical infant pain behavior self-regulation during and after the HL.

Conclusion: Our findings have implication for practice. We recommend inclusion of mothers with MDA and their infants in interventions that strengthen the early mother-infant interaction and mother's regulatory caregiving role. MDA and maternal caregiving behavior must be considered in future infant pain studies to examine if they confound effectiveness of mother driven caregiving interventions for neonatal pain. We highlight the importance of examining maternal mental health throughout the perinatal and postnatal trajectory, and particularly the newborn period.

(Continued on next page)

* Correspondence: fay.warnock@nursing.ubc.ca
[1]Developmental Neurosciences, Child and Family Research Institute, L408, 4480 Oak Street, Vancouver, BC, Canada
[2]University of British Columbia (BC), School of Nursing, Vancouver, BC, Canada
Full list of author information is available at the end of the article

(Continued from previous page)
Keywords: Prenatal depression, Prenatal anxiety, Maternal caregiving behavior, Infant pain, Infant pain behavior, Perinatal maternal mental health, Ethology

Abbreviations: MDA, Second-trimester prenatal maternal exposure to depression and/ or anxiety; HL, Infant heel lance pain procedure; Prop-T, The proportion of time that an individual or group spends in a particular behavior during an observation session(s); NAS, Neonatal abstinence syndrome; SSRIs, Selective Serotonin Re-uptake Inhibitor antidepressant medication; HPA, Hypothalamic–pituitary-adrenal axis

Background

Sensitive and responsive caregiving actions and interactions (typically provided by the mother) play a crucial role in protecting, buffering and strengthening infant ability to self-regulate to everyday stressors [1]. This is important because, throughout the perinatal period, the self-regulatory capacities of the human infant continue to develop with rapid changes also occurring in brain structure and function. It is also during the neonatal period when most infants are exposed to painful clinical procedures such as heel lance (HL) for necessary blood screening and monitoring. Established evidence suggests that early exposure to everyday stressors including routine HL can overtax and disrupt the still immature newborn's ability to self-regulate subsystems (autonomic, motor, state, attention, behavioral organization) [2], and confer damage to the structure and function of the developing pain system [3, 4]. This is particularly so if the infant is born at-risk (born with prenatal exposures, ill, developmentally compromised and/ or premature), and if the pain goes untreated [3, 4].

Currently, there are no analgesics that can be safely administered to infants to relieve procedural pain [5]. There is, however, substantial evidence that non-pharmacological pain treatments can effectively alleviate procedural pain in newborns based on a reduction in mean measures of pain behavior (primarily changes in facial movement), heart rate, and/or salivary cortisol levels [6, 7]. Examples include the use of oral sucrose as well as mother driven caregiving interventions (eg., kangaroo mother care, breastfeeding, facilitated tucking) [6, 7].

Growth in the number of maternal caregiving interventions for neonatal pain and their uptake into the clinical setting provides confidence in their reported effectiveness [6]. While in most of these interventions, the infant's mother is acknowledged to play a fundamental role in regulating the infant and that the mother drives/functions as the "intervention", there is limited reporting of the maternal sample beyond demographics (eg., age, socioeconomic status). Under-reporting precludes understanding as to whether the interventions are representative of the diverse population of mothers and infants for which they are intended. Furthermore, lack in examining maternal factors prevents early recognition/detection of perinatal factors and mechanisms that could hamper a mother's ability to regulate her infant, or that may function to confound effectiveness of the interventions. Findings of a recent narrative systematic review of 12 kangaroo maternal care intervention studies for neonatal pain [8], for example, show that none of the 12 studies provided information as to whether mothers with prenatal depression and/or anxiety were included in the sample. As well, none explicitly examined prenatal maternal depression and/or anxiety or maternal caregiving behavior as distinct study variables [8]. The consideration of these kinds of maternal factors in neonatal pain studies including mother driven interventions for neonatal pain is essential for the following reasons.

Depression and/or anxiety during pregnancy are considered some of the most serious and concerning issues confronting pregnant women and perinatal health practitioners [9]. Both often co-exist and confer increased risk for adverse maternal, pregnancy and infant outcomes [10]. Historically, the emphasis on prenatal assessment/ screening, epidemiology, and research has focused on depression [10]. For example, prenatal depression has been shown to increase the risk for preterm birth, low birth weight, and intrauterine growth restriction [9, 11]. Recent findings, however, indicate that prenatal anxiety and stress are also associated with adverse maternal and infant outcomes and that anxiety related to the current pregnancy (pregnancy anxiety) may be especially potent [9]. Although exact mechanisms underlying pregnancy anxiety remain unclear, it is thought that potent infant effects may be due to complex interactions between maternal vulnerabilities that predate the pregnancy (eg., insecure attachment, lack of psychosocial resources) and anxieties a mother may have concerning certain aspects of the pregnancy [9]. These interactions are thought to increase levels of maternal anxiety that, in turn, influence the maternal-fetal-placental stress and hormonal systems in a manner that may contribute to functional changes in fetal hypothalamic–pituitary-adrenal (HPA) axis and to increased risk for adverse fetal neurodevelopment and premature birth [9].

Systematic review studies estimate that major depression, during pregnancy, affects up to 12.7 % of pregnant women [12] and that the prevalence rates (95 % CI) of depression for the 1st, 2nd, and 3rd trimesters of pregnancy are 7.4 % (2.2, 12.6), 12.8 % (10.7, 14.8), and 12.0 % (7.4, 16.7), respectively [13]. The preceding findings contribute to increased understanding of the prevalence of depression and anxiety during the trimesters of pregnancy. More recently, interest has shifted to also examining how the course of depression and anxiety throughout and at each trimester may adversely impact maternal, fetal and infant outcomes. Findings of a recent systematic review, for example, suggest that depression occurring during mid to late pregnancy may have the greatest adverse effects on fetal growth and development, while anxiety associated with preterm birth may contribute to changes in fetal HPA axis [14].

Studies that have linked maternal psychopathology with maternal caregiving have mostly involved mothers with postnatal depression. Findings show that some of these mothers exhibit a range of inconsistent or atypical caregiving behaviors such as being less or overly responsive to their infant cues, intrusive, or they withdraw from interacting with their infants [15]. Currently, it has been suggested that maternal caregiving behavior (eg., sensitivity) is a likely mechanism that links prenatal maternal depression [16] and /or anxiety [17] to infant and child bio-behavioral outcomes (e.g., difficult emotion regulation, altered cortisol patterns).

The previous findings highlight the concerning implications of 2nd-trimester exposure to maternal depression and/or anxiety (hereafter referred to as MDA) on maternal and infant outcomes as well as pointing to the potential mediating effect of maternal caregiving behavior. As it pertains to maternal caregiving interventions for neonatal pain, improved reporting and targeted recruitment of mothers with MDA and their infants into the study will help ensure the interventions are representative. However, more research is needed to clarify the significance of MDA during the neonatal period and if it underlies atypical maternal caregiving behavior as well as neonatal pain outcomes during routine pain procedures.

To our knowledge, there have only been two independent studies that have examined some of the linkages between MDA, and/or postnatal maternal caregiving behavior and/ or newborn pain outcomes in full-term infants [18, 19]. Both were conducted by some of the authors of the current study (FW, KC, and RB). The first study [18] compared the proportion of time that mothers in three study groups [two groups of mothers with MDA (medicated with Selective Serotonin Re-uptake Inhibitor antidepressants (SSRIs) and not), and a control group] spent exhibiting atypical caregiving behavior as they held their infants while the infant had a routine HL. The findings showed that during the HL, both groups of mothers with MDA were more likely to be less responsive to their infant's pain cry and to engage their infant less, compared to maternal controls. The second study [19] quantified the temporal profile of the behavioral responses of infants with and without 2nd-trimester MDA exposure during the sub-phases of the actual HL procedure (HL, post-HL). In that study, the HL was performed with the infant laying on a cot. Findings showed no group differences in the magnitude of initial behavioral reactions to the actual HL, but during the post-HL sub-phase, MDA-exposed infants spent more time crying in a weak/exhausted manner and in exhibiting strained and erratic limb movement and immobility. The findings indicated that infant prenatal exposure to MDA might have contributed to delayed recovery and diminished capacities for self-regulation of noxious distress in those infants.

Taken together, findings from the two studies [18, 19] indicate that MDA may underlie the observed atypical expression of maternal caregiving behavior and infant pain behavior. They further suggest that MDA and maternal caregiving behavior are significant factors to consider in neonatal pain studies and maternal caregiving interventions for neonatal pain. However, the first study [18] was limited in that findings were based on the brief event of infant HL (eg., 2 min). Hence, it is unclear whether mothers with MDA would exhibit similar patterns of behavior for longer periods of the HL session. The second study [19] examined linkages between MDA and infant pain behavior self-regulation, but not maternal caregiving behavior. To further clarify the significance and potential underlying impacts of MDA, it is necessary to examine the relationships of MDA to maternal caregiving behavior and infant behavior self-regulation concurrently and to examine maternal caregiving behavior over longer durations during HL.

This study addresses gaps and builds on findings of the two preceding studies [18, 19]. The study is part of a large project on MDA and its potential underlying effects on the caregiving behavior of mothers and newborn pain behavior self-regulation from which findings of infant pain self-regulation behavior reported by Warnock et al. [19] originate.

The first aim was to examine association and group differences in caregiving behavior between mothers with and without MDA before and following infant HL. To do this behavioral data were generated from the pre-recorded videotapes of the caregiving behavior of 24 mothers that had been collected but never coded or analyzed in the Warnock et al. [19] study. On the basis of findings of the first study [18], we hypothesized that MDA (as measured by maternal mental health scores taken at 2nd trimester) would be associated with maternal atypical caregiving behavior during a 5 min observation session before the infant was placed in a cot to have the HL (Pre-HL phase), and during a 5 min observation session after the infant had the HL and was reunited with their mother (Post-HL phase). We also hypothesized that during each of these two study phases, that the proportion of time that mothers spend exhibiting atypical behavior would differ between MDA-exposed mothers and maternal controls.

The second aim was to examine associations between maternal MDA-exposure, time-based measures of maternal caregiving behavior and the three atypical patterns of infant pain behavior self-regulation previously reported (crying in a weak/exhausted manner, strained and erratic limb movement and immobility) [19], concurrently. Data were time-based measures of maternal caregiving behavior generated from the 24 maternal pre-recorded videotapes as well as time-based measures of the three atypical patterns of infant pain behavior self-regulation. The infant measures were drawn from the pool of pre-calculated time-based measures of the 21 infants who had participated in the Warnock et al. [19] study. From the total samples of 24 mothers and 21 babies, there was a matched subsample of 16 maternal-infant dyads with complete time-based behavioral data to undertake the second study aim. Extending prior research [18, 19], we hypothesized that in this matched subsample of 21 mothers and their infants, maternal atypical caregiving behavior during the 5 min Pre-HL phase would be associated with the three atypical patterns of infant pain behavior self-regulation during the sub-phases of the actual infant HL (HL, post-HL).

Methods

Study design

This was an ethological micro-analytic descriptive comparative study that made use of systematic observation methods and time-based analytic approaches. We chose these methods and approaches because unlike conventional approaches, they are capable of generating precise measures of the proportion of time (Prop-T) that an individual or group spends in a particular behavior during an observation session(s), and that can be compared [20]. Furthermore, they have a unique ability in distinguishing patterning in behavior from the co-occurring running streams of behavior as the normally unfold, and in explicating biological mechanisms, such as MDA, that may underlie observed behavior [20].

Main outcomes of the current study were Prop-T time scores of maternal caregiving behavior and infant pain behavior self-regulation for the 5 min Pre-HL, 2 min infant HL (including post-HL sub-phase), and 5 min Post-HL study phases. Prop-T scores were calculated by dividing the full duration of time a mother or infant spent in a particular behavior by the entire duration of the respective study phase. MDA was operationally defined as mild to severe symptoms of prenatal depression and/or anxiety based on mean scores of prenatal mental health measures that mothers completed at the 2nd trimester. Descriptions of maternal recruitment and data collection procedures that we provide below are summarized from Warnock et al. [19]. This is because mothers of the current study were mothers of some of the infants from the Warnock et al. [19] study and because measures of MDA were collected from mothers prenatally. A further reason is that measures of maternal caregiving and infant pain behavior self-regulation were collected at the same time.

Participants

As reported by Warnock et al. [19], mothers were recruited during the 2nd trimester of pregnancy (first visit) and then again on the day of their infant's scheduled HL, which occurred about 36 h after infant birth (second visit). The 2nd trimester was chosen because of the increased prevalence and impacts of depression and anxiety compared to the 1st and 3rd trimesters, as noted earlier. Four mothers with MDA, who volunteered their participation were referred to the study by their primary care physicians who had diagnosed them as depressed and/or anxious. The remaining mothers were those who responded to advertisements of the study posted in health clinics, prenatal classes or newspapers. To be included, women had to be proficient in the English language, have no birth complications, no bipolar disorder or Axis II disorders, and their infants had to be >37 weeks gestational age with a birth weight of > 2500 g. Excluded were infants with congenital heart disease, central nervous system malformations and neonatal abstinence syndrome (NAS). Of the 36 mothers who initially volunteered, all met study inclusion criteria and all completed a mental health assessment at 2nd trimester of pregnancy. There were no missing data on any of the mental health measures that mothers completed.

Twelve of the 36 mothers were not included in the current analysis because of loss to follow-up during pregnancy ($n = 1$) or because of insufficient data on maternal caregiving behavior ($n = 11$). Of the remaining 24 mothers, six had reported taking drugs during pregnancy (SSRIs ($n = 3$), crack cocaine ($n = 2$) or SSRI + crack cocaine ($n = 1$). Those six mothers were not excluded from the current analysis in recognition that in our region, 5 % of pregnant women are prescribed SSRIs antidepressant medications [21] and 3.5 % report taking crack cocaine during pregnancy [22]. A further reason was that none of the infants had NAS based on pre-study screening by a neonatologist. However, because little has been published on the effects of prenatal drug use on maternal caregiving behavior during neonatal pain, "prenatal maternal drug use" (SSRIs and/ or crack cocaine) was entered as a covariate in the analysis as appropriate.

The final sample, therefore, consisted of 24 mothers. On the basis of a-priori sample size calculations of the previous study that involved infants of study mothers [19] (for Type 1 error rate of 0.05, a power of .80 and effect size of .30, ((G-Power 3.1)), a total sample of 24 mothers was needed to examine change and group differences in Prop-T scores of maternal behavior before and following infant HL. Based on Stevens [23], the sample size for each of the simple regressions involving one predictor variable required 15 subjects. The larger study from which this study and the Warnock et al. [19] study originate, received ethical approved from the University of British Columbia Research Ethics Board and by the Children's and Women's Health Centre Research Review Committee. All mothers gave written informed consent for both themselves and their infants.

Procedures

Prenatal maternal mental health assessment

As reported by Warnock et al. [19], the prenatal assessment that the 24 study mothers completed at 2nd trimester and that took place during the first visit, included the well validated 10 item patient-rated Edinburgh Postnatal Depression Scale (EPDS), the well validated clinician-rated 21-item Hamilton Depression Scale (HAM-D) and the 14-item Hamilton Anxiety Scale (HAM-A). The three tools were administered to the mothers by a research assistant who was knowledgeable and trained in the tools, but not blinded to study aims. Mothers were assigned to the MDA-exposed group or the non-MDA-exposed group (control) on the basis of meeting predetermined cut-off scores on one or more of the mental health measures and that were capable of detecting symptoms of depression and/or anxiety or not. The cut-off scores were: HAM-D > 8 [24, 25], HAM-A > 8 [26], EPDS > 11 [27]. All three tools including same cut-off scores have been used in prior neonatal pain studies that involved mothers with MDA (medicated with SSRIs and not) [18, 19, 28–30].

Data collection: maternal and infant behavior

As per Warnock et al. [19], mothers and infants were assessed during the second visit in a quiet and heat regulated room in the hospital. Mothers were debriefed about the study procedures and advised that they could withdraw their participation at any time, or for any reason and to care for their infants as they normally would. Research staff did not interfere with the care that a mother chose to provide her infant during the HL procedure or with the routine hospital protocol for neonatal HL, which was performed with the infant laying on a cot. All HLs were performed by experienced lab technicians on infants who were awake and who did not have any HL in past 12 h. Also, data were based on a single HL.

Data collection commenced with mothers seated and holding their infants on their laps. One camera was positioned to capture full body views of the mother and the infant and to videotape continuously the behavioral responses a mother made to her infant for 5 min before the infant's HL (Pre-HL). Upon arrival of the lab technician, the infant who was clothed in a vest and diaper was gently placed supine onto a cot by the infant's mother or by the research assistant if the mother requested. A second camera captured body movements of the infant continuously for the duration of HL with crying simultaneously audio-recorded. All mothers remained in the room, and none chose to touch their infant. After the HL, the infant was reunited with their mother, and maternal behavioral responses to the infant were videotaped continuously for 5 min (Post-HL). The research assistant depressed a foot peddle to mark the beginning and end of each study phase and a running time was encoded on the study videotapes to enable second-by-second coding of maternal and infant behavior.

Maternal behavioral measures and coding procedures

In the current study, the pre-recorded videotaped cases of the 24 study mothers were each coded using the reliably established Maternal Behavior Coding System (MBCS) [18]. The MBCS is an ethologically based micro-analytic behavioral research coding tool that had been previously developed inductively for use with mothers with and without MDA during an infant pain event [18]. In a cross-validated sample, the MBCS distinguished typical from atypical caregiving behavior between two groups of mothers with MDA (medicated and not) and a control group of mothers [18]. The tool consists of main categories and subcategories of maternal caregiving behavior that are structured into two main domains–typical caregiving behavior and atypical caregiving behavior. We chose the MBCS because it enables trained coders to continuously code behavioral items second-by-second as the coders observe them to occur on pre-recorded videotapes from which precise Prop-T scores of behavior can be generated and compared (see Warnock et al. [18] for a copy of the MBCS for that study).

In this study, we drew on the coding procedures from the Warnock et al. [18] study to continuously code MBCS items from the 24 pre-recorded videotaped maternal cases. Two coders who were knowledge of the MBCS, trained in systematic coding, and who were blinded to maternal group and to study phase, coded the videotapes in random order, in terms of participants, using the MBCS. Starting with the first videotaped case and the first 60 s of the 5 min Pre-HL study phase, the coders examined each 1-s interval and coded the occurrence and duration of each maternal behavior described in the MBCS. Only when each of five 60 s time blocks was coded in succession for the Pre-HL session did the coders move to code the five 60 s time blocks of the Post-HL session. The same systematic steps were followed to code the two 5 min sessions for the remaining 23 maternal videotapes. Excluded from the analysis were behaviors that were not visible to coders for 20 s or more during any one 60 s time block (eg., due to the ill positioning of the video camera or when research staff walked in front of the camera) [20]. All of the 24 maternal videotapes used in the current analysis had complete data.

Of the 14,400 one-second intervals (~240 min) of coded maternal behavior (600 s for Pre-Hl + 600 s for Post-HL) (MDA group = 7000 s; control group = 7000 s) 20 % were randomly selected and subjected to inter-reliability testing, achieving k = 0.80 or better. Data were then entered into the General Sequential Querier for Windows (GSEQ 5.1). GSEQ5.1 is a unique data analysis program specially designed to calculate precise Prop-T measures of coded behavioral items by case, or by study group, or by study phase [20]. Next, we made use of GSEQ5.1 to combine Prop-T scores of coded MBCS items that were conceptually related, and that were then grouped into eight domains. Each domain was further structured into two mutually exclusive categories - the first representing typical maternal caregiving behavior and the other representing atypical behavior. Table 1 provides a summary of the eight MBCS main categories that were identified from this dataset, including definitions. Prop-T scores representing maternal atypical caregiving behavior and typical behavior for each maternal study case were then transferred to SPSS 21 to address study aims.

Infant behavioral measures and coding procedures

The systematic procedures that Warnock et al. [19] used to continuously code each of the 21 infant pre-recorded videotapes were the same as those described above for coding the 24 maternal pre-recorded videotapes. As reported by Warnock et al. [19], the reliably established and cross-validated Neonatal Distress Pain Related Behavioral Coding Schema (ND-BSC) was used to code the infant videotapes by four coders who were trained in the ND-BSC and who were blinded to infant group. However, coders were not blinded to study phase because the laboratory technician's hand, used to conduct the HL, was visible to the coder. The ND-BCS is an ethologically based behavioral coding schema that consists of items for coding continuously and concurrently infant motor movement, posture, respiration responsiveness and cry behavior. The procedures used to test for inter-reliability between coders, and to reduce and further analyze data in GSEQ 5.1 were also the same as those described above for coding the maternal videotaped cases. Inter-reliability between coders achieved k = 0.80 or better [19]. Sequential and comparative analysis of Prop-T scores of ND-BCS coded items led to identifying the

Table 1 Eight MBCS behaviors with definitions

	Definition/Description	
Coding Items	Typical maternal caregiving behavior	Atypical maternal caregiving behavior
Eye Gaze	Looking or seeking eye contact: Mother looking straight at baby's face, or mother seeking eye contact with baby.	Looking away: Mother looking away from baby.
Engages baby and responsive to baby cues/actions.	Interactive, engages baby: Mother makes frequent attempts to interact/engage infant. Mother directly or indirectly responds to infant cues (baby crying, looking at or touching mother),	Minimal or no responsiveness to infant cues. Mother makes minimal, or no attempt to interact or to engage with the infant. Mother not responsive - may appear detached.
Embracing (positioning) of the baby	Mother embracing baby: Close, protective. Baby's body is enclosed in mom's embrace	No embracing or cradling. Baby laying in unsafe position. Mother does not appear to notice baby may fall off her lap.
Direction of mother's attention	Attention directed to baby: Mother focuses attention on baby,	Attention not directed to baby. Mother seems self-absorbed, her attention is not directed to baby, to others, or to her environment.
Type and quality of facial expressions	Regular: Mother facial expression regular, smiling.	Not regular: Grimacing, crying quietly, crying excessively. Quality of facial expression is flat or mother appears disconnected or "checked out"
Comfort	Comfortable: Mother appears comfortable or she says she is comfortable.	Not comfortable: Mother appears uncomfortable (eg., mother sighs, rolls eyes) or says she is uncomfortable.
General affect	Unbothered: Mother's generally appears unbothered sad, or worried.	Bothered: Mother appears bothered, worried, sad, upset or very upset (distraught).
Anxiety	No such display: Mother does not appear anxious	Anxious: Mother bites nails, touches hair, repetitive nervous knee movement.

MBCS definitions from Ethogram of Maternal Behavior Coding System [18]

three temporal patterns of newborn pain behavior self-regulation that were suggestive of delay in pain recovery (crying in a weak/exhausted manner, strained/erratic limb movement and immobility).

Data analysis

Simple descriptive statistics were obtained for all study variables and distributions of continuous variables were inspected for normality. For the total sample of 24 mothers, Mann-Whitney and Wilcoxon Signed Rank test for non-normally distributed data were used to test the hypothesis that the proportion of time that study mothers spend exhibiting atypical behavior during the 5 min Pre-HL and the 5 min Post-HL study phases would differ between MDA-exposed mothers and maternal controls. For the later, Prop-T scores of maternal behavior were analyzed when six or more mothers in either group exhibited MBCS behaviors during Pre-HL or Post-HL. Separate simple linear regressions using adjusted R^2 were performed on the total sample of 24 mothers to test whether prenatal MDA (HAM-A, HAM-D and EPDS mean scores) would predict Prop-T scores of maternal atypical caregiving behavior during the 5 min Pre-HL and 5 min Post-HL study phases. For the matched subsample of 16 mothers and their infants, we also performed simple regressions to examine if Prop-T scores of types of maternal atypical behavior during the Pre-HL phase would predict Prop-T scores of the three atypical patterns of pain behavior self-regulation in infants previously reported [19] during the HL and post-HL sub-phases of infant HL. Finally, partial correlations were used to examine the potential contribution of prenatal maternal drug use (SSRI/SU) on study outcomes as appropriate. All analyses were two-tailed with alpha set at $p < .05$, as appropriate.

Results

Prenatal mental health measures and maternal and infant characteristics

Of the 24 mothers, 12 had scores that exceeded the predefined cut-off for the HAM-A (range, 8–29), or the HAM-D (range, 8–29) or the EPDS (range, 11–27). These 12 mothers were allocated to the MDA-exposed group, and the 12 mothers whose scores fell below the cut-offs were allocated to the non-MDA-exposed group (maternal controls). MDA-exposed mothers had significantly higher HAM-A, HAM-D and EPDS scores than did the non MDA-exposed group of mothers ($U = 14$, $p < .001$, $r = .75$; $U = 12$, $p < .001$, $r = .77$; $U = 11$, $p < .001$, $r = .78$, respectively). Of interest, we found that ten of 12 mothers allocated to the MDA-exposed group had comorbid anxiety and depression based on exceeding cut-off scores on two or more of the tools: HAM-A + HAM-D ($n = 5$) and HAM-A + HAM-D + EPDS ($n = 5$). In the subsample of 16 mothers, eight had scores that exceeded the predefined cut-offs, and eight had scores that fell below the cut-offs. Of the eight mothers whose scores exceeded the cut-offs, six had comorbid anxiety and depression: HAM-A + HAM-D ($n = 1$) and HAM-A + HAM-D + EPDS ($n = 5$).

The 24 mothers had a mean age of 34 years (SD = 5.6) and a mean of 17.46 years of education (SD = 4.9). Most were married (63 %), Caucasian (67 %), and first-time mothers (63 %). The mode of delivery was vaginal (58.1 %) or by C-section (41.7 %). As reported in the Warnock et al. [19] study, infants had a mean gestational age of 39.75 weeks (SD = 1.53), birthweight of 3436 g (SD = .3859), and 62 % were male. There were no statistically significant group differences on maternal characteristics or on factors considered as confounders to maternal caregiving behavior such as smoking, infant gender or number of children or on infant characteristics. The preceding findings were consistent for the subsample of 16 mothers and infants.

Association and group differences in types of caregiving behavior between mothers with and without MDA before and following infant HL

Initial analysis involving the 24 mothers, showed moderate positive correlation between prenatal maternal anxiety (HAM-A) and depression (HAM-D, EPDS), and total Prop-T scores of maternal atypical caregiving behavior during routine infant HL ($r = .604$, $p = .002$; $r = .447$, $p = .03$; $r = .631$, $p < .00$, respectively). Both groups of mothers (MDA-exposed and non-MDA-exposed) exhibited

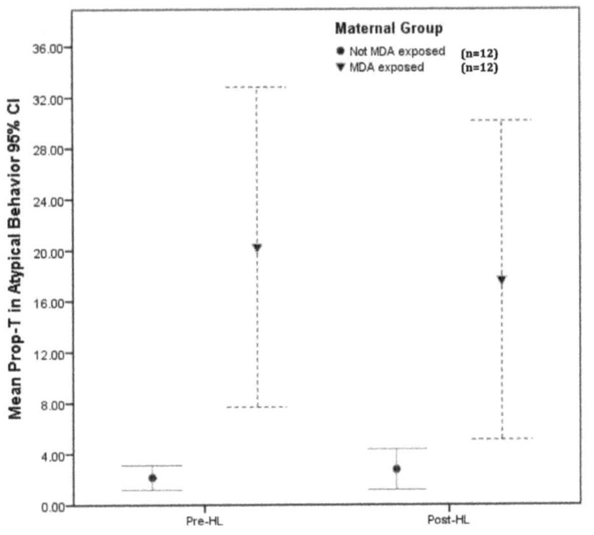

Fig. 1 Group differences and change in Mean proportion of time (total Prop-T score, 95 % CI) that the 24 mothers in the two study groups [(MDA-exposed ($n = 12$) and Non-MDA exposed ($n = 12$)] spent exhibiting atypical caregiving behavior to infant behavioral cues while with their infant for 5 min before the infant had the HL (Pre-HL) and for 5 min after the infant had the HL (Post-HL)

typical caregiving behavior to their infants, during the 5 min Pre-HL and 5 min Post-HL study phases. However, as Fig. 1 illustrates, during the two study phases, mean scores of atypical caregiving behavior were higher for MDA-exposed mothers compared to non-MDA exposed mothers with both groups showing little change from the Pre-HL phase to the Post-HL phase. Notably, the distributions of scores were considerably more varied for the MDA-exposure mothers than they were for the non-MDA exposed mothers.

The Mann-Whitney tests were conducted to examine group differences in Prop-T spent in varying types of atypical behavior when six or more mothers in either group (MDA-exposed (n = 12), non-MDA exposed (n = 12) exhibited MBCS behaviors during the 5 min Pre-HL or the 5 min Post-H study sessions. The results revealed that during the Pre-HL phase, MDA-exposed mothers were more likely than maternal controls to not embrace (U = 36, $p < .001$, r = .55), attend (U = 34, p = .028, r = .45) or engage and respond to the infant's behavioral pain cues (U = 36, p = .038, r = .42). Wilcoxon Signed Rank Test showed no change in Prop-T of atypical behavior between the two groups of mothers from the Pre-HL to Post-Hl study phase. However, the results showed, that although six MDA-exposed mothers spent a significant proportion of the Pre-HL phase not embracing, three of the six spent significantly less time in not embracing Post-HL (U = 40, p = .021, r = .51). Table 2 provides a summary of the preceding results. The table does not include results pertaining to atypical expression of MBCS comfort, or general affect and anxiety because the behaviors were not exhibited by enough mothers (six or more for the study phases).

Relationships between prenatal maternal mental health measures and maternal atypical caregiving behavior before and after infant HL

Separate simple linear regressions involving the 24 mothers were performed to determine if prenatal MDA (mean scores of HAM-D, or HAM-A or EPDS) would predict Prop-T scores of maternal atypical caregiving behavior during the Pre-HL and Post-HL study phases. Results showed HAM-D scores predicted Prop-T scores of atypical caregiving behavior during the Pre-HL (β = .46, t = 2.46, p = .022), but more so during the Post-HL phase (β = .66, t = 4.16, p = .01). HAM-A and EPDS scores also predicted Prop-T scores of maternal atypical caregiving behavior, but only during Post-HL: HAM-A (β = .64, t = 3.95, $p < .001$); EPDS (β = .64, t = 3.92, $p < .001$).

HAM-D scores accounted for a smaller proportion of variance in atypical behavior during Pre-HL [adjusted R^2 = .180, F (1, 22) = 6.05, p = .022] than during Post-HL [adjusted R^2 = .416, F (1, 22) = 17.35, p = .01]. HAM-A and EPDS scores also accounted for up to 38 % of the variance in atypical expression Post-HL: HAM-A [adjusted R^2 = .389, F (1, 22) = 15.66, $p < .001$], EPDS [adjusted R^2 = .385, F (1, 22) = 15.39, $p < .001$].

Relationship between maternal atypical caregiving behavior during Pre-HL and infant pain self-regulation behavior during the sub-phases of infant HL (HL and post-HL)

Results of the final simple linear regressions that involved the matched subsample of 16 mothers and their infants showed the Prop-T that mothers spent in not engaging/responding or attending to infant's behavioral cues during the 5 min Pre-HL phase, predicted the Prop-T that infant offspring spent exhibiting strained/erratic limb movements

Table 2 Proportion of time (Prop-T) study mothers spent in five MBCS atypical behavior Pre-HL and Post-HL

	Group	Phase						Z
		Pre-HL (5 min)			Post-HL (5 min)			
		n	M(SD)	Mdn	n	M(SD)	Mdn	
Looking away from baby.	Control	10	9.95 (13.89)	5.35	9	10.20 (9.49)	9.00	−314
	MDA-Exposed	12	22.67 (24.89)	15.50	12	18.72 (18.46)	12.80	−.235
Minimal or no responsiveness to baby cues/action. minimal, or no attempt to interact or to engage with the infant	Control	12	10.45 (13.70)	4.85	8	9.39 (8.86)	8.00	.000
	MDA-Exposed	12	28.72 (27.15)	20.50*	12	25.86 (38.86)	.110*	−1.34
Not embracing, cradling baby.	Control	0	.000 (.00)	.00	0	.000 (.00)	.00	.000
	MDA-Exposed	6	35.39 (45.11)	6.15*	3	9.14 (21.31)	.00	−.2.201**
Mothers attention not directed towards baby, others, or environment	Control	10	10.20 (13.88)	4.85	8	9.05 (8.56)	8.00	−.639
	MDA-Exposed	12	32.25 (33.30)	20.50*	10	20.77 (23.75)	12.65	.523
Type and quality of facial expression not regular.	Control	10	17.00 (28.29)	4.20	6	7.19 (14.96)	.50	−1.27
	MDA-Exposed	9	29.28 (36.26)	20.50	9	30.52 (36.65)	19.85	−.533

Values represent mean proportion of time (number of seconds behavior expressed/total number of seconds of the observation session) based on 24 mothers (12 in MDA-exposed grp, 12 in Control group), n total number of mothers in each group who exhibited the behavior (minimum of 6 required in either phase). *$p < .05$ Mann Whitney U test; **$p < .05$ Wilcoxon signed-rank test (β = .552, $t = 2.47$, $p = .027$) and immobility (β = .566, $t = 2.57$, $p = .022$) during the actual HL. Prop-T scores of these maternal behavior explained 25 % of the variance in infant strained/erratic limb movement [adjusted $R^2 = .255$, F (1, 14) = 6.14, $p = .027$] and 27 % in immobility [adjusted $R^2 = .272$, F (1, 14) = 6.60, $p = .022$] during the actual HL.

We also found the Prop-T the 16 mothers spent not engaging or attending during the 5 min Pre-HL phase, predicted the Prop-T their infants spent in weak/strained cry during the post-HL sub-phase (β = .690, t = 3.56, p = .003, and β = .518, $t = 2.26$, $p = .040$, respectively). The Prop-T the mothers spent in not engaging or attending Pre-HL explained up to 21 % of the variance in infant weak/strained cry post-HL subphase: [adjusted $R^2 = .216$, F (1, 14) = 5.132, $p = .040$].

Discussion

The overall goal of this basic observation study using time based analytic approaches was to clarify the significance of MDA and its potential underlying impact on maternal caregiving behavior and infant pain behavior self-regulation, in the first few days following infant birth. Acknowledging the complex and many multiple pathways of association possible, the precise and in-depth time-based findings generated in this study contribute robust foundational measures of maternal and infant behavior that could not have been generated using conventional approaches. Main findings suggest that MDA may underlie atypical maternal caregiving behavior and that maternal caregiving behavior may mediate infant pain behavior self-regulation.

As hypothesized, MDA-exposure was associated with type and temporal quality of atypical maternal caregiving behavior before and after infant HL. During the Pre-HL phase, MDA-exposed mothers were more likely than maternal controls to not engage /respond or attend to infant behavioral cues Pre-HL–with little change Post-HL. That three of the six MDA-exposed mothers spent less time in not embracing their infant Post-HL suggest change toward more responsive caregiving behavior. But given the very small number of mothers who exhibited change, further study is required before conclusion can be drawn. The considerable variability in Prop-T that the 12 mothers with MDA spent exhibiting atypical behavior may be because 83 % of these mothers had cut-off scores indicating moderate to severe comorbidity.

Our findings of association between MDA and time-based measures of maternal caregiving before and after routine infant HL are consistent with findings of a lack of responsiveness and insensitivity behavior in mothers with postpartum depression and/ or anxiety reported in studies that did not involve infant pain [31, 32]. They are also consistent with time-based findings of the Warnock et al. [18] study that showed a lack of engagement and responsiveness in mothers with MDA as they held their infants during the 2 min HL. Our findings extend those findings, in that our group of MDA-exposed mothers exhibited lack of engagement and responsive to infant cues while with their infants, 5 min before the 2 min HL and 5 min after the HL. Taken together, findings of the prior study [18] and this study suggest that MDA-exposed mothers may express atypical patterning in caregiving behavior over the course of infant HL.

In our study, factors that have been acknowledged to influence maternal atypical caregiving behavior such as the number of children, gender of an infant or maternal smoking did not present as confounders. However, one factor that we did not examine and that may have contributed to our findings of maternal atypical caregiving behavior is a lack of sleep or physical exhaustion in mothers, especially given that we sampled mothers within days of giving birth. In a recent study, mothers with an EPDS score of >12 at one week postpartum were significantly more likely to report being tired [33]. In addition, maternal fatigue in that study was strongly associated with new onset of depressive symptoms. These maternal variables may have interactive or confounding effects and therefore warrant consideration in future studies.

Our second and third hypotheses that MDA exposure (as measured by 2nd trimester HAM-D, or HAM-A or EPDS scores) would predict Prop-T scores of maternal atypical caregiving behavior and that maternal atypical caregiving behavior Pre-HL would be associated with the three patterns of atypical infant pain behavior self-regulation reported previously [19] were both supported. Similar to the findings reported by Warnock et al. [18], we found that prenatal depression and anxiety was positively associated with atypical expression of caregiving behavior. Our findings extend the prior findings [18] in that prenatal depression, and anxiety (based on independent analysis of HAM-A, HAM-D and /or EPDS scores) accounted for up to 41 % of the variance in atypical expression of caregiving behavior Post-HL. Controlling for prenatal maternal drug use (SSRIs, crack cocaine) had little impact on these findings. Our approach to examining the relationship of MDA to Prop-T scores of maternal caregiving contributed knowledge on the distinct contributions MDA during the 2nd trimester based on independent analysis of HAM-A, or HAM-D or EPDS scores. Future studies with large sample sizes will help determine which of the three measures best predict atypical maternal caregiving and the contributions of comorbidity and pregnancy anxiety at each trimester.

We also found that the Prop-T that the 16 mothers in the subsample spent in not embracing and in not engaging/responding or attending to infant behavioral cues during the 5 min Pre-HL phase were associated with the Prop-T their infants spent in immobility and in strained/erratic limb movement during actual HL, and in weak/strained cry during the post- HL sub-phase. These findings extend the findings by Warnock et al. [19] in that we included time-based measures of maternal caregiving in the concurrent analysis. While the prior findings [19] suggest that infant ability to self-regulate to and from painful stimuli may be impacted by prenatal exposure to MDA, the current findings suggest that type/quality of maternal caregiving behavior may play a mediatory role in this dynamic. However, these results were based on a sample of16 mothers and their infants. As such, the results are preliminary, but they warrant further study. If the maternal and infant findings are again observed in future studies, convergent findings may provide the basis for the development of early clinical interventions that promote the caregiving behavior and stress regulatory role of mothers with MDA. Newborn ability to behaviorally regulate to stressors is a marker of neurodevelopment [2], and early indication of sustained delay in self-regulation in the full-term necessitate early assessment and treatment.

The dearth of similar studies in the context of neonatal pain makes it difficult to compare our findings. Other studies that did not involve infant pain have reported linkages between prenatal maternal depression and/or anxiety and postnatal alteration in maternal caregiving behavior and later child outcomes. For example, findings have shown that prenatal anxiety predicts depressive symptoms during the postpartum [34] and that it accounts for 10–15 % of adverse behavioral, emotional, cognitive and mental health outcomes in later childhood [10, 35] such as low social competencies and adaptive functioning [36]. In contrast, other findings have shown that maternal insensitivity, but not antenatal psychiatric diagnosis, predicts infant responsiveness in a free play situation at four months post-partum [16]. Potential reasons for the discrepant findings between that study and our findings is that we examined caregiving behavior of mothers with MDA during the newborn period and because the findings were based on the use of ethologically driven methods that are specifically designed to help explain biological mechanisms underlying observed behavior.

The in-depth descriptions of the types and temporal qualities of maternal caregiving behavior that were elucidated in this study are clinically relevant. Clinicians with interests in mother driven interventions for neonatal pain may use the findings to consider inclusion of mothers with MDA and their infants. These mothers may represent the 36 % of women who decline participation [8], and it is unclear if these dyads would benefit from the regulatory properties of the interventions. There is, however, emerging evidence that maternal-infant skin-to-skin contact intervention for neonatal pain may have regulatory benefits for both mothers and infants regardless of maternal mental health status [37]. Clinical recruitment and future research of this kind will help support mothers with MDA and their infants and as noted, may provide the basis for potential modification of the interventions, as appropriate.

This study has limitations that necessitate cautious interpretation of study findings. Although this basic observation study yielded foundational data based on a huge amount of time-based measures, the small subject sample size limits the generalizability of the findings. Some of the study mothers had taken antidepressant medications and/or drugs (SSRIs, crack cocaine) during pregnancy. Although we controlled for these effects statistically, these mothers may exhibit a unique behavioral profile due to impacts of the drugs and chronic exposures to environmental adversity and stress. It was beyond the present study to have distinguished any behavioral differences, and this may be an area for future dedicated research. Findings were based on independent measures of prenatal depression and anxiety and the study focused on maternal and infant behavior. Targeting comorbidity at recruitment, making use of multivariate analysis and obtaining physiological and other measures (eg., measures of maternal and infant cortisol levels, heart rate variability) in future larger sized samples will help clarify pathways of association.

Conclusions

Sensitive and responsive maternal caregiving behavior strengthens infant self-regulatory capacities, but this powerful regulatory role may be diminished in some women with MDA. Our findings suggest that mothers and infants with 2nd trimester MDA exposure exhibit atypical behavior during a routine infant pain event and that MDA may underlie these atypical patterning in behavior. The findings are consistent with findings of studies that have examined associations between MDA, maternal caregiving behavior that did and did not involve infant pain, and that were conducted during the postpartum. We recommend early inclusion of mothers with MDA and their infants in interventions aimed to strengthen the early mother-infant interaction and a mother's caregiving regulatory role. MDA and maternal caregiving behavior must be considered in future infant pain studies and to examine potential confounding effects of MDA on effectiveness of mother driven interventions for neonatal pain. We highlight the importance of future research on maternal mental health throughout the trajectory of the perinatal period, particularly during the early newborn period, and on development and implementation of early strength-based interventions.

Acknowledgements

We would like to thank all of the mothers and infants who participated in this study.

Funding
This study was supported by the Michael Smith Foundation for Health Research (Scholar award to FW) and by an operating grant from Canadian Institutes of Health Research (MOP 77769 to FW). The funding bodies did not play any role in the design of the study or in data collection, interpretation of data or in writing of the manuscript.

Authors' contributions
FW, RB and KC contributed to conception and study design. FW coordinated the study and contributed to recruitment, acquisition of study data and training of coders. FW and TC performed data analysis. FW, RB, KC, TC and JM all participated in the interpretation of study data and to the drafting and critical revision of the manuscript making contributions to the content. All authors read and approved the final manuscript.

Competing interests
The authors declare that they have no competing interests.

Author details
[1]Developmental Neurosciences, Child and Family Research Institute, L408, 4480 Oak Street, Vancouver, BC, Canada. [2]University of British Columbia (BC), School of Nursing, Vancouver, BC, Canada. [3]Department of Psychology, University of British Columbia (BC), Vancouver, BC, Canada. [4]Georgia State University, Atlanta, Georgia 30303, USA. [5]University of Goiás Faculty of Nursing, Goiânia, GO, Brazil. [6]School of Nursing and Midwifery, Tehran University of Medical Sciences, Tehran, Iran.

References

1. Gunnar MR, Quevedo KM. Early care experiences and HPA axis regulation in children: a mechanism for later trauma vulnerability. Prog Brain Res. 2007;167:137–49.
2. Als H, Duffy FH, McAnulty GB, Rivkin MJ, Vajapeyam S, Mulkern RV, et al. Early experience alters brain function and structure. Pediatrics. 2004;113(4):846–57.
3. Grunau RE, Tu MT. Long-term consequences of pain in human neonates. In: Anand KJ, Stevens B, McGrath PJ, editors. Pain in neonates and infants. 3rd ed. Amsterdam: Elsevier; 2007. p. 45–55.
4. Fitzgerald M, Walker SM. Infant pain management: a developmental neurobiological approach. Nat Clin Pract Neurol. 2009;5(1):35–50.
5. Carbajal R, Lenclen R, Jugie M, Paupe A, Barton BA, Anand KJS. Morphine does not provide adequate analgesia for acute procedural pain among preterm neonates. Pediatrics. 2005;115(6):1494–500.
6. Campbell-Yeo M, Fernandes A, Johnston CC. Procedural pain management for neonates using nonpharmacological strategies: part 2: mother-driven interventions. Adv Neonatal Care. 2011;11(5):312–8.
7. Fernandes A, Campbell-Yeo M, Johnston CC. Procedural pain management for neonates using nonpharmacological strategies: Part 1: sensorial interventions. Adv Neonatal Care. 2011;11(4):235–41.
8. Warnock FF, Castral TC, Brant R, Sekilian M, Leite AM, de la Presa Owens S, Scochi CGS. Brief report: maternal kangaroo care for neonatal pain relief: a systematic narrative review. J Pediatr Psychol. 2010;35(9):975–84.
9. Schetter CD, Tanner L. Anxiety, depression and stress in pregnancy: implications for mothers, children, research, and practice. Curr Opin Psychiatry. 2012;25(2):141–8.
10. Glover V. Maternal depression, anxiety and stress during pregnancy and child outcome; what needs to be done. Best Pract Res Clin Obstet Gynaecol. 2014;28(1):25–35.
11. Grote NK, Bridge JA, Gavin AR, Melville JL, Iyengar S, Katon WJ. A meta-analysis of depression during pregnancy and the risk of preterm birth, low birth weight, and intrauterine growth restriction. Arch Gen Psychiatry. 2010;67(10):1012–24.
12. Gavin NI, Gaynes BN, Lohr KN, Meltzer-Brody S, Gartlehner G, Swinson T. Perinatal depression: a systematic review of prevalence and incidence. Obstet Gynecol. 2005;106(5 Pt 1):1071–83.
13. Bennett HA, Einarson A, Taddio A, Koren G, Einarson TR. Prevalence of depression during pregnancy: systematic review. Obstet Gynecol. 2004;103(4):698–709.
14. Accortt EE, Cheadle AC, Schetter CD. Prenatal depression and adverse birth outcomes: an updated systematic review. Matern Child Health J. 2015;19(6):1306–37.
15. Jones NA, Field T, Fox NA, Davalos M, Malphurs J, Carraway K, et al. Infants of intrusive and withdrawn mothers. Infant Behav Dev. 1997;20(2):175–86.
16. Kaplan LA, Evans L, Monk C. Effects of mothers' prenatal psychiatric status and postnatal caregiving on infant biobehavioral regulation: can prenatal programming be modified? Early Hum Dev. 2008;84(4):249–56.
17. Grant K, McMahon C, Austin M, Reilly N, Leader L, Ali S. Maternal prenatal anxiety, postnatal caregiving and infants' cortisol responses to the still-face procedure. Dev Psychobiol. 2009;51(8):625–37.
18. Warnock FF, Bakeman R, Shearer K, Misri S, Oberlander T. Caregiving behavior and interactions of prenatally depressed mothers (antidepressant-treated and non-antidepressant-treated) during newborn acute pain. Infant Mental Health J. 2009;30(4):384–406.
19. Warnock FF, Craig KD, Bakeman R, Castral T. Self-regulation (recovery) from pain: association between time-based measures of infant pain behavior and prenatal exposure to maternal depression and anxiety. Clin J Pain. 2014;30(8):663–71.
20. Bakeman R, Quera V. Sequential analysis and observational methods for the behavioral sciences. 1st ed. New York: Cambridge Univ Press; 2011.
21. Oberlander TF, Warburton W, Misri S, Aghajanian J, Hertzman C. Effects of timing and duration of gestational exposure to serotonin reuptake inhibitor antidepressants: population-based study. Br J Psychiatry. 2008;192(5):338–43.
22. Lussier P, Tzoumakis S, Healey J, Corrado R, Reebye P. Pre/perinatal adversities and behavioural outcomes in early childhood: preliminary findings from the Vancouver longitudinal study. Int J Child Youth Fam Stud. 2011;2(1&2):36–64.
23. Stevens JP. Applied multivariate statistics for the social sciences. 3rd ed. Mahwah: Lawrence Erlbaum Associates; 1996.
24. Cusin C, Yang H, Yeung A, Fava M. Rating scales for depression. In: Baer L, Blais MA, editors. Handbook of clinical rating scales and assessment in psychiatry and mental health. New York: Humana Press, Springer; 2010. p. 7–35.
25. Hamilton M. A rating scale for depression. J Neurol Neurosurg Psychiatr. 1960;23(1):56–62.
26. Hamilton M. The assessment of anxiety states by rating. Br J Med Psychol. 1959;32(1):50–5.
27. Cox J, Holden J. Perinatal Mental Health: a guide to the Edinburgh Postnatal Depression Scale. 1st ed. Glasgow: RCPsych Publications; 2003.
28. Oberlander TF, Grunau R, Mayes L, Riggs W, Rurak D, Papsdorf M, Misri S, Weinberg J. Hypothalamic-pituitary-adrenal (HPA) axis function in 3-month old infants with prenatal selective serotonin reuptake inhibitor (SSRI) antidepressant exposure. Early Hum Dev. 2008;84(10):689–97.
29. Oberlander TF, Weinberg J, Papsdorf M, Grunau R, Misri S, Devlin AM. Prenatal exposure to maternal depression, neonatal methylation of human glucocorticoid receptor gene (NR3C1) and infant cortisol stress responses. Epigenetics. 2008;3(2):97–106.
30. Oberlander TF, Reebye P, Misri S, Papsdorf M, Kim J, Grunau RE. Externalizing and attentional behaviors in children of depressed mothers treated with a selective serotonin reuptake inhibitor antidepressant during pregnancy. Arch Pediatr Adolesc Med. 2007;161(1):22–9.
31. Beck CT. The effects of postpartum depression on maternal-infant interaction: a meta-analysis. Nurs Res. 1995;44(5):298–305.
32. Feldman R, Granat A, Pariente C, Kanety H, Kuint J, Gilboa-Schechtman E. Maternal depression and anxiety across the postpartum year and infant social engagement, fear regulation, and stress reactivity. J Am Acad Child Adolesc Psychiatry. 2009;48(9):919–27.
33. Dennis C, Ross L. Relationships among infant sleep patterns, maternal fatigue, and development of depressive symptomatology. Birth. 2005;32(3):187–93.
34. Heron J, O'Connor TG, Evans J, Golding J, Glover V. The course of anxiety and depression through pregnancy and the postpartum in a community sample. J Affect Disord. 2004;80(1):65–73.
35. Kingston D, Tough S. Prenatal and postnatal maternal mental health and school-age child development: a systematic review. Matern Child Health J. 2014;18(7):1728–41.
36. Luoma I, Tamminen T, Kaukonen P, Laippala P, Puura K, Salmelin R, Almqvist F. Longitudinal study of maternal depressive symptoms and child well-being. J Am Acad Child Adolesc Psychiatry. 2001;40(12):1367–74.

16

Measuring progress in maternal and newborn health care in Mexico: validating indicators of health system contact and quality of care

Ann K. Blanc[1*], Claudia Diaz[2], Katharine J. McCarthy[1] and Karla Berdichevsky[2]

Abstract

Background: The majority of births in Mexico take place in a health facility and are attended by a skilled birth attendant, yet maternal mortality has not declined to anticipated levels. Coverage estimates of skilled attendance and other maternal and newborn interventions often rely on women's self-report through a population-based survey, the accuracy of which is not well established.

Methods: We used a facility-based design to validate women's report of skilled birth attendance, as well as other key elements of maternal, newborn intrapartum, and immediate postnatal care. Women's reports of labor and delivery care were collected by exit interview prior to hospital discharge and were compared against direct observation by a trained third party in a Mexican public hospital ($n = 597$). For each indicator, validity was assessed at the individual level using the area under the receiver operating curve (AUC) and at the population level using the inflation factor (IF).

Results: Five of 47 indicators met both validation criteria (AUC > 0.60 and 0.75 < IF < 1.25): urine sample screen, injection or IV medication received during labor, before the birth of the baby (i.e., uterotonic for either induction or augmentation of labor), episiotomy, excessive bleeding, and receipt of blood products. An additional 9 indicators met criteria for the AUC and 18 met criteria for the IF. A skilled attendant indicator had high sensitivity (90.1 %: 95 % CI: 87.1–92.5 %), low specificity (14.0 %: 95 % CI: 5.8–26.7 %) and was suitable for population-level estimation only.

Conclusion: Women are able to give valid reports on some aspects of the content of care, although questions regarding the indication for interventions are less likely to be known. Questions that include technical terms or refer to specific time periods tended to have lower response levels. A key aspect of efforts to improve maternal and newborn health requires valid measurement of women's access to maternal and newborn health interventions and the quality of such services. Additional work on improving measurement of population coverage indicators is warranted.

Keywords: Maternal and newborn health, Quality of care, Intervention coverage, Validation, Measurement, Indicators, Skilled birth attendance

* Correspondence: ablanc@popcouncil.org
[1]Population Council, New York, NY, USA
Full list of author information is available at the end of the article

Background

The maternal mortality ratio in Mexico has declined by less than 7 % in the past two decades [1]. As part of its efforts to improve maternal health, the Mexican government has emphasized increasing access to skilled obstetric care as a central focus of the national health plan [2, 3]. To scale-up access, government-led initiatives have sought to promote contact with the health system and skilled birth attendance, establishing policies such as universal health coverage for pregnant women and no-cost emergency obstetric services [3].

To track such efforts, the Mexican government has emphasized monitoring women's contact with the health system [4]. Indicators routinely collected as proxy measures for skilled obstetric care include the proportion of births delivered in health facilities and the proportion of births attended by a skilled birth attendant. In the absence of health monitoring systems that can provide accurate data on population coverage, these indicators often rely on women's self-reports collected in household surveys such as the National Health and Nutrition Survey (Encuesta Nacional de Salud y Nutrición) in Mexico or international programs including the Demographic and Health Surveys (DHS) and Multiple Indicator Cluster Survey (MICS). However, the accuracy of women's reports on these indicators is not well understood [5].

Insufficient progress in improving maternal health in Mexico and elsewhere has called into question reliance on indicators of health system contacts, rather than the content and quality of care. For example, researchers have noted that while physician-attended births were reported to be near universal in Mexico in 2012 (96 %), maternal deaths have not declined to the anticipated level [6–9].

A small, but emerging evidence base has sought to validate which aspects of maternal and newborn care women are able to report with accuracy. Validation research to date has largely taken place in settings where maternal mortality rates are low and often relies on hospital records, which often are subject to incomplete and inaccurate reporting as the reference standard. Although three rigorous studies were recently published in this area, to our knowledge, one of the most widely used indicators of health service contact – skilled attendance at birth– remains to be empirically validated [10–12]. In addition, apart from research by Tuncalp and colleagues which focused on validating women's reports of cesarean section in the Dominican Republic [11], we know of little research to validate indicators of the quality and content of maternal and newborn health care in the Latin America and Caribbean region.

This study responds to the need for enhanced data related to the measurement of maternal and newborn health intervention coverage. We assessed the validity of a set of intrapartum and immediate postnatal indicators among women who delivered in a large Mexican public hospital. Our goal is to inform which aspects of intrapartum and immediate postnatal care women are able to report with accuracy and have the potential to be included in routine population-based surveys to monitor the coverage of lifesaving maternal and newborn health interventions.

As part of this work, a parallel study validated a set of quality of care indicators in Kenya [13]. Given variation in the status of maternal health and the organization of maternal health services, these results are reported separately.

Methods

Study design

Data for the validation analysis were drawn from women's reports on the maternal and newborn health services they received during labor and delivery gathered by exit interviews prior to their discharge from the hospital. Women's reports were compared against observations by a trained third party using a structured checklist. Direct observation was chosen as the reference standard as it was considered to yield the most accurate reflection of all facets of the care-giving process. In the event that clarification was needed (e.g., in a few instances the newborn and mother were taken into separate rooms and the observer remained with the mother) observations were supplemented by checking medical records or by consulting providers.

Study setting and population

The study took place in a large public hospital in Mexico City where approximately 4,000 deliveries (54 % vaginal) take place annually. Hospital services include comprehensive obstetric care to women with normal pregnancies who are self-referred for admission, in combination with women with high-risk pregnancies who are referred from other public primary or secondary health care institutions. The population served by the study hospital tends to have a lower-than-average socioeconomic status and characteristically lacks health insurance. Patients may travel large distances to arrive at the study hospital with a large proportion from the neighboring State of Mexico (37 %) and 5 % from the rest of the country.

All pregnant women aged 15–49 who were admitted for delivery at the study hospital and were able to provide consent were eligible for participation. Women were excluded if they were unable to provide consent, if they presented with a complication, or if their stage of labor was considered too advanced by medical personnel. Study observation was discontinued if a cesarean section was indicated at any point.

Ethical approval and consent

Written informed consent was obtained from all participants prior to observation. For women under the age of 18, written consent was also obtained from their spouse/common law partner or parent (as responsible parties) in accordance with local ethical guidelines [14]. Provider consent was obtained to observe health care workers in the labor and delivery ward. A list of providers who gave their consent was provided to observers before they commenced observation. Very few providers refused participation.

The study protocol was approved by the Population Council's Institutional Review Board and the Ethics and Research Committee of the participating hospital prior to participant enrollment.

Data collection

Data collection took place between November 2013 and April 2014 and occurred over a 24-h period, using three daily observation shifts. Observations included all interactions between women and provider (s) upon admission to the labor ward until one hour following delivery. Client exit-interview questionnaires reflected the same elements of care and patient-provider interactions as the observation checklist (Additional files 1, 2, 3 and 4). Observers were general medical practitioners or nurses with sufficient clinical training to accurately record delivery room practices. Interviewers were social workers and psychologists with prior research experience. To minimize the potential for bias, study interviewers and observers were not the same individuals and all data collectors were external to the study facility. We recruited only female interviewers to facilitate rapport with participating women and interviews were conducted in Spanish. Data collectors received intensive training on the study protocol, including detailed explanation of each aspect of the client questionnaire and observation checklist to ensure full understanding, how to record responses, and the procedures for ethical research.

Indicator selection

Indicators selected for validation were identified through a landscaping scan of published and grey literature conducted between April and July 2012, a detailed description of which is published elsewhere [13]. Inclusion criteria for indicator selection were: reflection of the content or quality of maternal and newborn health services relating to the early labor and immediate postnatal period (up to one hour following delivery) [15], current or proposed use in household survey programs (e.g., DHS or MICS) or the ability to reflect critical elements of care and be recalled by women. A total of 82 indicators were selected for validity testing (Additional file 5: Table S1).

Interview questionnaires were translated into Spanish and underwent minor modifications to improve participant understanding.

Sample size

The target sample size for this study was 600 women. Since no information on the coverage of maternal and newborn interventions in the facility was available, we assumed 50 % prevalence for all indicators, with 60 % sensitivity ± 6 % precision, 70 % specificity ± 6 % precision, and with $\alpha = 0.05$ assuming normal approximation to the binomial distribution. Using these assumptions, a target sample size of 500 was calculated. To allow for non-response, the sample size was increased to approximately 600 women.

Data analysis

Analyses were performed using Stata Version 12 (StataCorp, College Station, TX). We assessed two aspects of indicator validity, accuracy at the individual level and population level. To measure individual level reporting accuracy, we compared women and observer responses to a single or combination of questions computed for each indicator by constructing two-by-two tables. Missing and "Don't Know" responses were excluded from the analysis. Where there was sufficient sample size (i.e., at least five counts per cell), we plotted the receiver-operating curve for each indicator. Receiver operating curve (ROC) analysis provides a global statistic of indicator accuracy by plotting the tradeoff between indicator sensitivity (i.e., the true positive rate), against its false positive rate (or 1 – specificity) [16]. To summarize the average accuracy of each indicator, we calculated the area under the receiver-operating curve (AUC). AUC scores range from 0 to 1, with an AUC of 0.5 representing a random guess and an AUC of 1 representing perfect diagnostic accuracy. For the purposes of this study we used an AUC of 0.6 or greater as an a priori benchmark of validity [12]. We present estimates of sensitivity, specificity and the AUC with accompanying 95 % confidence intervals (CIs) assuming a binomial distribution.

To estimate the prevalence that would be obtained for each indicator if assessed in a population-based survey (Pr), we applied the sensitivity (SE) and specificity (SP) calculated for each indicator to its true prevalence (P) (i.e., observer report) using the following equation: $Pr = P \times (SE + SP\text{-}1) + (1\text{-}SP)$ [17]. We then calculated the inflation factor (IF), or the ratio of the survey-based prevalence to the true prevalence, to estimate the degree to which each indicator would be over or underestimated if assessed at the population level. A priori validation criteria for the IF was set at 0.75 < IF < 1.25 [12].

We defined overall acceptable indicator performance in terms of meeting both the individual (AUC) and population-level (IF) criteria (0.60 < AUC and 0.75 < IF < 1.25). However, we note that indicator validity criteria should be weighed according to the indicator's intended use. For example, an indicator with low accuracy at the individual-level may produce an acceptable estimate of population-level coverage if the false positive reports and false negative reports yield a ratio of approximately one. Given this, we refer readers to the full validation results.

Results

Sample descriptive characteristics

In total, 779 women admitted for labor gave consent to participate. Due to hospital policies that allowed complete observation of women who underwent vaginal deliveries only, data collection for women who delivered by cesarean section was discontinued at the time of indication. Six hundred and sixteen women who consented to participate delivered by vaginal birth (Fig. 1). Of these women, 597 (97 %) were observed throughout labor and delivery and completed an exit interview before hospital discharge. The age, marital status, parity and education for women are presented in Table 1.

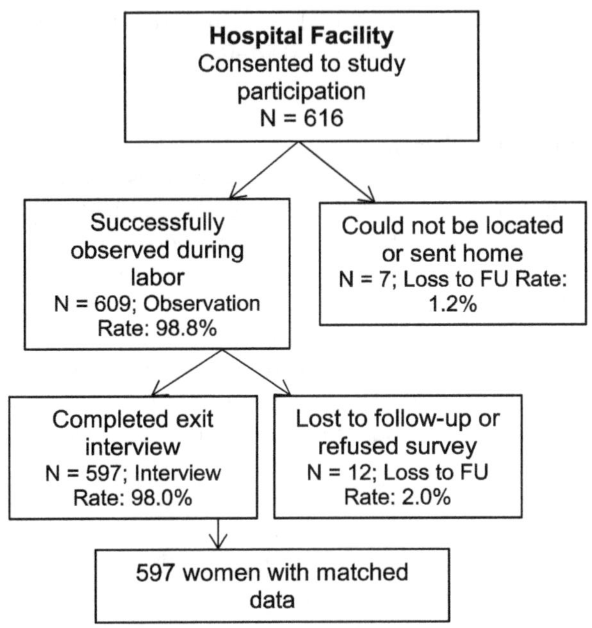

Fig. 1 Participant response rates. Enrollment and response rates reflect women who delivered by vaginal birth only

Table 1 Percent distribution of women by background characteristics

Variable	Percentage (%) $N = 597$
Age	
15-19	27.5
20-24	36.2
25-29	19.1
30-34	9.7
35-39	5.9
40+	1.7
Prior parity (Total number live births)	
0	47.7
1	29.3
2	14.4
3	5.4
4 or more	3.5
Educational attainment	
None	0.2
Primary	8.4
Secondary	42.3
Higher	49.2
Marital status	
Single, never married	25.6
Married	17.9
Living together	55.4
Separated	1.0
Widowed	0.0

Validation results

The full list of indicators selected for validity testing as well as the prevalence of each indicator as reported by women and observers is presented in Additional file 5: Table S1. For all survey questions, women could respond "I Don't Know". Across indicators, "Don't Know" responses were generally minimal. Greater than 5 % of women responded "Don't Know" to 9 indicators (Table 2).

The highest percentage of women responded "Don't Know" to questions regarding administration of oxytocin (i.e., uterotonic for the prevention of post-partum hemorrhage) at any time or before the delivery of the placenta (53 % and 38 %, respectively). An alternate proxy indicator regarding receipt of a uterotonic for prevention of postpartum hemorrhage – whether, immediately after delivery, *"anyone [gave] medication intravenously through a tube in your arm"* – also exceeded 5 % (8 %) "Don't Know" responses. High percentages of "Don't Know" responses were also recorded for several immediate postnatal interventions for the mother and newborn. In addition,

Table 2 Percentage of women who responded "Don't Know" to survey questions

Client question	N^a	% "Don't Know"
Immediately after the delivery of your baby, did anyone give you a medication or injection called oxytocin to help your uterus contract/become firm?	592	38.3
Did anyone give you medication or an injection called 'oxytocin' before you delivered the placenta?	414	52.9
While you were at the health facility for the birth of your baby, did you receive a HIV test?	596	23.7
Did you or anyone else give anything to the baby to eat or drink within the first hour after delivery?	593	21.4
Did the health provider(s) wash their hands with soap and water or use antiseptic before examining you?	592	19.4
Just after the delivery of your baby, in the first few minutes after the delivery of your baby, did anyone give you medication intravenously (through a through a tube in your arm)?	547	7.7
Was your baby dried off with a towel immediately, within a few minutes after his/her birth ?	593	6.6
About how long after birth was your baby bathed for the first time?	573	19.7
In your first physical examination/check after delivery, did a health provider check your belly to see whether your womb was becoming firm after the birth of your baby?	597	5.9

[a]Sample sizes vary by question due to the number of women who responded to each question. Note: In "Don't Know" responses were excluded in the validation analysis. High 'Don't Know' indicators were considered to be those questions to which greater than 5 % of women responded "I Don't Know"

nearly one-quarter of women did not know whether they received an HIV test. Anecdotal evidence from data collectors indicated that many women did not know what HIV was, or confused it with human papillomavirus (HPV).

There was adequate cell size to validate 47 indicators: five of which met both validation criteria (Table 3). These were: urine sample screen (i.e., check for preeclampsia), injection or IV medication received during labor and before the birth of the baby (i.e., proxy for uterotonic for either induction or augmentation of labor), episiotomy, hemorrhage, and receipt of blood products. An additional 27 indicators met either the criteria for individual-level classification (AUC) (9 indicators) or population-level coverage (IF) (18 indicators). We discuss the results below in relation to: (1) contact with the health system, (2) content and quality of maternal and immediate newborn health care, and (3) maternal health outcomes.

Contact with the health system

Indicators of contact with the health system were: the type of provider involved in labor and delivery care and the type of facility where the delivery took place.

Skilled birth attendance

To assess skilled birth attendance, women were asked, *"Who was the main provider assisting you during delivery?"* Cross-tabulation results of observer and women's reports of provider type showed that most women reported attendance by a doctor (either a general provider or a doctor with specialization in obstetrics and gynecology (ob-gyn)), while most observers reported attendance by a medical resident (Table 4). In Mexico, there is little distinction between the type of care doctors and medical residents are legislated to provide. However, while doctors and medical residents are considered 'skilled', medical interns are not. To assess the accuracy of women's reports of a 'skilled' attendant, we assessed a combined doctor and medical resident indicator. The true prevalence of skilled attendance during delivery (i.e., the main provider who 'caught' the baby was a doctor or medical resident) was 91 % and the reported prevalence was 90 %. This indicator had high sensitivity (90 %, 95 % CI: 87–93), low specificity (14 %, 95 % CI: 6–27 %) and met the IF criterion only (AUC: 0.52, 95 % CI: 0.48–0.56; IF 0.98).

Institutional delivery

Although this study was not designed to assess recall of the type of institution for delivery given that it took place in one facility only, for exploratory purposes women were asked to identify where they gave birth and whether it was a public or private sector facility. Replicating the methodology of the DHS and MICS surveys, women were also asked to specify the facility type (e.g., hospital, health clinic/center, health post, or other location). If women were unable to provide this information, they were asked to name the place.

Among women who responded to the question on whether the facility was classified as public or private sector and then specified its type, 85 % were correct. Among women who responded to the open-ended component of the question only: 83 % correctly named the facility, 9 % identified the facility as a hospital but did not identify the sector, and four percent identified both

Table 3 Validation results for maternal and newborn intrapartum and immediate postnatal care indicators †

Indicator	Total N	True Prev[a] (%)	Sensitivity[b] (95 % CI)	Specificity[c] (95 % CI)	Self-report survey estimate (%), Based on sensitivity and specificity[d]	AUC (95 % CI) (>0.60)	IF[e] (0.75 to 1.25)	Criteria Met[f]
Indicators of Health Service Contacts								
Main provider labor- doctor or medical resident	580	96.2	82.3 (78.8-85.3)	27.3 (10.7-50.2)	81.9	0.55 (0.51-0.59)	0.85	IF
Main provider delivery– doctor or medical resident	563	91.1	90.1 (87.1-92.5)	14.0 (5.8-26.7)	89.7	0.52 (0.48-0.56)	0.98	IF
Indicators of Content of Care								
Takes urine sample	572	25.2	50.0 (0.63-0.71)	84.4 (80.6-87.7)	24.3	0.67 (0.63-0.71)	0.97	Both
Injection or IV[g] medication received at some time during labor, before birth of baby (general)	571	76.0	70.1 (65.5-74.3)	56.9 (48.2-65.4)	63.6	0.63 (0.59-0.68)	0.84	Both
Episiotomy performed	580	67.8	97.7 (95.7-98.9)	63.1 (55.8-70.0)	78.1	0.80 (0.77-0.84)	1.2	Both
Blood products given	582	2.41	35.7 (12.8-64.9)	98.4 (97.0-99.3)	2.4	0.67 (0.63-0.71)	1.0	Both
Receives injection or IV[g] medication for induction or augmentation of labor	476	76.1	59.1 (53.9-64.2)	79.8 (71.3-86.8)	49.8	0.69 (0.65-0.74)	0.65	AUC
Augments labor with uterotonic	472	75.2	49.6 (44.3-54.9)	81.2 (72.9-87.8)	42.0	0.65 (0.61-0.70)	0.56	AUC
Membranes ruptured (labor induction or augmentation)	356	57.0	38.4 (31.7-45.5)	88.2 (82.0-92.9)	27.0	0.63 (0.58-0.68)	0.47	AUC
Breastfeeding initiated within first hour of birth[i]	449	34.7	81.4 (74.4-87.2)	44.1 (38.3-49.9)	64.8	0.63 (0.58-0.67)	1.9	AUC
First post-delivery exam, provider checks for involution	556	81.7	84.6 (80.9-87.8)	21.6 (14.0-30.8)	83.5	0.53 (0.49-0.57)	1.0	IF
Palpates uterus after delivery of placenta	580	82.4	79.5 (78.4-85.5)	19.6 (9.7-25.4)	79.7	0.50 (0.45-0.54)	0.97	IF
Uterotonic received 1-3 min after birth	580	64.0	61.5 (56.3-66.4)	40.7 (33.9-47.7)	60.7	0.51 (0.47-0.55)	0.95	IF
3 AMTSL[h] elements: prophylactic uterotonic + controlled cord traction + uterine massage following delivery of placenta	549	81.2	75.7 (71.5-79.6)	24.0 (16.0-33.6)	75.7	0.50 (0.46-0.54)	0.93	IF
HIV status checked	569	69.8	54.9 (49.9-59.9)	47.7 (40.0-55.4)	54.1	0.51 (0.47-0.55)	0.78	IF
Induces labor with uterotonic	559	11.6	27.7 (17.3-40.2)	89.1 (86.0-91.7)	12.9	0.58 (0.54-0.62)	1.1	IF
Woman received pain relief medication	581	79.4	89.4 (86.2-92.0)	20.0 (13.3-28.3)	87.4	0.55 (0.51-0.59)	1.1	IF
First post-delivery exam, provider ask/checks for bleeding	590	80.5	87.4 (84.0-90.2)	12.2 (6.8-19.6)	87.5	0.50 (0.46-0.54)	1.1	IF
First post-delivery exam, provider examines perineum	586	75.1	90.2 (87.1-92.8)	10.3 (5.9-16.4)	90.1	0.50 (0.46-0.54)	1.2	IF
First post-delivery exam, provider takes temperature	586	66.9	94.4 (91.6-96.4)	8.8 (5.2-13.7)	93.4	0.52 (0.47-0.56)	1.4	
Encourages/assists woman to ambulate during labor	580	22.2	7.8 (3.8-13.8)	91.6 (88.6-94.0)	8.3	0.50 (0.46-0.54)	0.37	
Woman asked for pain relief medication at some time	575	44.7	32.7 (27.0-38.8)	78.9 (74.0-83.3)	26.3	0.56 (0.52-0.60)	0.59	
Something other than breastmilk given to baby within first hour of birth[i]	438	21.7	71.6 (61.4-80.4)	46.1 (40.7-51.5)	57.8	0.59 (0.54-0.64)	2.7	
Uterotonic received 1-3 min after delivery of placenta	576	20.0	95.7 (90.1-98.6)	6.3 (4.3-8.9)	94.1	0.51 (0.47-0.55)	4.7	
Baby given to mother immediately after birth[i]	580	10.3	63.3 (49.9-75.4)	40.6 (36.3-44.9)	59.8	0.52 (0.48-0.56)	5.8	

Table 3 Validation results for maternal and newborn intrapartum and immediate postnatal care indicators † *(Continued)*

Maternal Complications								
Severe bleeding (hemorrhage)	593	8.1	50.0 (35.2-64.8)	95.2 (93.1-96.9)	8.4	0.73 (0.69-0.76)	1.0	Both
High blood pressure/convulsions (eclampsia)	594	2.4	57.1 (28.9-82.3)	79.5 (76.0-82.7)	21.4	0.68 (0.64-0.72)	9.1	AUC
Complication (yes to any)	595	13.6	60.5 (50.3-72.3)	65.4 (61.3-69.7)	38.2	0.64 (0.60-0.68)	2.8	AUC
None	595	86.4	65.6 (61.3-69.7)	61.7 (50.3-72.3)	61.8	0.64 (0.60-0.68)	0.72	AUC

†Validation analysis based on matched data, excluding 'Don't Know' and missing responses. Sensitivity and specificity analysis was not performed for indicators that had fewer than 5 counts per cell of constructed two-by-two tables

[a]True prevalence refers to prevalence of intervention or event as measured by direct observation by a trained third party in the study hospital facility; [b]True positive rate; [c]True negative rate; [d]Estimated prevalence that would be obtained through women's self-report in a household survey (Pr), calculated using the following equation where P = true prevalence, SE = sensitivity, SP = specificity, Pr = P*(SE + SP-1) + (1-SP); [e]IF = Pr/P, or ratio of survey-based prevalence to the true prevalence; [f]AUC > 0.60 and 0.75 < IF < 1.25; [g]IV refers to intravenous medication; [h]Refers to active management of the third stage of labor; [i]Questions asked of mothers whose infants were breathing at birth

*Note: For full description of study indicators, please see Additional file 5: Table S1

elements (e.g., reporting "Hospital público", "Hospital federal", or "Hospital de asistencia pública"); the open-ended probe elicits additional correct information not captured initially in the categorical response.

Content of care

We validated 21 indicators related to interventions received throughout labor and the immediate postnatal period. Indicators of content of care with the highest individual-level accuracy were episiotomy (AUC: 0.80, 95 % CI: 0.77–0.84), followed by receiving an injection for the induction or augmentation of labor (AUC: 0.69, 95 % CI: 0.65–0.74), urine sample screen upon hospital admission, (AUC: 0.67, 95 % CI: 0.67–0.71) and receipt of blood products (AUC: 0.67, 95 % CI: 0.63 – 0.71). Indicators related to the third stage of labor, including receiving an injection or medication following delivery (i.e., uterotonic for the prevention of postpartum hemorrhage) and immediate postnatal care for the mother had moderate or low overall individual level validity.

Population-level accuracy for 13 content of care indicators were within 25 % of the true prevalence (0.75 < IF < 1.25). Overestimation was nearly double or greater the observed prevalence for four indicators: the infant was placed with the mother immediately after birth (5.8), receipt of an injection or medication following delivery of the placenta (i.e., uterotonic for the prevention of postpartum hemorrhage) (4.7), something other than breastmilk was given to the infant within the first hour of birth (2.7), and breastfeeding initiated in the first hour of birth (1.9).

Uterotonic for prevention of postpartum hemorrhage

A critical component of maternal health care is receipt of a uterotonic for the prevention of hemorrhage, a leading cause of maternal death in Mexico and globally [18, 19]. Women were asked whether, *"Immediately after the delivery of your baby, did anyone given you"* (1) *"an injection in your thigh or buttocks"*, (2) *"medication intravenously (through a tube in your arm"*, or (3) *"tablets to swallow or hold in your mouth", or* (4) *"tablets placed in your rectum".* As the standard of care in the study facility was administration of the uterotonic via intravenous injection (100 % of cases observed), there was insufficient sample size to assess each of these indicators independently. Given this, we compared a combined indicator comprised of women who

Table 4 Cross-tabulation of women's response and observer report of the main provider during delivery

Self- report (Number)	Observer report (Number)					
	Doctor /Ob-gyn	Medical resident	Medical intern	Nurse	Student nurse	Self-report total
Doctor /Ob-gyn	14	487	40	1	0	542
Medical resident	0	17	0	0	0	17
Medical intern	0	11	2	0	0	13
Nurse	0	11	0	1	0	12
Student nurse	0	0	0	0	0	0
Don't Know	0	9	2	0	0	11
Observer Total	14	535	44	2	0	595

reported "Yes" to any method of uterotonic administration within the first few minutes of birth against the observer report of whether the woman received a uterotonic within three minutes of birth. The observed prevalence was 61 % and the reported prevalence was 64 %. The indicator did not meet the AUC (0.51, 95 % CI: 047–0.55) but did meet the IF criterion (0.95).

Women were asked the same set of questions about the first few minutes after the delivery of the placenta. A combined indicator constructed from women's reports of whether she received a uterotonic via any method met neither criteria (AUC 0.51, 95 % CI: 0.47–0.55; IF 4.7). The specificity of this indicator (6 %, 95 % CI: 4–9 %) was low.

We attempted to validate an alternative indicator that used the name of the uterotonic drug and its purpose. Women were asked whether, *"Immediately after the birth of your baby, did anyone give you a medication or injection called oxytocin to help your womb contract/become firm?"* In the study facility, oxytocin was the standard uterotonic (administered in 97 % of cases). However, of women who reported "Yes" to any of the methods of uterotonic administration, 62 % responded either "Don't Know" or "No" to the oxytocin question. While there was insufficient sample size to robustly analyze this indicator, descriptive results show that, among women who were observed to receive oxytocin and who gave a valid response to the question, 50 % accurately reported receiving the medication by its name.

Maternal complications

Women were asked whether they had experienced a list of several obstetric complication symptoms (e.g., excessive bleeding, prolonged labor, high blood pressure, convulsions). There was sufficient sample size to assess the validity of four indicators based on these questions. One indicator- excessive bleeding (hemorrhage), met both acceptability criteria (IF 1.0, AUC 0.73, 95 % CI: 0.69–0.76). This indicator high specificity (95.2 %, 95 % CI: 93.1–96.9) but moderate sensitivity (50.0 %, 95 % CI: 35.2–64.8 %); nearly half of women who experienced excessive bleeding would not be captured in a survey question. The other three indicators met the individual criteria only and were overreported by women at the population level. For example, experiencing high blood pressure and convulsions (eclampsia) was overestimated by over 9 times at the population level (IF 9.1), although the low prevalence means that even slightly less than perfect reporting can lead to large overestimation.

Discussion

Indicators that measure contact with the health system in addition to the quality of received care are critical for measuring progress in improving maternal and newborn health. This is the first study to empirically validate indicators related to the contact, quality and outcomes of maternal and immediate newborn postnatal care in Mexico. A strength of this study is the use of direct observation as the reference standard.

Few indicators assessed in the present study met both study validity criteria. This occurred in part because many interventions were routine practice and there was insufficient variation in the observed prevalence for robust analysis. However, an additional 9 indicators met the individual-level criteria and 18 met the population-level criteria. Indicators that did not meet both criteria are not necessarily invalid for all measurement purposes, but should be used in accordance with the rationale for their use. For example, indicators that do not meet criteria for the AUC but do meet the IF criterion may be suitable to measure intervention coverage at the population-level as false positive and negative reporting balance each other at the aggregate level.

Our findings also highlight the challenges of measuring low prevalence indicators accurately. Given that the calculation of the IF depends upon the indicator's observed prevalence, even a small number of false positive responses can result in overestimation as measured by the IF. The implications of varying 'true' prevalence rates on the estimated prevalence that would be obtained from women in a household survey is illustrated in a previous article [13]. Additional validation work is needed to identify appropriate strategies for measuring low prevalence indicators, such as maternal complications and non-indicated practices.

The consistency of our results with prior findings is mixed. For example, the moderate sensitivity and high specificity for reported symptoms of hemorrhage (excessive bleeding) corresponds with levels found among women delivering in Indonesia, Benin and the Philippines [20–22]. However, these results differ from women's reporting in Taiwan and Ghana [23]. We also found high sensitivity and low specificity for an indicator of whether or not the woman received a uterotonic within the first few minutes of birth; which differs from the low sensitivity and moderate specificity documented in a study conducted in Mozambique [12]. Taken together, these findings suggest that women's understanding and recall of interventions received and obstetric complications experienced may vary by clinical and cultural context, and reinforces the importance of validating women's reporting in different settings.

No contact with care indicators that we were able to assess (i.e., indicators of skilled birth attendance) met both validation criteria. However, a combined indicator of whether the primary birth attendant during delivery was a doctor/ob-gyn or medical resident did meet the criteria for valid estimation at the population level. Given that broad categorizations of provider types are likely to be more programmatically meaningful than the ability of women to delineate between finer categories of qualified health professionals (e.g., doctors versus medical residents), a composite indicator is likely to have utility for assessing population-level coverage. It is important to recognize, however, that skilled attendance is not synonymous with receiving appropriate care. Even a competent provider may not be able to provide high quality care if necessary supplies and other aspects of the enabling environment are inadequate [24, 25]. When possible, self-reported data should be triangulated with other data sources, such as stock-outs of essential medicines [26, 27].

Given that "skilled attendance" cannot be used reliably as a proxy for quality of care, indicators that measure the content of care administered by providers should also be assessed. Across content of care indicators assessed in this study, however, we observed a tendency for women to overreport some standard prevention practices, particularly related to the initial client assessment and immediate postnatal care for the mother and newborn. The high sensitivity and low specificity of many of these indicators suggests that in the few instances when an intervention was not administered, women tended to falsely report that it had occurred.

One potential explanation for this pattern is facility bias, or the assumption by women that they received quality care due to the fact that they delivered in a health facility [10, 13]. For example, more careful probing of some indicators of care, such as whether an injection or IV medication was received before birth (i.e., uterotonic for induction or augmentation of labor), or following delivery (i.e., uterotonic for prevention of postpartum hemorrhage) suggests that women did not know the specific indication for the care received, just that an intervention occurred. Validation results for the uterotonic indicators may reflect more general knowledge women had about having an IV line set, which was standard hospital practice for all women entering the labor and delivery ward, rather than knowledge of which medication was given or why. For example, neither an indicator of whether "an injection or IV medication was received to speed up labor" (i.e., uterotonic induction of labor) or whether "an injection or IV medication was received to strengthen labor" (i.e., uterotonic for augmentation of labor) met both validation criteria, while a general indicator of receiving an injection or IV medication at some time before the birth of the baby did. Similarly, most women correctly reported receipt of a uterotonic within the first few minutes after delivery of the baby, but also falsely reported the receipt of a uterotonic within the first few minutes after the delivery of the placenta, suggesting women may be able to report that some intervention occurred, but not be able to report accurately on aspects of its timing or purpose.

In light of the tendency for overreporting in a facility setting, high specificity for an indicator of receipt of a uterotonic may be favored at the cost of sensitivity. The near universal administration of oxytocin limited our ability to determine if an alternate uterotonic indicator that used the name of the drug and its purpose would achieve higher specificity as opposed to an indicator that asks women about the route of drug administration. Our descriptive results, however, did show that use of an indicator that uses the drug name captured substantially fewer true cases and fewer women were able to answer the question at all. This suggests that asking about receipt of a uterotonic using the drug name and reason for its use may not be a better alternative to asking women about whether they received an injection or some other method of drug administration.

An alternate explanation for positive reporting bias by women is that mothers misunderstood or conceptualized the meaning of questions differently than the observer definitions. For example, indicators with the highest "Don't Know" responses generally included (1) technical terms, such as medication or disease names, related to the (2) timing of interventions received (including the sequence of newborn thermal care), or (3) the immediate postnatal period. Anecdotal evidence from study interviewers shows that additional explanation was needed to describe the difference between HIV vs. HPV, intravenous vs. intramuscular drug administration, and to define epidurals. Questions to which a substantial percentage of women responded "Don't Know" (e.g. 20 % or more) are unlikely to yield valid information via self-reports and are not recommended for inclusion in population-based surveys.

Our findings highlight the importance of a two-part question with an open-ended component to improving reporting for complex indicators, such as the type of institution where the woman delivered. The fact that additional women could identify key facility attributes in an open-ended format suggests that providing the opportunity for women to name the specific facility, as is done in both the DHS and MICS surveys, is advantageous for capturing information on institutional deliveries.

While the study provides useful insight regarding the validity of contact and content of care indicators, there were some limitations. Due to budget limitations, the validation exercise took place in one type of facility only. Our study results are therefore reflective of women who delivered in a large public hospital. For example, although institutional delivery is near universal in Mexico (94 %), it is higher among women who reside in urban relative than rural areas (96 % and 88 %, respectively) and our results may be more reflective of this type of population [28]. The minimal variation in standard hospital procedures limited our ability to assess all indicators, which may have otherwise been proven valid. Additionally, in the study setting relatively few women experienced complications such as eclampsia, a leading cause of maternal death in Latin America and the Caribbean. It is possible that with a greater sample size, different combinations of questions regarding the symptoms of eclampsia could be validated to identify question wording with the highest accuracy.

Another limitation it that, due to hospital policy, it was not possible to include women who became indicated for a cesarean section delivery in the study. Future research should extend this work to a broader range of types of health facilities, including health centers and clinics, and may have the potential to validate the reporting accuracy of women who underwent a cesarean delivery. Validation research in other types of facilities may also reduce the potential for positive facility bias in reporting. Finally, exit interviews with women occurred shortly following delivery, prior to hospital discharge. The short recall time may cause women's self-reports to be more accurate than in population level surveys such as the DHS and MICS when women are typically interviewed about a birth that took place one to three years prior. As part of an overall program of work on indicator validation, a separate follow-up study is underway to re-interview women approximately one year following delivery in Kenya.

Conclusion

As attention in maternal health shifts to a new emphasis on ending preventable maternal mortality (EPMM) and addressing inequities, the tracking of progress will remain important [29]. A key aspect of these future efforts will require the valid measurement of not only *contact* with maternal and newborn health services but also *coverage* of key interventions that reflect the quality of services received. Until recently, however, little attention has been paid to improving the measurement of intervention coverage and quality at the population level. This information is needed to set programmatic priorities and to allocate resources effectively. Given the effect that this information can have on improvements in the lives of women and newborns, priority should be given to work that ensures that indicators of progress are selected, measured, and interpreted accurately.

Additional files

Additional file 1: Client Exit Interview Questionnaire (English).

Additional file 2: Client Exit Interview Questionnaire (Spanish).

Additional file 3: Observation Checklist (English).

Additional file 4: Observation Checklist (Spanish).

Additional file 5: Table S1. List of Maternal and Newborn Care Indicators Assessed and Reported Prevalence.

Acknowledgements

We acknowledge Hannah Taboada, who developed the data collection tools used in the study. We also thank Tahilin Karver and Alberto Martinez Polis who provided oversight for the facility-based data collection. We appreciate the advice of the maternal health experts who advised on the study and are grateful to the women and providers who allowed us to share their experiences. This study was supported by the Maternal Health Task Force through a grant from the Bill & Melinda Gates Foundation.

Authors' contributions

Conceived of the study design and selected indicators for analysis: AKB, CD. ICMJE criteria for authorship read and met: AKB CD KM KB. Agree with manuscript and conclusions: AKB CD KM KB. Collected the data: CD KB. Analyzed the data: KM. Wrote the paper: AKB KM KB. All authors read and approved the final manuscript.

Competing interests

The authors declare that they have no competing interests.

Author details

[1]Population Council, New York, NY, USA. [2]Population Council, Mexico City, Mexico.

References

1. Lozano R, Wang H, Foreman KJ, Rajaratnam JK, Naghavi M, Marcus JR, Dwyer-Lindgren L, Lofgren KT, Phillips D, Atkinson C, et al. Progress towards millenium development goals 4 and 5 on maternal and child mortality: an updated systematic analysis. Lancet. 2011;378:1139–65. doi:10.1016/S0140-6736(11)61337-8.
2. Frenk J, Gómez-Dantés O, Langer A. A comprehensive approach to women's health: lessons from the Mexican health reform. BMC Womens Health. 2012;12:42. doi:10.1186/1472-6874-12-42.
3. Secretaría de Salud. El Convenio General de Colaboración Interinstitucional para la Atención de la Emergencia Obstétrica, un camino hacia la universalización de los servicios de salud. Mexico City. 2012. http://www.ccinshae.salud.gob.mx/descargas/Atencion_de_la_Emergencia_Obstetrica.pdf. Accessed 21 Jan 2015.
4. Evidence and Lessons from Latin America (ELLA): Observatory of maternal mortality in Mexico: a civil society-led initiative. 2013. https://www.gov.uk/dfid-research-outputs/ella-policy-brief-observatory-ofmaternal-mortality-in-mexico-a-civil-society-led-initiative. Accessed 25 May 2015.
5. Bryce J, Arnold F, Blanc A, Hancioglu A, Newby H, Requejo J, Wardlaw R, CHERG Working Group on Improving Coverage Measurement. Measuring coverage in MNCH: New findings, new strategies and recommendations for action. PLoS Med. 2013;10(5):e1001423. doi:10.1371/journal.pmed.1001423.
6. Gutiérrez JP, Rivera-Dommarco J, Shamah-Levy T, Villalpando-Hernández S, Franco A, et al. Encuesta Nacional de Salud y Nutrición 2012. Resultados Nacionales. Instituto Nacional de Salud Publica. 2012. http://ensanut.insp.mx/informes/ENSANUT2012ResultadosNacionales.pdf. Accessed 21 Jan 2015.
7. United Nations, Population Division: World Population Prospects, The 2012 Revision. (2014). http://esa.un.org/wpp/. Accessed 24 Nov 2014.
8. Walker D, De María L, Campero L, González D, Suárez L, et al. El uso y rol de proveedores no-médicos para la atención prenatal y obstétrica en México: parteras profesionales técnicas y enfermeras obstetras. Evidencias y áreas de oportunidad. Cuernavaca, Mexico: Instituto Nacional de Salud Pública; 2011.
9. Demaria LM, Campero L, Vidler M, Walker D. Non-physician providers of obstetric care in Mexico: Perspectives of physicians, obstetric nurses and professional midwives. Hum Resour Health. 2012;10:6. doi:10.1186/1478-4491-10-6.

10. Liu L, Li M, Yang L, Ju L, Tan B, Walker N, Bryce J, Campbell H, Black RE, Guo Y. Measuring coverage in MNCH: A validation study linking population survey derived coverage to maternal, newborn and child health care records in rural China. PLoS One. 2013;8(5):e60762. doi:10.1371/journal.pone.0060762.
11. Tuncalp O, Stanton C, Castro A, Adanu R, Heymann M, Adu-Bonsaffoh K, Lattof SR, Blanc A, Langer A. Measuring coverage in MNCH: Validating women's self-report of emergency cesarean sections in Ghana and the Dominican Republic. PLoS One. 2013;8(5):e60761. doi:10.1371/journal.pone.0060761.
12. Stanton CK, Rawlins B, Drake M, dos Anjos M, Cantor D, Chongo L, Chavane L, da Luz VM, Ricca J. Measuring coverage in MNCH: Testing the validity of women's self-report of key maternal and newborn health interventions during the peripartum period in Mozambique. PLoS One. 2013;8(5):e60694. doi:10.1371/journal.pone.0060694.
13. Blanc AK, Warren C, McCarthy KJ, Kimani J, Ndwiga C, RamaRao S. Assessing the validity of indicators of the quality of maternal and newborn health care in Kenya. J Glob Health. 2016;6(1):010405.
14. Secretaría de Salud, Mexico. Programa de acción específico 2007-2012: salud sexual y reproductiva para adolescentes. Mexico City. 2008. http://www.cdi.salud.gob.mx:8080/BasesCDI/Archivos/Saludsexualyreproductiva/110801_pae_adolescentes.pdf. Accessed 12 Apr 2014
15. Austin A, Salam RA, Lassi LS, Das JK, Bhutta ZA. Approaches to improve the quality of maternal and newborn health care: an overview of the evidence. Reprod Health. 2014;11 Suppl 2:S1. doi:10.1186/1742-4755-11-S2-S1.
16. Eng J. Receiver operating characteristic analysis: a primer. Acad Radiol. 2005;12:909–16.
17. Vecchio TJ. Predictive value of a single diagnostic test in unselected populations. N Engl J Med. 1966;274(21):1171–3.
18. Schiavon R, Tronsco E, Polo G. Analysis of maternal and abortion-related mortality in Mexico over the last two decades, 1990-2008. Int J Gynaecol Obstet. 2012;118 Suppl 2:S78–86. doi:10.1016/S0020-7292(12)60004-6.
19. Say L, Chou D, Gemmill A, Tuncalp O, Moller AB, Daniels J, Gulmezoglu AM, Temmerman M, Alkema L. Global causes of maternal death: a WHO systematic analysis. Lancet Glob Health. 2014;2:e323–33. doi:10.1016/S2214-109X(14)70227-X.
20. Ronsmans C, Achadi E, Cohen S, Zazri A. Women's recall of obstetric complications in South Kalimantan, Indonesia. Stud Fam Plann. 1997;28(3):203–14.
21. Filippi V, Ronsmans C, Gandaho T, Graham W, Alihonou E, Santos P. Women's reports of severe (near-miss) obstetric complications in Benin. StudFam Plann. 2000;31(4):309–24.
22. Stewart KM, Festin M. Validation study of women's reporting and recall of major obstetric complications treated at the Philippine General Hospital. Intl J Gynaecol Obstet. 1995;48:S53–66.
23. Souza JP, Parpinelli MA, Amaral E, Cecatti JG. Populations surveys using validated questionnaires provided useful information on the prevalence of maternal morbidities. J Clin Epidemiol. 2008;61:169–76. doi:10.1016/j.jclinepi.2007.04.009.
24. Hussein J, Bell J, Nazzar A, Abbey M, Adjei S, Graham W. The skilled attendance index: proposal for a new measure of skilled attendance at delivery. Reprod Health. 2004;12(24):160–70.
25. Harvey S, Wong Blandon YC, McCaw-Binns S. Are skilled birth attendants really skilled? A measurement method, some disturbing results and a potential way forward. Bull World Health Organ. 2007;85(10):783–90.
26. Winter R, Pullum T, Florey L, Hodgins S. Impact of scale-up of maternal and delivery care on reductions in neonatal mortality in USAID MCH priority countries, 2000-2010. Rockville, Maryland: ICF International; 2014. http://dhsprogram.com/publications/publication-as46-analytical-studies.cfm Accessed 12 Apr 2015.
27. Hodgins S. Achieving better maternal and newborn outcomes: coherent strategy and pragmatic, tailored implementation. Glob Health Sci Pract. 2013;1(2):146–53. doi:10.9745/GHSP-D-13-00030.
28. UNICEF Global Database: Delivery care: institutional deliveries-percentage. 2014. http://Data.unicef.org/maternal-health/delivery-care. Accessed 19 May 2015
29. World Health Organization: Strategies toward ending preventable maternal mortality (EPMM). 2015. http://who.int/reproductivehealth/topics/maternal_perinatal/epmm/en/. Accessed 4 June 2015.

17

Community and provider perceptions of traditional and skilled birth attendants providing maternal health care for pastoralist communities in Kenya

Abbey Byrne[1], Tanya Caulfield[1], Pamela Onyo[2], Josephat Nyagero[2], Alison Morgan[1], John Nduba[2] and Michelle Kermode[1*]

Abstract

Background: Kenya has a high burden of maternal and newborn mortality. Consequently, the Government of Kenya introduced health system reforms to promote the availability of skilled birth attendants (SBAs) and proscribed deliveries by traditional birth attendants (TBAs). Despite these changes, only 10 % of women from pastoralist communities are delivered by an SBA in a health facility, and the majority are delivered by TBAs at home. The aim of this study is to better understand the practices and perceptions of TBAs and SBAs serving the remotely located, semi-nomadic, pastoralist communities of Laikipia and Samburu counties in Kenya, to inform the development of an SBA/TBA collaborative care model.

Methods: This descriptive qualitative study was undertaken in 2013–14. We conducted four focus group discussions (FGDs) with TBAs, three with community health workers, ten with community women, and three with community men. In-depth interviews were conducted with seven SBAs and eight key informants. Topic areas covered were: practices and perceptions of SBAs and TBAs; rewards and challenges; managing obstetric complications; and options for SBA/TBA collaboration. All data were translated, transcribed and thematically analysed.

Results: TBAs are valued and accessible members of their communities who adhere to traditional practices and provide practical and emotional support to women during pregnancy, delivery and post-partum. Some TBA practices are potentially harmful to women e.g., restricting food intake during pregnancy, and participants recognised that TBAs are unable to manage obstetric complications. SBAs are acknowledged as having valuable technical skills and resources that contribute to safe and clean deliveries, especially in the event of complications, but there is also a perception that SBAs mistreat women. Both TBAs and SBAs identified a range of challenges related to their work, and instances of mutual respect and informal collaborations between SBAs and TBAs were described.

Conclusions: These findings clearly indicate that an SBA/TBA collaborative model of care consistent with Kenyan Government policy is a viable proposition. The transition from traditional birth to skilled birth attendance among the pastoralist communities of Laikipia and Samburu is going to be a gradual one, and an interim collaborative model is likely to increase the proportion of SBA assisted deliveries, improve obstetric outcomes, and facilitate the transition.

Keywords: Maternal health, Newborn health, Skilled birth attendants, Traditional birth attendants, Health systems, Pastoralist communities, Kenya

* Correspondence: mkermode@unimelb.edu.au
[1]Nossal Institute for Global Health, University of Melbourne, 161 Barry St, Carlton, VIC 3010, Australia
Full list of author information is available at the end of the article

Background

Traditional birth attendants (TBAs) are lay community members, mostly women, who assist with childbirth, and who are commonplace in many low-income settings. The story of TBAs in global maternal health programming has been characterised by both engagement and exclusion. In the 1970s and 1980s the efforts to reduce maternal mortality focused on training TBAs to provide safer delivery care. However, the impact of this strategy on maternal mortality was negligible as TBAs are not equipped to manage maternal complications, and risk screening for complicated deliveries is poorly predictive of outcomes [1]. Consequently, the focus in the 1990s was on scaling up access to skilled birth attendants (SBAs), who are trained health workers such as nurses, midwives and doctors, able to manage complicated deliveries and resuscitate newborn babies, and who mostly work in health facilities [2]. The shift to SBAs as the preferred provider of maternal health care was clearly reflected in the Millennium Development Goals, which nominated the proportion of deliveries attended by SBAs as the primary indicator of progress in maternal mortality reduction [3]. The practices of TBAs were subsequently ignored, and in some places even proscribed by government. For complex reasons, many women in low-income settings are still cared for by TBAs rather than SBAs at the time of pregnancy and delivery [4–6]. TBAs are valued by communities because they are accessible, inexpensive, and well-respected; abide by local traditions; and provide services that SBAs do not, such as in-home postpartum care [4–10]. In recent years there has been some reassessment of the TBA role, and the potential for SBAs to collaborate with them to improve maternal and newborn health outcomes [10, 11].

Kenya experiences a high burden of maternal and newborn mortality with a maternal mortality ratio of 488 deaths per 100,000 live births (95 %CI 333, 643), and a neonatal mortality rate of 30 deaths per 1000 live births [12, 13]. As these rates were not improving with the passage of time, the Government of Kenya instituted health system reforms aiming to have 90 % of deliveries assisted by SBAs by 2015, a doubling from the 2008 level of 43 % [12]. To achieve this goal, beginning in 2009, the Government deployed SBAs to level two health facilities (commonly referred to as dispensaries), which are mostly located in remote areas such as those populated by pastoralist communities. The Government also actively discourages TBA supported births. However, despite these initiatives, uptake of SBA services remains low, and inequitably distributed; for example, 89 % of women giving birth in Nairobi were attended by an SBA during 2008–09, while fewer than one in ten women birthing in remote pastoralist communities had an SBA present in 2012 [12, 14]. A 2012 survey among the remote semi-nomadic pastoralist communities of Laikipia and Samburu counties in the Rift Valley region revealed that 92 % of births took place at home, and 57 % were assisted by a TBA. The remaining home deliveries were attended by family members or the woman delivered alone [14].

Providing women in remote semi-nomadic pastoralist communities with maternal health care from SBAs is particularly challenging. Barriers include: more remote settings with fewer health facilities; mobile populations for whom static health services are less accessible; and strong traditions of using TBAs [10].

The Government proscription of TBA assisted deliveries means that health planners no longer engage with TBAs, so little is understood about their current roles and practices in remote communities. The objectives of this qualitative study were to investigate and describe the: 1) roles and practices of TBAs and SBAs serving pastoralist communities in Laikipia and Samburu counties, Kenya; 2) attitudes of TBAs and SBAs regarding their own practices and those of one another; 3) communities' attitudes in relation to care provided by TBAs and SBAs.

Methods

In order to better understand practices and perceptions of TBAs and SBAs providing maternal care in remote pastoralist communities in Kenya we undertook a descriptive mixed methods study. This paper reports on the qualitative phase of the study.

Study setting

This work was undertaken by a partnership between the Nossal Institute for Global Health at the University of Melbourne, Amref Health Africa, the Mothers Union of the Anglican Church in Kenya (MUACK), and the relevant County Health Ministries. The study builds on the existing health and development projects of MUACK with the pastoralist communities of Laikipia and Samburu counties of Kenya. These pastoralist counties are sub-divided into group ranches that consist of several villages, and each of these consist of a small number of homesteads (*manyattas*). The study sites were five group ranches in Laikipia (Chumvi, Morupusi, Makurian, Naibor, Tiamamut), and three in Samburu (Kirimon, Kisima, Longewan). Participating communities are mostly semi-nomadic; men migrate with cattle during dry seasons while women and children remain at home for most of the year caring for goats and sheep. The predominant language is Maa, although Kiswahili, English and other tribal languages and dialects of Maa are spoken. The health system comprises: dispensaries located in group ranches, which serve as primary care facilities mostly staffed by solo nurses; health centres and sub-district hospitals where medical officers and basic emergency obstetric care can be provided; and the district hospital where comprehensive emergency obstetric care is available.

Sampling

The qualitative data collection involved: focus group discussions (FGDs) with TBAs, community health workers (CHWs), and community women and men (Table 1). CHWs are local women and men who have received brief intensive training as part of the Ministry of Health's 'Community Strategy'; each group ranch has its own CHWs. A component of their role is to link pregnant women with health facilities. CHWs are ideally positioned to understand the perspectives of communities, TBAs and SBAs, hence their inclusion in the study. The number and range of FGDs was anticipated to be sufficient to achieve data saturation. We conducted individual semi-structured in-depth interviews (IDIs) with SBAs and key informants. IDIs were conducted with the seven SBAs (all dispensary level nurses) from the study sites because it was not logistically feasible to bring them all together in one place for an FGD; most would have to travel a long distance to participate in an FGD, which would involve leaving the dispensaries unattended. Purposive sampling was used to select the group ranches for the various FGD categories based on background knowledge of the sites. Specifically, the sampling approach ensured inclusion of people residing in places with and without a local health facility and SBA, and people who were close to and far away from health facilities. Sampling the FGD participants from within each study site was largely opportunistic.

A total of seven IDIs were conducted with SBAs (five female and two male; all were based in dispensaries) and eight IDIs with key informants i.e., dispensary managers (2), staff from the County Departments of Health (2), and male (2) and female (2) Community Development Committee (CDC) members. The topic areas discussed during the SBA interviews were similar to those identified for the FGDs with TBAs (see Table 1); and the topic areas for the key informant interviews were roles and relationships of SBAs and TBAs, and options for improved collaboration.

Data collection was undertaken from October 2013 to March 2014. The project commenced with engagement of stakeholders and permission from community leaders to proceed with the study in each of the group ranches. Interview guides for the FGDs and IDIs were drafted in English by the researchers based on the study objectives and the literature, and reviewed with the local data collection team who had in-depth knowledge of the communities. Interview guides were translated into Maa or Kiswahili language by local research team members, and back translated to English, piloted and revised. Pictures representing pregnancy, birth, birth complications, and the different types of health facilities were created by a local artist and used as prompts to stimulate discussion during the FGDs with TBAs and community women.

Data were collected by local research team members (two females, one male; two Maa speakers, one Kiswahili speaker) trained in FGD facilitation and IDI techniques, and supervised by study investigators. FGDs and IDIs were conducted in Maa, Kiswahili and English languages dependent on the preference of the participants. Participants were reimbursed for transport and lunch expenses, typically to the value of 400 Kenyan Shillings (approx. USD 4), consistent with the standard payment dispensed by NGOs active in the sites. All FGDs and IDIs were digitally audio-recorded.

Table 1 Summary of FGD participants and content

Category	Number FGDs	Total no. participants	Topic areas investigated during FGDs
Traditional birth attendants (TBAs)	4	46	Experience & training; perceptions of quality care; rewards & challenges; managing complications; community preferences for care; options for TBA/SBA collaboration.
Community health workers (CHWs)	3	45	Community preferences for care; reasons for this; decision making about care; accessibility of services; managing complications; perceptions of TBAs and SBAs.
Women who have delivered with an SBA in the past two years	3	27	Care seeking choices and decision making; practitioner preferences; reasons for this; experiences of care; characteristics of good quality care; options for SBA/TBA collaboration.
Women who have delivered with a TBA in the past two years	5	59	As above.
Women who have delivered unattended in the past two years	2	30	As above.
Husbands of women who have delivered in the past two years	2	25	Care seeking choices and decision making; practitioner preferences; reasons for this; characteristics of good quality care; options for SBA/TBA collaboration.

Data analysis

All FGDs and IDIs were translated and transcribed verbatim by local team members and cross-checked for accuracy. The transcriptions were inductively and deductively thematically analysed by two of the researchers independently (AB & TC), and subsequently assessed for consistency and divergence [15]. Analysis was undertaken manually by one researcher, and using NVivo 10 software by the other. The final themes were those that emerged from the data i.e., what participants said in response to questions from the interview guide, questions asked in order to probe responses, and questions asked to obtain clarity on what was being said. Our approach was more emic than etic in orientation. Following data analysis, interim findings were shared with representatives of group ranches to ensure that they resonated with the varied experiences and perceptions of the communities. The topic areas and themes relevant to this paper are summarised in Table 2.

Ethics

Ethics approval was granted in June 2013 from the Ethics and Scientific Review Committee of Amref Health Africa Kenya, and the Human Research Ethics Committee of The University of Melbourne, Australia. Informed consent was obtained from all participants, using written or verbal methods dependent on the participant's level of literacy.

Results

Practices of TBAs

Traditional birth attendants are predominantly older women who gain their skills through experience and working alongside other TBAs. In this way, knowledge is passed across generations. TBAs are seen as the repository of knowledge regarding traditional birth practices and associated herbal treatments. Additionally, they mediate between the pregnant or labouring woman and her husband, provide advice about care required, including diet, when to slaughter an animal, and if referral to a health centre is necessary.

> *The woman tells the TBA what she wants, she cannot tell the husband. I [the TBA] also ask her if there is anything she needs, then I tell the husband. If she needs meat, then we* [TBAs] *tell the husband and a goat is slaughtered.* [FGD with TBAs, Laikipia]

Table 2 Themes that emerged from FGDs, semi-structured interviews, and key informant interviews

Topic area	Themes
TBA practices	
- antenatal	Dietary and workload advice; abdominal massage; linking with SBAs.
- delivery	Receiving the baby; giving comfort to mother; mediating with the husband; administration of special foods and herbs; abdominal massage; observing traditions.
- post-partum	Keeping mother and baby warm; preparing special foods; cleaning the woman; disposal of placenta; assistance with domestic chores; encouraging breast feeding.
- complications	Administration of herbs; food supplementation; inducing vomiting; referral to health facility.
- challenges	Fear of becoming infected with HIV when women are 'sick'; managing complications; difficulty obtaining transport for referrals
SBA practices	
- antenatal	Checking vital signs of woman and baby; administration of medications/immunisation; making a birth plan; referral for laboratory testing; dietary and workload advice; promotion of bed nets.
- delivery	Monitoring the mother and baby; encouraging the woman.
- post-partum	Monitoring baby and mother; care of episiotomy/tear; encouraging breastfeeding; dietary advice; family planning.
- complications	Transfer to higher level facility.
- challenges	Trying to get women to attend health facility for delivery; doing deliveries at home; difficulty getting an ambulance in case of complications; lack of necessary equipment at health facility; being a lone practitioner.
Perceptions of TBAs	
- strengths	Accessible and available; assistance with domestic chores; referral and accompanying to health facility; trusted and respected by community; valued traditional knowledge; courage.
- concerns	Inability to manage complications; poor hygiene; unsafe practices.
Perceptions of SBAs	
- strengths	Valuable technical knowledge & skills; provision of safety; access to equipment, medications & injections; ability to manage complications; able to refer easily.
- concerns	Negative attitudes and behaviours towards women; leaving women alone; cold facilities; unwanted clinical procedures; staff absenteeism; restricted visitors; lack of equipment.

Antenatal care by TBAs

TBAs advise women to reduce their workload to avoid miscarriage during the early stages of pregnancy, and in some group ranches this advice extends throughout pregnancy. In many but not all group ranches, TBAs and other women assist pregnant women in their first trimester with their domestic chores such as collecting firewood, cooking, and washing clothes. They also recommend that women eat foods of their choosing at this stage of pregnancy, although advice concerning the quantity of food intake varied; some TBAs said that women should avoid eating too much while others believed the woman would become sick if she did not eat enough. TBAs consistently advocated that pregnant women should not consume fresh milk or eggs because the child may grow too large. Many TBAs said they advised women to consult SBAs for antenatal care, and some actually accompanied them to the dispensary.

During the second trimester, TBAs massage the pregnant woman's abdomen with oil. Most TBAs recommend food restriction during the second trimester and some TBAs take this to the extreme of instructing women to vomit after eating, with the intention of preventing the baby from becoming too large. Related to this, TBAs also recommend that women recommence domestic work and avoid resting.

> *A child can become so big in the womb, the mother will have difficulties during her delivery. That's why we make her vomit and we don't give fresh milk or eggs, because the child will become big.* [FGD with TBAs, Laikipia]

In the third trimester, the size of the baby remains a key concern for TBAs so they continue to recommend women take on a high workload, induce vomiting by drinking fermented milk and fat, and in some sites encourage running. If the baby is thought to be large, the TBA may refer the woman for a facility-based delivery. A common practice of TBAs during late stage pregnancy is abdominal massage in the belief that it will correctly position the baby for the birth.

Delivery care by TBAs

The role of a TBA during delivery was primarily described by TBAs as *"receiving the baby"* and comforting the mother by *"holding her until she delivers"*. Other women from the community may be present, but the TBA instructs them on what to do. TBAs traditionally feed labouring women oil or animal fat, then herbs, followed by porridge. Women are offered clean water or milk to drink for sustained energy. Abdominal palpation during delivery is practiced by most TBAs to hasten the birth process. Most TBAs allow any birthing position, and women typically express a preference for the squatting position.

Post-partum care by TBAs

During the post-partum period, the TBA focuses on thermal care of the mother and newborn, and oversees a rather strict dietary regime for the mother. It is common practice for TBAs to apply a layer of fat to the skin of the mother and the newborn, and wrap them with a cloth to protect from the cold. It is especially important to maintain a warm home as cold is believed to be dangerous for both mother and baby. Immediately after delivery, the TBA ensures that the *"house of the baby"* (placenta) is removed. Following delivery of the placenta, the TBA boils water and bathes the mother, changes her clothing, cooks tea and/or porridge that is fed to the woman, and holds the baby so the mother can rest. TBAs often take over the new mother's domestic chores such as collecting firewood, managing domestic animals and washing clothes for up to 2–3 weeks after delivery.

The mother's dietary regime is a cornerstone of the TBA's traditional knowledge and practice. TBAs usually cook for the woman for the first week or so post-delivery. During the first four days post-partum, women are given meat and soup, tea with milk and sugar, fat and porridge, and every morning and evening are given fresh animal blood to drink. Water is generally withheld and 'hard foods' such as rice or beans are not allowed. After one week, the woman is allowed to consume other foods. One TBA described that:

> *On the fifth day we give her a traditional herb that cleans the stomach then the following day a ram is slaughtered and (she) is given fat, we give fat to give her diarrhoea and clean out the stomach – it helps her to stop bleeding and after that she is given any hard* [dense/solid] *food.* [FGD with TBAs, Laikipia]

The baby is rubbed with oil, and bathing is delayed for one month or until the umbilical cord stump falls off. In Samburu, some communities reported smearing the cord stump with a mixture of herbs and ashes to stop it from bleeding. Several TBAs said they instruct women to breastfeed immediately after birth, and help them to establish breastfeeding over the ensuing days. Occasional supplementary feeding of the newborn was mentioned; this involved giving water with herbs, and one TBA reported administering boiled water with salt and sugar to a baby for four days when the mother was perceived to have insufficient milk.

TBA care in the event of obstetric complications

It is common for TBAs to palpate the woman's abdomen to assess the term of the pregnancy, predict the sex, and identify potential birth complications such as multiple births, large baby size, or poor positioning of the baby. It is custom in some group ranches for TBAs to tie a "*traditional thread*" loosely around the woman's waist for spiritual protection if the pregnancy is judged to be high risk. In terms of antepartum complications, bleeding is the main concern noted by TBAs, for which they prescribe herbs and animal fat.

For most complications TBAs administer locally collected herbs prepared as a soup or with milk, often combined with fat or animal blood. If this fails, then the mother, reported by TBAs in all group ranches, is referred to a health facility. TBAs identified that some women are "*weak*" or "*do not have enough blood*" (possibly referring to anaemia), and therefore considered to be at high risk of obstetric complications because they may not have the strength to push during labour. Such women are given cow's blood and often referred for facility-based deliveries.

Retained placenta is a major concern for TBAs. When this occurs they generally induce vomiting by giving the woman large volumes of water to drink.

> *We make the woman vomit as this will help the placenta to come out easily and fast. These days, to prevent the placenta from retaining... before cutting the umbilical cord, we make the woman vomit to push the placenta out.* [FGD with TBAs, Laikipia]

For prolonged labour, women are given herbs believed to accelerate labour, and food for additional energy. For breech deliveries, generally referred to as the "*baby sitting in a wrong position*", TBAs most often refer to a health facility, although in one site TBAs advise women to walk until the baby turns, and the TBAs manage the delivery themselves.

> *Children are also delivered by the legs coming out first. There is a way we handle this. Sometimes one leg comes out, you push it back, one hand comes again, you push it back, this way we try because there is no hospital near* [FGD with TBAs, Samburu]

TBAs may refer women to an SBA before labour begins for a range of reasons including when the woman is anaemic, very young, giving birth for the first time, expecting twins, experiencing bleeding or has a history of complications or pre-term delivery; or the baby is judged to be too large. More commonly though, referral is only after the TBA attempts to treat the complication herself but is "*defeated*" and realises she cannot manage the situation. All TBAs described referring women for facility-based deliveries for complications occurring during labour. The husband is usually instructed to take the woman to a health facility, at which time the family begins the (often difficult) search for a vehicle. The main indications for referral are prolonged labour (sometimes for days at home), breech presentation, haemorrhage, retained placenta, premature rupture of membranes, cord prolapse, or maternal exhaustion. TBAs often accompany the woman to the health facility, where the majority introduce themselves as a relative rather than identify as a TBA, fearing judgement for not adhering to the Government policy proscribing their practice.

Challenges for TBA practice

Managing complications, especially retained placenta, was a major challenge frequently identified by TBAs who commonly acknowledged that SBAs are best at dealing with such problems. Also challenging for TBAs is the difficulty of obtaining transport for women requiring referral to a health facility. Many TBAs expressed concerns about becoming infected with HIV, and consequently conducted deliveries wearing polythene bags on their hands, in lieu of gloves, to protect themselves from becoming "*sick*" (referring to HIV). Several TBAs also mentioned the danger they face when called to attend a delivery that requires them to travel through areas inhabited by wild animals.

> *We have to leave our work to help women to deliver. Diseases are many, and if you touch the blood you can be infected. Sometimes we are called at night and there is a lot of wildlife.* [FGD with TBAs, Samburu]

> *When we want to take someone to the hospital it is difficult because we don't have a vehicle. We use polythene bags as gloves, and sometimes you are called far from home at night and you might meet wild animals on your way.* [FGD with TBAs, Laikipia]

Practices of SBAs in dispensaries

Antenatal care by SBAs

SBAs provide a range of services for pregnant women including: assessment of maternal weight, blood pressure, fundal height, foetal heart rate, and foetal positioning. Mothers are issued an antenatal record card, given iron-folic acid supplements and tetanus toxoid injections, and a birth plan is developed. Some health facilities also provide a full antenatal work-up, which includes ultrasound, urinalysis, haemoglobin, blood grouping and HIV testing. Laboratory services are not available at dispensary level, although the nurse may send blood samples to higher level facilities for analysis if the family is able and willing to pay the related costs. SBAs advise women to undertake light work only, increase rest, sleep with an insecticide treated bed net, and consume a balanced healthy diet. From the perspective of community members, antenatal care with SBAs involves administration of injections and medicines, identification of possible complications, and estimation of the delivery date. Several SBAs described involving TBAs in antenatal care – for example in Samburu:

> *The moment I meet a mother who is pregnant, I go and tell the TBA "so and so is pregnant, so you monitor her, check if she is coming to the clinic... bring her to the hospital."* [Interview with SBA, Samburu]

Delivery care by SBAs

When a woman presents at a health facility in labour, SBAs assess the status of the mother and baby, determine the stage of labour, and document the woman's birthing history. SBAs also see it as part of their role to encourage women through the various stages of labour. They try to convince women to deliver in the lithotomy position, a position the women generally dislike. One SBA reported that partographs are used in sub-district hospitals, but are not available at dispensary-level health facilities.

During FGDs with community members, it became clear that in several group ranches, women and their husbands had limited understanding of the practices and services offered by SBAs. It was perceived that SBAs focused mainly on the technical aspects of delivery, and less on supportive care for women. Women who had delivered with SBAs described that they "*make you lie backwards, then tell you to push out, and she makes a lot of noise for you until you give birth, while she is just standing there looking at you*" [FGD with community women, Laikipia].

SBAs working at dispensary level attempt to manage obstetric complications, but readily call a vehicle and escort the mother to a higher level facility (district hospital) if indicated. Some SBAs also informally collaborate with TBAs at the time of delivery.

> *We must have the TBAs here* [in the dispensary]. *They accompany the women so they can feel at least I have someone of my own with me – I have a TBA around. So we encourage them – if you are in labour, come to the hospital and let the TBA accompany you.* [Interview with SBA, Laikipia]

Post-partum care by SBAs

After birth, SBAs routinely examine the newborn, wash the mother, and show her the baby. A woman typically remains in the facility for 24 h following delivery, with both mother and baby receiving a check-up prior to discharge. SBAs monitor the woman for post-partum bleeding, provide breast feeding advice, counsel her regarding family planning, and explain the necessary care of episiotomy wounds or vaginal tears. Women are advised to eat plenty of food, and if a mother is underweight she may be given flour and beans to supplement her diet. Family visits are restricted to visiting hours only, unless there is a complication, in which case the family is allowed greater access. Some SBAs arrange for CHWs to provide home visits for post-partum women.

Challenges for dispensary-based SBA practice

SBAs identified a number of challenges in relation to their work. Many found it particularly difficult to convince women to deliver in the health facility. Even women who are willing to attend for antenatal care, prefer to labour and deliver at home, only using the health facility if they experience complications. Many SBAs described requests to deliver women in their own homes and felt duty-bound to respond. This involves finding a means of transport or walking long distances, sometimes through areas inhabited by wild animals, and the health facility is left unattended while the SBA attends the home birth.

> *They call us to go and deliver them at the manyattas, which are very far away, and the mode of transport is very poor, and we come across wild animals on our way.* [Interview with SBA, Laikipia]

Several SBAs expressed concern regarding the infection risks for mother and baby in the relatively unclean home environment, and the frustration of being called to attend a woman at home who is already in advanced labour and experiencing complications.

Another major challenge for SBAs is obtaining an ambulance for women who urgently need to be transferred to higher level facilities. When phoning for an ambulance, sometimes no-one answers, the SBA is told that there is no driver or no fuel available, or advance payment for fuel is demanded from the woman's family before the ambulance will be dispatched. Several SBAs reported that their dispensaries lacked basic essential equipment and medicines, making it very difficult for them to practice in a skilled and safe way. Being a lone practitioner with no colleagues to double-check assessments or share decision-making was concerning for several SBAs, especially in the event of obstetric emergencies. Others mentioned the challenge of one person having to fulfil a number of different roles, and deliver on both government and community expectations.

Dispensaries are left unattended when SBAs travel for work-related or personal reasons. When labouring women arrive at the facility seeking skilled birth attendance and the SBA is absent, they and their family members become (understandably) very annoyed, and do not always understand that the nurse's absenteeism may be legitimate.

> *I am the only one there. If I go for a seminar the facility is left unattended. So that is one of the challenges – the workforce is very low... We have a lot of work, we are the clinical nurse, we are everything... We are given accounts, we are the manager of the whole facility, and we have to work with the community... The community does not understand... If they find that the nurse is not in the facility, they just say she is not at work. Even though I am at a seminar or have taken some official things to town, they will just say 'the nurse is not there.'* [Interview with SBA, Samburu]

Perceptions of TBAs

Strengths of TBAs

According to TBAs, their primary strength is their availability to the community. They are always available to assist, and commented that they had delivered many of the people in their communities over a long period of time, including those who are now SBAs. They see themselves as particularly useful for young mothers, and when nurses are not available. They value their own traditional knowledge, particularly their expertise regarding herbs and foods that should be consumed (or not) around the time of pregnancy and childbirth. They see this as knowledge that doctors do not possess. Many community members and TBAs described how it is necessary to have courage to be a TBA.

From the perspective of SBAs, the strength of TBAs is the emotional and practical support they provide to mothers. SBAs report that some TBAs advise women to attend the health facility for antenatal care, accompany them for facility-based deliveries, and promote immunisations. TBAs are considered particularly important in remote areas where health facilities are inaccessible, particularly if they have delivery kits and are able to assist women unable to otherwise reach facilities. Some SBAs perceived the traditional knowledge of TBAs as an admirable attribute. Several SBAs mentioned that TBAs are widely trusted, and have a very comfortable communication style with the women. Overall, SBAs perceive TBAs as an asset to the health system because of their influence in the community.

Community members were very affirming of the TBA role, and clearly trusted them and held them in high regard.

> *Women want to deliver at home because they see that a TBA will deliver them well. She is the one who will light a good fire, she will clean her well, so you find that the majority like to deliver at home.* [Interview with female CDC member, Samburu]

The fact that TBAs are available, accessible and affordable was particularly valued by community members. Additionally, there are no transport challenges or transport costs incurred when women are cared for by TBAs. Community members mentioned that TBAs accompany women to health facilities where possible, and are essential in remote communities where health facilities are inaccessible. The traditional knowledge held by TBAs was considered a valuable asset. Women and their husbands trusted TBAs' abilities to determine the position and sex of the baby, massage the women's abdomen to position the baby for birth, and administer herbal remedies. Community leaders said that TBAs were particularly helpful for first-time mothers who were less likely to fear a TBA, and would not feel shy about sharing the *"secrets of the body"*.

Concerns regarding TBAs

The main concern regarding TBAs was their inability to manage the complications of childbirth. This was echoed by all categories of participants, although the views expressed varied somewhat. Community members were of the opinion that TBAs do know about likely complications, but are unable to manage them because they lack the training and equipment. In contrast, SBAs maintained that TBAs are not competent to recognise complications such as prolonged labour, anaemic mothers, and premature separation of the placenta, and therefore delay referring women to health facilities. SBAs and CHWs both pointed out that TBAs cannot manage postpartum complications such as retained placenta and haemorrhage, nor can they administer injections or undertake any surgical procedures.

Unhygienic practices of TBAs were frequently mentioned as a major concern, voiced by TBAs themselves, women, SBAs and community leaders. This was linked to the TBAs' lack of training and resources (delivery kits), making it difficult for them to provide sanitary care. The absence of hand washing and gloves, dirty utensils used for cord cutting, and the generally unclean delivery environment were noted as potential causes of disease affecting both mothers and newborns.

> *Some are dirty and they don't even wash their hands. Some don't have the knowledge, and they can use anything to cut the umbilical cord, they force you to push out the baby before time.* [FGD with women delivered with no TBA or SBA, Samburu]

SBAs identified several TBA practices as dangerous including: encouraging women to push before the cervix was fully dilated; allowing delivery in the squatting position (which SBAs linked to complications); neglecting the delivery of the placenta and postpartum haemorrhage;

administration of herbs; inducing vomiting; and instituting restrictive ante- and post-partum dietary regimes. SBAs were of the firm opinion that TBAs should not attempt to deal with complications as this only delays subsequent referral for assistance, and some SBAs believed that delays in referral are in part because TBAs want to avoid loss of payment for the delivery.

Perceptions of SBAs

Strengths of SBAs

From their own perspective, the primary strength of SBAs is their technical knowledge, skills and experience. They see themselves as able to detect women and newborns at risk of complications, and having the skills and medicines to manage them. Beyond the skills of individual SBAs, being a part of the health system was considered valuable because it provides a safe environment for conducting deliveries, and means that SBAs are more easily able to refer women to higher level facilities if unable to handle the situation themselves.

From the perspective of TBAs, the strengths of SBAs lie in the resources and skills they have. TBAs respect SBAs' training, and appreciate it when they are willing to share information and advice. They admire SBAs' ability to remove retained placenta, manage multiple births and determine if a woman is HIV positive. SBAs are seen to have an advantage because they possess medicines and equipment (such as gloves), are able to administer injections, and can perform caesarean section if indicated (although this is not actually available at dispensary level or even sub-district level).

Community members were of the view that SBAs possess specialised knowledge and are particularly valuable for complicated deliveries such as twins, retained placenta or if the mother is "*sick*" (HIV positive). Community members also identified the injections given by SBAs following delivery as a strength, although there were varied opinions regarding the benefit of these injections. For instance, they were thought to prevent bleeding, reduce labour pain, prevent the woman from feeling cold, "*wash the womb*" and prevent "*stomach problems*". Other strengths identified were the capacity to perform caesarean section, dispense medications, and refer to higher level facilities.

> *When you go there with different problems, they [SBAs] can treat you. It's good they help if you have difficulty with the first child. You are given injections to prevent bleeding. You don't bleed like at home.* [FGD with women delivered by TBAs, Samburu]

Dispensary-level services were preferred over sub-district and district health facilities as they are nearer, and dispensary nurses are considered to be more attentive than nurses in hospitals, as they do not have too many patients at one time. Across group ranches, community members welcomed the fact that SBAs, unlike TBAs, allowed women to eat any food they want. The SBAs were said to have brought hope, as one community leader said:

> *If the nurse is not near...these people, how will they be? They will just die. We see the goodness of the doctors and nurses being near the community. The community has hope.* [Interview with female CDC member, Samburu]

Concerns regarding SBAs

Concerns about SBAs, mentioned by TBAs, community women and even by SBAs themselves, pertained to the negative attitudes and behaviours of some SBAs. Experiences of poor quality care and dissatisfaction with care were reported by several women – some accounts were of personal experiences and others were descriptions based on anecdote. Women reported verbal and physical abuse by SBAs including insults, slapping, pinching and being clipped with scissors. These experiences were mainly associated with higher level health facilities (not dispensaries), where they described being left unattended, abandoned, and neglected.

> *Only those who are courageous go to the hospital. I can't go because I am afraid. I deliver at home so I can get someone to hold me. In hospital you are beaten, at home you get someone who comforts you until you deliver.* [FGD with TBAs, Laikipia]

> *Women are not comforted, you are left alone. Doctors keep a distance and keep watching you. You are also tied. During labour pains you meet a doctor who slaps you seriously. At home you say let me stay where nobody beats me up. Some don't want to be stitched and you are told to remove your clothes.* [FGD with TBAs, Samburu]

Some SBAs were considered to be arrogant and unmotivated, and appeared to treat women's presence in their health facility as an inconvenience. Some women fear health facilities, particularly large hospitals, citing concerns that: children can be swapped or exchanged; women and babies don't return from there (because they have died); unfamiliar medicines are administered; birthing beds are too high; and facilities are too cold, which is considered to be dangerous to the health of mothers and babies. Some women do not attend SBAs because they want to avoid certain clinical procedures, especially episiotomy and suturing, vaginal examination, surgery, being forced to deliver in the lithotomy position, and being without clothing.

These negative perceptions of SBAs were at odds with SBA's views of themselves. Without exception, the SBAs readily recognised that good quality care is characterised not only by technical competence but also by kind, respectful and patient communications with people they care for.

> *You have to be patient and tolerant. Then you must be friendly to them... Talk to them, share some stories, make them laugh. Share some experiences you have had.* [Interview with SBA, Laikipia]

> *You just have to be gentle. You just have to be tender and caring. Not just standing there, you should be attending to that woman.* [Interview with SBA, Laikipia]

Discussion

The findings from this qualitative study describe the practices of traditional and skilled birth attendants providing care for pastoralist communities in Laikipia and Samburu counties, Kenya, as well as the perceptions of the value and limitations of SBAs and TBAs from a range of perspectives including those of the practitioners themselves, the communities they serve, and key informants from the formal health system and from the Community Development Committees.

TBAs are described as familiar, trusted and respected repositories of traditional knowledge, who are actively engaged with pastoralist women during pregnancy, birth, and especially post-partum. Several TBAs have built links with SBAs in their areas, and are encouraging women to attend the dispensary. However, despite these positive attributes, it is probable that some routine TBA practices are potentially harmful to women and their babies, especially dietary advice involving food restrictions, induction of vomiting, abdominal palpation/massage, administration of herbs, and inadequate personal and environmental hygiene. It is widely acknowledged by participants (including TBAs) that TBAs do not possess the knowledge, skills, or equipment required to recognise and manage obstetric and neonatal complications. When complications occur at home, arranging referral and transport to the health facility is a challenging process for all involved, likely to result in substantial delays.

SBAs are recognised by all categories of participants to have the technical skills and resources required to provide safe and hygienic deliveries. However, SBAs regularly encounter a number of challenges that potentially compromise the quality of care they provide. Clearly, many pastoralist women remain reluctant to deliver in the health facilities, even if they have engaged with antenatal care. The health facilities are thought to be cold, unfriendly and even frightening, which possibly deters women from attending. Similarly, the reputation of SBAs as uncaring, and even abusive, is likely to negatively influence the uptake of health facility services. There is growing international awareness of this problem and the urgent need to address it in order to increase the proportion of births attended by SBAs, as evidenced by the 2014 WHO statement on 'The prevention and elimination of disrespect and abuse during facility-based childbirth' [16].

The SBAs are often practicing alone, which makes it difficult for them to staff the dispensaries at all times, and occasional absenteeism can be judged harshly by the community. Managing complicated deliveries as a solo practitioner is stressful, and arranging transfers to higher level facilities is not always a smooth process. Additionally, dispensaries are not always adequately equipped with essential items such as birthing kits and medicines. Despite these issues, there is ample evidence of mutual respect between SBAs and TBAs, and it is clear that some are already collaborating for collective benefit in the provision of care for women and babies in these remote settings. Creating greater collaboration between SBAs, TBAs and communities may maximise the strengths, fill the gaps and address the concerns regarding both SBA and TBA practices.

The development of a model for SBA/TBA collaborative care is likely to increase the uptake of SBA services [4, 10, 17]. For example, in a rural county of Kenya, TBAs were trained to provide birth planning advice and given a financial incentive for referrals to SBAs, which resulted in a 113 % increase in facility-based deliveries [18]. Evidence suggests that more collaborative models of care that collectively engage SBAs, TBAs and communities can improve the quality of maternal and newborn care and the utilisation of health services, as well as avert obstetric complications and perinatal, newborn and maternal mortality [11, 18–21].

However, it is critical to recognise that other persistent barriers such as distance and accessibility, staff availability, cost of services and transport, informed decision making, social and cultural preferences, must also be addressed [11, 19].

In the context of the pastoralist communities in Laikipia and Samburu, TBAs could, and in some places already do, escort women to dispensaries for antenatal care, refer them to the SBA at the onset of labour, provide them with support and comfort during delivery, and assist with domestic chores pre- and post-partum. Women may be more inclined to attend health facilities for maternal care if they are accompanied by a trusted, respected member of their own community, and the provision of continuous support to women in labour results in better obstetric outcomes and a more positive birth experience [22]. Additionally, TBAs could assist SBAs, who are predominantly solo practitioners, at the time of delivery. TBAs would require basic training to facilitate this new role, and to eliminate some of their more unsafe practices. If TBAs escort labouring women to health facilities, their presence will ensure that women are not left alone. The approach of engaging female birth companions from local communities, such as TBAs, has been assessed in 13 randomised controlled trials and found to reduce the incidence of adverse birth events and improve satisfaction with facility-based delivery among mothers [23].

This study has certain limitations that should be considered when interpreting the findings. Although data collection was designed to capture a range of perspectives from the sampled communities, as with all qualitative research, the findings are not representative of these communities, and cannot be generalised. Social desirability bias may have influenced some responses i.e., what participants actually believe, would do or have done may differ from what they reported. The SBAs in our study were based at dispensary level health facilities and therefore quite familiar with the communities and TBAs. Their views about TBAs may not be shared by SBAs based in higher level facilities such as district hospitals.

Conclusion

These findings suggest that a collaborative model of care involving both TBAs and SBAs is a viable proposition. While the Government of Kenya's goal is 90 % skilled birth attendance, the current reality among the semi-nomadic pastoralist communities in Laikipia and Samburu is that the majority of births are occurring at home with TBAs in attendance. The transition from predominantly traditional birth to skilled birth attendance in these communities is going to be a gradual one, and an interim collaborative model has the potential to maximise the safety of pastoralist women and babies during the transition phase, as well as facilitating the transition itself.

Abbreviations

CDC: Community Development Committee; CHW: community health worker; FGD: focus group discussion; IDI: in-depth interview; MUACK: Mothers' Union of the Anglican Church Kenya; SBA: skilled birth attendant; TBA: traditional birth attendant.

Competing interests

The authors declare that they have no competing interests.

Authors' contributions

AB contributed to study design, data collection, data analysis, and led the first draft of the manuscript; TC contributed to data collection, data analysis, and development of the manuscript; PO contributed to data collection and development of the manuscript; JN contributed to data collection and development of the manuscript; AM contributed to study design and development of the manuscript; JN contributed to study design and development of the manuscript; MK contributed to study design, managed the project, and led revisions of the manuscript. All authors have given final approval for this version of the manuscript.

Acknowledgments

Mothers' Union of the Anglican Church Kenya, Health Ministries of Laikipia and Samburu counties, Lillian Piroris, John Ole Tingoi, Florence Nderitu, Phillip Walker, Natalie Stephens, Jamie Han Chu. This study was funded by the Australian government's Department of Foreign Affairs and Trade. The views expressed are those of the authors and not necessarily those of the Commonwealth of Australia. The Commonwealth of Australia accepts no responsibility for any loss, damage or injury resulting from reliance on any of the information or views contained in this publication.

Author details

[1]Nossal Institute for Global Health, University of Melbourne, 161 Barry St, Carlton, VIC 3010, Australia. [2]Amref Health Africa, PO Box 27691-00506, Nairobi, Kenya.

References

1. Rosenfield A, Maine D. Maternal mortality-a neglected tragedy: Where is the M in MCH? Lancet. 1985;2(8446):83–5.
2. AbouZahr C. Safe motherhood: a brief history of the global movement 1947–2002. Br Med Bull. 2003;67(1):13–25.
3. United Nations. Millennium Development Goals and Beyond 2015. http://www.un.org/millenniumgoals Accessed 22 May 2015.
4. Kruske S, Barclay L. Effect of shifting policies on traditional birth attendant training. J Midwifery Womens Health. 2004;49(4):306–11.
5. Bergström S, Goodburn E. The role of traditional birth attendants in the reduction of maternal mortality. In: De Brouwere V, Van Lerberghe W, editors. Safe motherhood strategies: a review of the evidence. Belium: ITG Press; 2001. p. 77–99.
6. Saravanan S, Turrell G, Johnson H, Fraser J. Birthing practices of traditional birth attendants in South Asia in the context of training programmes. J Health Manag. 2010;12(2):93–121.
7. Kaingu C, Oduma J, Kanui T. Practices of traditional birth attendants in Machakos district, Kenya. J Ethnopharmacol. 2011;137:495–502.
8. Cotter K, Hawken M, Temmerman M. Low use of skilled attendants' delivery services in rural Kenya. J Health Popul Nutr. 2006;24(4):467–71.
9. The Safe Motherhood Demonstration Project. Traditional birth attendants in maternal health programmes. Nairobi: Ministry of Health Kenya, University of Nairobi and Population Council; 2003.
10. Roggeveen Y, Birks L, van Kats J, Manyama M, Hatfield J, Bunders J, et al. Low untilization of skilled birth attendants in Ngorongoro Conservation Area, Tanzania: a complex reality requiring action. Health. 2013;5:71–83.
11. Byrne A, Morgan A. How the integration of traditional birth attendants with formal health systems can increase skilled birth attendance. Int J Gynaecol Obstet. 2011;115(2):127–34.
12. Kenya National Bureau of Statistics (KNBS) and ICF Macro. Kenya Demographic and Health Survey 2008-09. Calverton, Maryland: KNBS and ICF Macro; 2010.
13. World Health Organization. World health statistics 2012. Geneva: WHO; 2012.
14. Nossal Institute for Global Health, Mothers Union of the Anglican Church of Kenya, Anglican Overseas AID. The Road Less Travelled: Maternal and child health baseline survey among Maasai and Samburu nomadic pastoralist communities in Laikipia and Samburu, Kenya. Kenya: Anglican Overseas Aid; 2012.
15. Braun V, Clarke V. Successful qualitative research: a practical guide for beginners. London: Sage; 2014.
16. World Health Organization. The prevention and elimination of disrespect and abuse during facility-based childbirth. Geneva: WHO/RHR/14.23, WHO; 2014.
17. Falle T, Mullany L, Thatte N, Khatry S, LeClerq S, Darmstadt G, et al. Potential role of traditional birth attendants in neonatal healthcare in rural southern Nepal. J Health Popul Nutr. 2009;27(1):53–61.
18. Tomedi A, Tucker K, Mwanthi M. A strategy to increase the number of deliveries with skilled birth attendants in Kenya. Int J Gynaecol Obstet. 2013;120:152–5.
19. Vieira C, Portela A, Miller T, Coast E, Leone T, Marston C. Increasing the use of skilled health personnel where traditional birth attendants were providers of childbirth care: a systematic review. PLoS ONE. 2012;7(10), e47946.
20. Wilson A, Gallos ID, Plana N, Lissauer D, Khan KS, Zamora J, et al. Effectiveness of strategies incorporating training and support of traditional birth attendants on perinatal and maternal mortality: meta-analysis. BMJ. 2011;343:d7102. doi:10.1136/bmj.d7102.

21. Ray A, Salihu H. The impact of maternal mortality interventions using traditional birth attendants and village midwives. J Obstet Gynaecol. 2004;24(1):5–11.
22. van Roosmalen J, Walraven G, Stekelenburg J, Massawe S. Integrating continuous support of the traditional birth attendant into obstetric care by skilled midwives and doctors: a cost-effective strategy to reduce perinatal mortality and unnecessary obstetric interventions. Trop Med Int Health. 2005;10(5):393–4.
23. Hofmeyr G, Haws R, Bergström S, Lee A, Okong P, Darmstadt G, et al. Obstetric care in low-resource settings: What, who, and how to overcome challenges to scale up? Int J Gynaecol Obstet. 2009;107(Suppl):S21–45.

18

The impact of a community driven mass media campaign on the utilisation of maternal health care services in rural Malawi

Collins O. F. Zamawe[1,2*], Masford Banda[3] and Albert N. Dube[1,4]

Abstract

Background: Mass media is critical in disseminating public health information, improving health knowledge and changing health behaviours. However, most of the mass media public health interventions do not sufficiently engage the local people; they are externally determined. Due to this, very little is known about the effects of locally instigated mass media promotion. Therefore, the aim of this study was to examine the impact of a community driven mass media campaign called Phukusi la Moyo (tips of life) on the utilisation of maternal health care services.

Methods: A community-based cross-sectional study involving 3825 women of reproductive age (15–49 years) was conducted in rural Malawi to evaluate the Phukusi la Moyo (PLM) campaign. To do this, we compared the utilisation of maternal health care services between women who were exposed to the PLM campaign and those who were not. Respondents were identified using a multistage cluster sampling method. This involved systematically selecting communities (clusters), households and respondents. Associations were examined using Pearson chi square test and a multivariable logistic regression model.

Results: The likelihood of using contraceptives (AOR = 1.61; 95 % CI = 1.32–1.96), sleeping under mosquito bed-nets (AOR = 1.65; 95 % CI = 1.39–1.97), utilising antenatal care services (AOR = 2.62; 95 % CI = 1.45–4.73) and utilising postnatal care services (AOR = 1.59; CI = 1.29–1.95) were significantly higher among women who had exposure to the PLM campaign than those who did not. No significant association was found between health facility delivery and exposure to the PLM campaign.

Conclusion: Women exposed to a community driven mass media campaign in rural Malawi were more likely to utilise maternal health care services than their unexposed counterparts. Since, the use of maternal health care services reduces the risk of maternal morbidity and mortality, community-led mass media could play a significant role towards improving maternal health outcomes in low-and-middle-income countries. Therefore, we recommend the use of locally driven mass media in disseminating public health information in limited resource settings.

Keywords: Women's health, Community intervention, Radio campaign, Phukusi la Moyo

* Correspondence: fzamawe@gmail.com
[1]Parent and Child Health Initiative (PACHI), Research Centre, Amina house, Off Chilambula Road, P.O. Box 31686, Capital City, Lilongwe 3, Malawi
[2]The Ministry of Health, Lilongwe, Malawi
Full list of author information is available at the end of the article

Background

Many people needlessly die every day due to lack of access to health information which would have allowed them or health workers to make appropriate decisions [1]. Thus, access to reliable health information is a cornerstone of improved and sustainable health outcomes [2]. In low-and-middle-income countries (LMIC), poor access to health information, especially among rural women is a major public health problem [3, 4]. It undermines efforts to bring health care services closer to the people. Hence, innovative strategies are required to meet the goal of 'Health Information For All' (HIFA) campaign [1].

Mass media is one of the popular and cost-effective public health promotion tools globally [2, 5, 6]. It is the main source of health information in many parts of the world, especially in LMIC. In Nigeria, for example, mass media is one of the major sources of information about malaria [7], women's health, HIV/AIDS and family planning among others [3]. Likewise, access to information in rural Tanzania is mainly through mass media (radio, television, newspapers), cell-phones and face to face communication [5]. Moreover, mass media interventions have been at the centre of maternal health and HIV prevention in Malawi [4, 8].

A growing body of evidence shows that mass media impacts public health knowledge, attitudes, beliefs and behaviours [9–11]. In Zambia, for example, exposure to radio and television programs about condom and HIV/AIDS was associated with higher condom use [12]. Similarly, a behaviour change communication media campaign in Uganda improved knowledge of six months as the ideal period for exclusive breastfeeding [13]. In addition, media exposure significantly improved dietary diversity and meal frequency among infants and children in Ethiopia [14]. Further, a host of HIV media campaigns implemented between 1998 and 2007 in 23 countries effectively stimulated behaviour change [15].

In particular, the effects of mass media on maternal health behaviours have long been recognised in LMIC, where most of the maternal deaths occur [6, 16, 17]. In Nepal, exposure to mass media increased utilization of antenatal care services among rural women [18]. Comparable observations were made in Ghana, where exposure to mass media was recognized as a significant predictor of the likelihood that a woman would utilize antenatal care services and opt for childbirth assisted by a skilled provider [19]. Moreover, mass media impact men's involvement in maternal health. For example, Malawian women exposed to a specific media campaign reported higher participation of men in antenatal, postnatal and delivery care services [20].

Evidently, mass media is critical in disseminating public health information, improving health knowledge and changing health behaviours. Nonetheless, mass media campaigns have had inconsistent outcomes [3, 21]. A review of media campaigns on contraceptive use in LMIC demonstrated that most of the interventions had short-term effects, to the extent that demand for contraceptives would fall back to the initial level [22]. At country level, radio communication campaigns in Malawi had limited effect on condom use [4]. Likewise, media campaigns in Bangladesh appear to have no impact on contraceptive use [23].

Unreliable outcomes of mass media interventions in public health could be down to three factors: (a) media messages do not address cultural and practical barriers to behaviour change, (b) use of inappropriate media platforms to reach rural target audiences and (c) programs focus on one issue in the face of other related problems [24]. In short, most of the mass media interventions do not sufficiently engage the local people or community members [6, 25]. Usually, what is branded as 'community-based mass media' merely specifies that the "unit of intervention is at the community level" [3, 6, 7, 18]. To be truly community grounded, an intervention is supposed to be developed and spearheaded by and for the communities it aims to serve [6]. Such interventions are more likely to be acceptable, sustainable and cost-effective [26–28].

Lack of community involvement implies that most of the public health mass media interventions are externally determined [6, 29, 30]. Owing to this, very little is known about the effects of locally instigated mass media promotion. For this reason, the aim of this study was to examine the impact of a mass media campaign (Phukusi la Moyo), which was initiated and led by the community members, on the utilisation of maternal health care services. The study will provide critical insights into the role of the community members in public health mass media interventions. This would help to inform and strengthen designs of future media interventions in maternal health and other global health areas.

Methods

A synopsis of the Phukusi la Moyo campaign

The Malawi Ministry of Health in collaboration with the Institute for Global Health (University College London) established a project called MaiMwana (mother and child) in 2003. The aim of the project was "to build capacities of communities in rural Malawi to take control of mother and child health issues that affect them" [31, 32]. The project was set up in Mchinji district, which was divided into 48 clusters. Of these, 24 received the women's group intervention [31]. Women in treatment clusters formed 207 groups to facilitate learning, sharing of lessons and to provide a platform for dealing with maternal health problems locally. The intervention was divided into four phases, with each having its main objective as follows: (a) to identify priority problems affecting women during pregnancy, delivery and postpartum; (b) to plan for the solutions of the problems identified and prioritised; (c) to implement the locally driven solutions to the problems and (d) to evaluate the solutions [31].

One of the major priority problems that most of the groups identified during phase one of the project was that health information was not accessible in some parts of the district due to shortage of community health workers. As a result, during phase two, the groups identified the feasibility of using a community radio to bring knowledge about maternal and child health issues to a large population. The groups agreed to lobby for a maternal health education program to be aired on the district's community radio station called "Mudziwanthu" (our community). Following that, a weekly radio program called "Phukusi la Moyo" (tips of life) was born. The intervention was implemented between 2009 and 2011.

As a radio campaign, the focus of Phukusi la Moyo (PLM) was to provide comprehensive maternal health information to women of reproductive age (15–49 years). The ultimate goal of the PLM campaign was to help reduce maternal and child mortality through improving utilisation of maternal health care services [31, 32]. The PLM's emphasis was on raising awareness of the risks associated with pregnancy, the importance of antenatal and postnatal care, and the advantages of delivering at the health facility. The campaign also aimed to promote (a) men's engagement in maternal health, (b) the use of mosquito bed-nets and (c) uptake of malaria prophylaxis among pregnant women.

The PLM campaign messages were delivered by means of different activities. These included panel discussions, community discussions, drama and songs. Members of the women's groups developed the radio programs with the technical support of the MaiMwana project and the Mudziwanthu radio station. The communities formed radio listening clubs, where women could listen to the program in groups and discuss the key messages afterwards.

The study design

A community-based cross-sectional study was conducted to evaluate the PLM interventions. This involved comparing the utilisation of maternal health care services between women who were exposed to the PLM campaign and those who were not. In the absence of the baseline data, this design was considered appropriate for the evaluation.

The study setting

The study was implemented in Mchinji, one of the 28 districts in Malawi. It is a typical rural district located in the central region of Malawi. Mchinji was particularly chosen because it was the catchment area of the PLM campaign, which this study intended to evaluate. The MaiMwana project divided the district into 48 equal clusters based on population size. This study was conducted in 24 of these 48 clusters, which were selected using a simple random sampling method.

Population of the study and sample size

Women of reproductive age (15–49 years) who gave birth or fell pregnant at least 12 months after the implementation of the PLM campaign were the target population of this study. The study engaged women only because the objective was to examine the utilisation of maternal health care services. Other inclusion criteria included: stayed continuously in the community between 2009 and 2013, willingness to participate and ability to provide informed consent. To allow meaningful analysis at cluster-level, the study included statistically reasonable number of respondents from each cluster. This was computed using G*Power version 3.1 program [33]. The minimum cluster sample size was 143 (effect size = 0.3; power = 0.80; alpha < 0.05). Overall, data were collected from 3825 women.

Data collection and sampling methods

The data collection period was from July to December 2013. A team of 14 local research assistants conducted the fieldwork. They received a short training in research ethics and data collection. Data were collected using pre-tested structured electronic questionnaires, which were put in the Personal Digital Assistants (PDAs). Among other things, the questionnaire captured demographic details, exposure to the PLM program and utilisation of maternal health care services during the last pregnancy.

Respondents were systematically identified through a multistage cluster sampling method. In the first stage, the clusters were chosen using a simple random sampling technique. This was followed by selection of households through a systematic sampling approach. The sampling frame for each cluster was 160. Finally, a single respondent was identified from each household using a simple random sampling method. The study registered 100 % response rate.

Description of study variables

Five outcome variables were examined in this study. These were (a) utilisation of antenatal care services, (b) use of mosquito bed nets during pregnancy, (c) delivery at the health facility, (d) utilisation of postnatal care services and (e) use of contraceptives. All outcome variables were dichotomous (yes/no). Exposure to the PLM campaign was the main independent variable of this study. Respondents were either exposed or not (no/yes). The following covariates were also measured: highest education level, occupation, marital status and participation in the women's group intervention.

Data analysis

The level of missing values in all relevant variables was below 5 %. As a result, all cases with missing values were discarded ($n = 386$) [34]. The final sample size of the study was 3439. Stata (version 12) was used for analysis. Descriptive statistics were used to describe variables. Then, we examined the relationships between independent and outcome variables using the Pearson chi-square (χ^2) test of independence. Finally, a multivariable logistic regression model was fitted to determine the direction and degree of the associations between the independent and outcome variables. Each outcome variable was examined twice against the independent variable: first, without adjusting for covariates and then, after controlling for marital status, age, occupation, participation in women's groups and education level. The relationships were estimated using crude and adjusted odds ratios and a 95 % confidence interval. We used alpha (α) of $p < 0.05$ to determine statistical significance.

Ethical clearance and consent

The protocol of this study was reviewed and approved by Malawi's National Health Sciences Research Committee (NHSRC). Participation in this study was voluntary and written informed consent was obtained from all the participants. Data collectors explained relevant details of the study to each potential respondent and asked if she would be interested in participating. Participants were required to sign or thumb-stamp the consent form. For participants under 18 years old (minors), additional written consent was obtained from their parents or guardians.

Results

Characteristics of the participants

Table 1 presents descriptive and bivariate results. Overall, the study engaged 3439 women residing in Mchinji district. The largest subgroup of the respondents were young women aged between 20 and 29 (47 %) followed by those between 30 and 39 years old (34 %). Very few teenage girls (7 %) and older women over the age of 40 (12 %) were involved. Most of the respondents at least attended primary education (72 %), but none had gone beyond secondary school. A small number of participants (15 %) had no formal education. Most of the participants (74 %) were subsistent farmers. Regarding marital status, most of the respondents were married (90 %). Additionally, many participants were members of the women's groups (68 %).

Sources of maternal health information and use of maternal health services

Different sources of maternal health information were reported by our respondents. Most of them mentioned antenatal clinics followed by community health workers and radio (Fig. 1). Moreover, most participants (70 %) acknowledged that they had access to the radio. In particular, around 60 % of the participants were exposed to the PLM campaign (Table 1). We also assessed utilisation of maternal health care services. Women were asked about utilisation of maternal health care services during their last pregnancy. Almost all the women (98.4) attended antenatal care clinics, even though it was not certain if they fulfilled the recommended minimum of four visits. Similarly, most of the participants used contraceptives, delivered at the health facility, used postnatal care, and were sleeping under mosquito bed-net during pregnancy.

Impact of the PLM campaign

We examined the association between exposure to the PLM campaign and the utilisation of maternal health care services. The results indicate that there was a significant association between exposure to the PLM campaign and use of contraceptives ($p \leq 0.001$), utilisation of antenatal care ($p \leq 0.001$), sleeping under mosquito bed-nets ($p \leq 0.001$) as well as utilisation of postnatal care ($p \leq 0.001$). No significant association was found between exposure to the PLM program and delivery at the health facility ($p = 0.209$).

The results further show that the likelihood of using contraceptives (OR = 1.72; 95 % CI = 1.43–2.07), mosquito bed-nets (OR = 1.88; 95 % CI = 1.59–2.22), antenatal care services (OR = 2.90; 95 % CI = 1.65–5.10), and postnatal care services (OR = 1.64; CI = 1.35–1.99) were significantly higher among women who had exposure to the PLM campaign than those who did not. After adjusting for potential confounders (i.e. age, education, occupation, marital status, participation women's groups), women who had exposure to the PLM campaign were still significantly more likely to use contraceptives (AOR = 1.61; 95 % CI = 1.32–1.96), mosquito bed-nets (AOR = 1.65; 95 % CI = 1.39–1.97), antenatal care services (AOR = 2.62; 95 % CI = 1.45–4.73), and postnatal care services (AOR = 1.59; CI = 1.29–1.95) than those who were not exposed; although with some reductions (Table 2). No significant association was found between health facility delivery and exposure to the PLM campaign.

Discussion

A community driven mass media campaign in rural Malawi was associated with improved utilisation of maternal health care services among women who were exposed to it. Specifically, exposure to the PLM campaign increased the likelihood of using contraceptives by 61 %, utilising antenatal care services by 162 %, sleeping under mosquito bed nets during pregnancy by 65 % and utilising postnatal care by 59 %. This suggests that community driven mass media interventions are effective

Table 1 Characteristics of the participants and bivariate results ($n = 3439$)

Variable	n (%)		Exposure to PLM program				*p*-value
			No (%)		Yes (%)		
Total	3439	(100.0)	1349	(39.2)	2090	(60.8)	
Age (years)							
15–19	224	(6.5)	102	(45.5)	122	(54.5)	<0.003*
20–29	1628	(47.3)	590	(36.2)	1038	(63.8)	
30–39	1183	(34.4)	480	(40.6)	703	(59.4)	
40–49	404	(11.8)	177	(43.8)	227	(56.2)	
Education							
None	529	(15.4)	261	(49.3)	268	(50.7)	<0.001*
Primary school	2463	(71.6)	964	(39.1)	1499	(60.9)	
Secondary school	447	(13.0)	124	(27.7)	323	(72.3)	
Marital status							
Never married	99	(2.9)	53	(53.5)	46	(46.5)	<0.001*
Currently married	3094	(90.0)	1180	(38.1)	1, 914	(61.9)	
Formerly married	246	(7.2)	116	(47.1)	130	(52.9)	
Occupation							
Farmers	2559	(74.4)	1033	(40.4)	1526	(59.6)	<0.001*
Self employed	514	(15.0)	159	(30.9)	355	(69.1)	
Casual worker	273	(7.9)	119	(43.6)	154	(56.4)	
Others	93	(2.7)	38	(40.9)	55	(59.1)	
Women's group member							
No	2341	(68.1)	1090	(46.6)	1251	(53.4)	<0.001*
Yes	1098	(31.9)	259	(23.6)	839	(76.4)	
Used contraceptives							
No	529	(15.4)	267	(50.5)	262	(49.5)	<0.001*
Yes	2910	(84.6)	1082	(37.2)	1828	(62.8)	
Utilised antenatal health care services							
No	54	(1.6)	35	(64.8)	19	(35.2)	<0.001*
Yes	3385	(98.4)	1314	(38.8)	2071	(61.2)	
Sleeping under bed-nets during pregnancy							
No	710	(20.6)	365	(51.4)	345	(48.6)	<0.001*
Yes	2729	(79.4)	984	(36.1)	1745	(63.9)	
Delivered at health facility							
No	271	(7.9)	116	(42.8)	155	(57.2)	0.209**
Yes	3168	(92.1)	1233	(38.9)	1935	(61.1)	
Utilised postnatal health care services							
No	469	(13.6)	233	(49.7)	236	(50.3)	<0.001*
Yes	2970	(86.4)	1116	(37.6)	1854	(62.4)	

PLM phukusi la moyo
*Significant ($p < 0.05$); **Not significant ($p > 0.05$)

in improving uptake of maternal health care services in limited resource settings.

The main focus of PLM was to raise awareness of the maternal health complications and the importance of family planning, antenatal care, postnatal care and delivering at the health facility. Therefore, increased utilisation of maternal health care services among women exposed to the PLM campaign was likely due to improved knowledge of maternal health issues. This is consistent with other studies in LMIC that have shown that mass

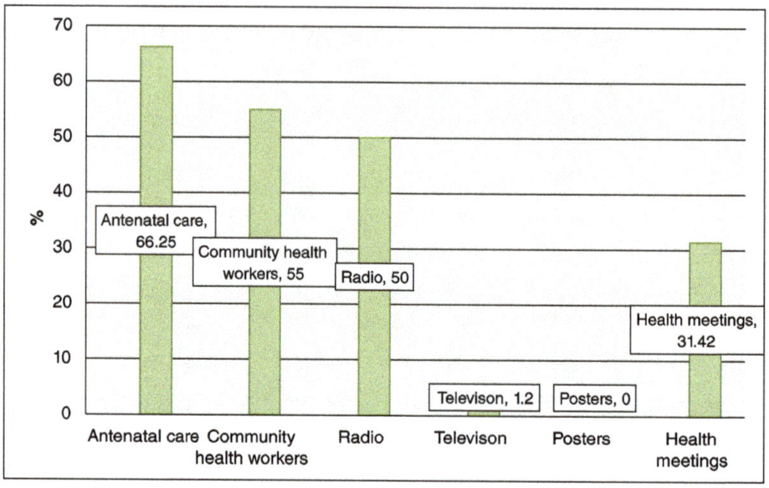

Fig. 1 Sources of maternal health information (multiple responses)

media campaigns influence knowledge and behaviours [35, 36]. However, most of the earlier mass media promotions were externally developed with no input from the targeted communities [6, 8, 18]. The PLM campaign was different; it employed a bottom-up approach. Therefore, the results of this study add a new dimension to the literature of mass media in global health.

Moreover, our outcomes demonstrate that a true community centred approach is conceivable in mass media. Like other health programs, we believe that the benefits of mass media would be maximised if the campaigns are grounded in the targeted communities. For instance, apart from the intended outcomes, community involvement in public health mass media interventions would probably promote self-reliance/ownership, encourage the use of locally available resources and address priority health needs [37, 38]. To this effect, where appropriate, a bottom-up approach should be prioritised in media interventions

Table 2 Exposure to the PLM campaign and the utilisation of maternal health care services (logistic model) ($n = 3439$)

Outcome variables	OR	(95 % CI)	*p*-value	AOR	(95 % CI)	*p*-value
Used contraceptives						
No (Rc)	1.00					
Yes	1.72	(1.43–2.07)	<0.001*	1.61	(1.32–1.96)	<0.001*
Utilised antenatal care services						
No (Rc)	1.00					
Yes	2.90	(1.65–5.10)	<0.001*	2.62	(1.45–4.73)	0.001
Slept under bed-net						
No (Rc)	1.00					
Yes	1.88	(1.59–2.22)	<0.001*	1.65	(1.39–1.97)	<0.001*
Delivered at a health facility						
No (Rc)	1.00					
Yes	1.17	(0.91–1.51)	0.209**	1.11	(0.85–145)	0.44**
Utilised postnatal care services						
No (Rc)	1.00					
Yes	1.64	(1.35–1.99)	<0.001*	1.59	(1.29–1.95)	<0.001*

OR Odds ratio
AOR Adjusted odds ratio
CI Confidence interval
Rc Reference category
*Significant ($p < 0.05$)
**Not significant ($p > 0.05$)

targeting the rural masses. In the meantime, however, there is a need to compare the impact of the community driven and externally determined media interventions.

In particular, community driven media campaigns could be critical in improving maternal health outcomes in LMIC. Although the utilisation of maternal health care services reduces the risk of maternal morbidity and mortality, some of the women continue to shun these health care services [17, 39, 40]. The findings of this research reveal that locally driven mass media could be a reliable instrument for enhancing uptake of maternal health care services.

The findings of this study further indicate that mass media is or could be an essential platform for transmitting health information in rural areas. Over 70 % of the participants had access to the radio and about 50 % of the women also indicated that the radio was the main source of maternal health information. Similar findings have also been observed elsewhere [3, 5, 41]. Since the shortage of community health workers makes it impossible to reach every woman (especially in rural areas) with maternal health information [42], community driven mass media campaigns could be a reliable alternative.

While recommending community driven mass media campaigns, we would like to recognise the need for the community members to adequately engage professional health care workers in the production of campaign materials. This would ensure that correct information is made available. Besides, more community radio stations should be set up in rural places. This would allow broadcasting of tailor-made programs like the PLM that meet the specific needs of the people in a particular setting. Equally, it is logical to expand the signal radius of the existing community radio stations to reach out to more people living in the remote areas.

This study had some limitations and strengths. Due to the cross-sectional design, we could not establish causal-effect relationships. Besides, owing to the self-reporting of both exposure and health behaviours, we cannot rule out the recall and social desirability biases. Nonetheless, the statistical significance was robust due to relatively large sample size.

Conclusion

Women exposed to a community driven mass media campaign in rural Malawi were significantly more likely to utilise maternal health care services than their unexposed counterparts. Since, the use of maternal health care services reduces the risk of maternal morbidity and mortality, community driven mass media could play a significant role towards improving maternal health outcomes in LMIC. To this end, community driven mass media interventions should be promoted, especially in limited resource settings.

Abbreviations

AOR: adjusted odds ratio; CI: confidence interval; LMIC: low-and-middle-income-countries; NHSRC: National Health Sciences Research Committee; PDA: Personal Digital Assistants; PLM: Phukusi la Moyo.

Competing interests

The authors declare that they have no competing interests.

Authors' contributions

CZ designed the study, contributed to the fieldwork, performed statistical analysis and drafted the manuscript. MB designed the study, contributed to the fieldwork and performed statistical analysis. AD designed the study, contributed to the fieldwork, performed statistical analysis. All the authors read and approved the final manuscript.

Acknowledgements

We would like to recognise the support, which we received from all the members of the Phukusi la Moyo steering committee. We also acknowledge the contribution of Fatsani Kusamula, Mark Manyau, Tambosi Phiri, Bright Singini and Florida Malamba during data collection. The Commonwealth of Learning (CoL) funded both Phukusi la Moyo radio program and the current study. However, the funder played no part in the designing of this study and did not influence our decision to publish these results.
We are also grateful to Masautso Chimombo (Lilongwe University of Agriculture and Natural Resources), Neo Kazembe (Dignitas International) and Aggie Wizi (Catholic University of Malawi) for editing our draft manuscript.

Author details

[1]Parent and Child Health Initiative (PACHI), Research Centre, Amina house, Off Chilambula Road, P.O. Box 31686, Capital City, Lilongwe 3, Malawi. [2]The Ministry of Health, Lilongwe, Malawi. [3]MaiMwana Project, P.O. Box 2, Mchinji, Malawi. [4]The University of Malawi, College of Medicine, School of Public Health, Blantyre, Malawi.

References

1. A global campaign: healthcare information for all by 2015 [http://www.hifa2015.org/about/why-hifa2015-is-needed/]. Accessed date 2 Jun 2015.
2. Godlee F, Pakenham-Walsh N, Ncayiyana D, Cohen B, Packer A. Can we achieve health information for all by 2015? Lancet. 2004;364:295–300.
3. Nwagwu WE, Ajama M. Women ' s health information needs and information sources: a study of a rural oil palm business community in South-Western Nigeria. Ann Libr Inf Stud. 2011;58:270–81.
4. Meekers D, Van Rossem R, Silva M, Koleros A. The reach and effect of radio communication campaigns on condom use in Malawi. Stud Fam Plann. 2007;38:113–20.
5. Mtega WP. Access to and Usage of Information among Rural Communities: a Case Study of Kilosa District Morogoro Region in Tanzania. Can J Libr Inf Pract Res. 2013;7:1–9.
6. Sood S, Shefner-Rogers C, Skinner J. Health Communication Campaigns in Developing Countries. J Creat Commun. 2014;9:67–84.
7. Umeano-Enemuoh JC, Uzochukwu B, Ezumah N, Mangham-Jefferies L, Wiseman V, Onwujekwe O. A qualitative study on health workers' and community members' perceived sources, role of information and communication on malaria treatment, prevention and control in southeast Nigeria. BMC Infect Dis. 2015;15:437.
8. Reijer P, Chalimba M, Nakwagala AA. Malawi goes to scale with anti-AIDS clubs and popular media. Eval Program Plann. 2002;25:357–63.
9. LaCroix JM, Snyder LB, Huedo-Medina TB, Johnson BT. Effectiveness of mass media interventions for HIV prevention, 1986–2013: a meta-analysis. J Acquir Immune Defic Syndr. 2014;66 Suppl 3:S329–40.
10. Naugle DA, Hornik RC. Systematic Review of the Effectiveness of Mass Media Interventions for Child Survival in Low- and Middle-Income Countries. J Health Commun. 2014;19:190–215.
11. Robinson MN, Tansil KA, Elder RW, Soler RE, Labre MP, Mercer SL, et al. Mass Media Health Communication Campaigns Combined with Health-Related Product Distribution. Am J Prev Med. 2014;47:360–71.

12. Van Rossem R, Meekers D. The reach and impact of social marketing and reproductive health communication campaigns in Zambia. BMC Public Health. 2007;7:352.
13. Gupta N, Katende C, Bessinger R. An evaluation of post-campaign knowledge and practices of exclusive breastfeeding in Uganda. J Health Popul Nutr. 2004;22:429–39.
14. Beyene M, Worku AG, Wassie MM. Dietary diversity, meal frequency and associated factors among infant and young children in Northwest Ethiopia: a cross- sectional study. BMC Public Health. 2015;15:1007.
15. Noar SM, Palmgreen P, Chabot M, Dobransky N, Zimmerman RS. A 10-year systematic review of HIV/AIDS mass communication campaigns: Have we made progress? J Health Commun. 2009;14:15–42.
16. Tsawe M, Moto A, Netshivhera T, Ralesego L, Nyathi C, Susuman AS. Factors influencing the use of maternal healthcare services and childhood immunization in Swaziland. Int J Equity Health. 2015;14:32.
17. United Nations. The Millennium Development Goals Report 2014. New York; 2014. http://www.who.int/woman_child_accountability/ierg/reports/2012_15S_MassMediaEvidenceBase.pdf. Accessed date 20 May 2015.
18. Acharya D, Khanal V, Singh JK, Adhikari M, Gautam S. Impact of mass media on the utilization of antenatal care services among women of rural community in Nepal. TT -. BMC Res Notes. 2015;8:4–9.
19. Asmah EE, Twerefou DK, Smith JE. Health Campaigns and Use of Reproductive Health Care Services by Women in Ghana. Am J Econ. 2013;3:243–51.
20. Zamawe C, Banda M, Dube A. The effect of mass media campaign on Men's participation in maternal health: a cross-sectional study in Malawi. Reprod Health. 2015;12:31.
21. Asp G, Pettersson KO, Sandberg J, Kabakyenga J, Agardh A. Associations between mass media exposure and birth preparedness among women in southwestern Uganda: A community-based survey. Glob Health Action. 2014;7:1–9.
22. Hornik R, McAnany E. Theories and Evidence: Mass Media Effects and Fertility Change. Commun Theory. 2001;11:454–71.
23. Raut MK. Interpersonal communication and contraception: Insights and evidences from Bangladesh demographic and health survey, 2011. Indian J Public Health. 2015;59:220–4.
24. Snell W. Mass Media: The Evidence Base. London; 2012. http://www.who.int/woman_child_accountability/ierg/reports/2012_15S_MassMediaEvidenceBase.pdf. Accessed date 19 Apr 2015.
25. Creel AH, Rimal RN, Mkandawire G, Böse K, Brown JW. Effects of a mass media intervention on HIV-related stigma: "Radio Diaries" program in Malawi. Health Educ Res. 2011;26:456–65.
26. Colbourn T, Nambiar B, Bondo A, Makwenda C, Tsetekani E, Makonda-Ridley A, et al. Effects of quality improvement in health facilities and community mobilization through women's groups on maternal, neonatal and perinatal mortality in three districts of Malawi: MaiKhanda, a cluster randomized controlled effectiveness trial. Int Health. 2013;5:180–95.
27. Manandhar DS, Osrin D, Shrestha BP, Mesko N, Morrison J, Tumbahangphe KM, et al. Effect of a participatory intervention with women's groups on birth outcomes in Nepal: cluster-randomised controlled trial. Lancet. 2004;364:970–9.
28. More NS, Bapat U, Das S, Alcock G, Patil S, Porel M, et al. Community mobilization in Mumbai slums to improve perinatal care and outcomes: A cluster randomized controlled trial. PLoS Med. 2012;9.
29. Kane TT, Gueye M, Speizer I, Pacque-margolis S, Baron D. The Impact of a Family in Campaign Planning Bamako, Multimedia Mali. Stud Fam Plann. 1998;29:309–23.
30. Davis J, Luchters S, Holmes W. Men and Maternal and Newborn Health: Benefits, Harms, Challenges and Potential Strategies for Engaging Men. Melbourne; 2013. http://www.wchknowledgehub.com.au/sites/default/files/BP_Davis_FEB13.pdf. Accessed date 30 May 2015.
31. Rosato M, Mwansambo C, Lewycka S, Kazembe P, Phiri T, Malamba F, et al. MaiMwana women's groups: A community mobilisation intervention to improve mother and child health and reduce mortality in rural Malawi. Malawi Med J. 2010;22:112–9.
32. Lewycka S, Mwansambo C, Rosato M, Kazembe P, Phiri T, Mganga A, et al. Effect of women's groups and volunteer peer counselling on rates of mortality, morbidity, and health behaviours in mothers and children in rural Malawi (MaiMwana): A factorial, cluster-randomised controlled trial. Lancet. 2013;381:1721–35.
33. Faul F, Erdfelder E, Lang A-G, Buchner A. G*Power 3: a flexible statistical power analysis program for the social, behavioral, and biomedical sciences. Behav Res Methods. 2007;39:175–91.
34. Baraldi AN, Enders CK. An introduction to modern missing data analyses. J Sch Psychol. 2010;48:5–37.
35. Mashreky SR, Rahman F, Rahman A, Talab A, Rahman Z. Role of mass media in increasing knowledge and practices of mothers on IYCF: findings from a community trial in rural Bangladesh. South East Asia J Public Heal. 2015;5:18.
36. Mishra SR, Adhikari S, Khanal V. Role of mass media on knowledge generation and countering misconceptions about tuberculosis transmission in Nepal. Asian Pac J Trop Biomed. 2014;4:S610–5.
37. Jimba M, Poudel-Tandukar K, Poudel KC. School and community health project: Part 1: A community development and health project in Nepal. Japan Med Assoc J. 2008;51:225–34.
38. Rosato M, Laverack G, Grabman LH, Tripathy P, Nair N, Mwansambo C, et al. Community participation: lessons for maternal, newborn, and child health. Lancet. 2008;372:962–71.
39. Ahmed S, Li Q, Liu L, Tsui AO. Maternal deaths averted by contraceptive use: An analysis of 172 countries. Lancet. 2012;380:111–25.
40. Yego F, D'Este C, Byles J, Williams JS, Nyongesa P. Risk factors for maternal mortality in a Tertiary Hospital in Kenya: a case control study. BMC Pregnancy Childbirth. 2014;14:38.
41. Bosompra K. Sources of Health Information Among Rural Dwellers in Africa: A Case Study of Two Ghanaian Villages. African media Rev. 1987;1:120–33.
42. Warren C. Care seeking for maternal health: challenges remain for poor women. Ethiop J Heal. 2010;24:100–4.

19

eRegistries: Electronic registries for maternal and child health

J. Frederik Frøen[1,2*], Sonja L. Myhre[1], Michael J. Frost[1,3], Doris Chou[4], Garrett Mehl[4], Lale Say[4], Socheat Cheng[1,5], Ingvild Fjeldheim[1], Ingrid K. Friberg[1], Steve French[1], Jagrati V. Jani[1,2], Jane Kaye[6], John Lewis[7,8], Ane Lunde[1], Kjersti Mørkrid[1], Victoria Nankabirwa[1,9], Linda Nyanchoka[1], Hollie Stone[1], Mahima Venkateswaran[1,2], Aleena M. Wojcieszek[10,11], Marleen Temmerman[3] and Vicki J. Flenady[10,11]

Abstract

Background: The Global Roadmap for Health Measurement and Accountability sees integrated systems for health information as key to obtaining seamless, sustainable, and secure information exchanges at all levels of health systems. The Global Strategy for Women's, Children's and Adolescent's Health aims to achieve a continuum of quality of care with effective coverage of interventions. The WHO and World Bank recommend that countries focus on intervention coverage to monitor programs and progress for universal health coverage. Electronic health registries - eRegistries - represent integrated systems that secure a triple return on investments: First, effective single data collection for health workers to seamlessly follow individuals along the continuum of care and across disconnected cadres of care providers. Second, real-time public health surveillance and monitoring of intervention coverage, and third, feedback of information to individuals, care providers and the public for transparent accountability. This series on eRegistries presents frameworks and tools to facilitate the development and secure operation of eRegistries for maternal and child health.

Methods: In this first paper of the eRegistries Series we have used WHO frameworks and taxonomy to map how eRegistries can support commonly used electronic and mobile applications to alleviate health systems constraints in maternal and child health. A web-based survey of public health officials in 64 low- and middle-income countries, and a systematic search of literature from 2005–2015, aimed to assess country capacities by the current status, quality and use of data in reproductive health registries.

Results: eRegistries can offer support for the 12 most commonly used electronic and mobile applications for health. Countries are implementing health registries in various forms, the majority in transition from paper-based data collection to electronic systems, but very few have eRegistries that can act as an integrating backbone for health information. More mature country capacity reflected by published health registry based research is emerging in settings reaching regional or national scale, increasingly with electronic solutions. 66 scientific publications were identified based on 32 registry systems in 23 countries over a period of 10 years; this reflects a challenging experience and capacity gap for delivering sustainable high quality registries.

Conclusions: Registries are being developed and used in many high burden countries, but their potential benefits are far from realized as few countries have fully transitioned from paper-based health information to integrated electronic backbone systems. Free tools and frameworks exist to facilitate progress in health information for women and children.

Keywords: Health systems, eRegistries, Women's, Children's and Adolescent's Health, health surveillance, eHealth, mHealth

* Correspondence: frederik.froen@fhi.no
[1]Department of International Public Health, Norwegian Institute of Public Health, Pb 4404 Nydalen, N-0403 Oslo, Norway
[2]Centre for Intervention Science in Maternal and Child Health (CISMAC), University of Bergen, Bergen, Norway
Full list of author information is available at the end of the article

Background

Electronic health (eHealth) solutions, including mobile health technologies (mHealth), have the potential to improve quality of healthcare by addressing technical shortcomings embedded in health systems (Frame 1). Many eHealth initiatives in low and middle income countries (LMIC) have been fragmented [1, 2]. Now, global health agencies are moving towards more sustainable and holistic approaches for institutionalizing e- and mHealth into healthcare systems [1, 3–5].

The new World Bank/WHO/USAID Roadmap for Health Measurement and Accountability Post-2015 (MA4Health) underlined that *"Public health and clinical care cannot be delivered safely, with high quality, and in a cost-effective manner, without seamless, sustainable, and secure data and information exchanges at all levels of the health system"* [5]. An effective healthcare system must therefore entail a seamless common or interoperable digital thread for health information so that the full range of uses can be driven by, or contribute to, an *integrated backbone system* [4, 5]. In line with this, MA4Health has outlined the importance of having all health information system (HIS) development initiatives aligned with a single operational country platform for data and indicators by 2020.

With the new United Nation's Global Strategy for Women's, Children's and Adolescent's Health (UN Global Strategy) [6], the global community for mothers' and children's health is converging on post-2015 policies for integrated care for the health and survival of the mother and her baby alike. This brings together multiple recent initiatives such as *Strategies toward Ending Preventable Maternal Mortality* [7] and the *Every Newborn Action Plan* [8], representing an integrated continuum of community and facility health promotion and care from family planning, thru periconception, pregnancy, childbirth and postpartum, to the newborn and child. The potential of health systems focusing on the continuum of care cannot come to fruition without integrated eHealth solutions [9]. When any isolated silo keeps its information separate, potential synergies within the system are being squandered. eHealth is the most frequently mentioned emerging opportunity for maternal health among international researchers [10].

Better data on health status and quality of healthcare are crucial to address bottlenecks in achieving universal health coverage (UHC) and producing better policies for health. Traditional measures of points of contact, such as attending antenatal care or having a skilled birth attendant, are far from sufficient measures of having received quality care [11, 12]. Pertaining to this, the WHO and the World Bank accentuate that in monitoring UHC, the coverage of health interventions should be at the center of countries' attention [13–15].

In the maternal and child health context, primary data on coverage of interventions is typically created when a woman is booked for antenatal care, and data on her health and the services she receives is subsequently added, retrieved and reported from her personal file over a continuum of community and facility services. But without eHealth in many settings, paper registers and patient folders make no timely and actionable data available for program management and policy development, and subsequent extraction of data from paper files results in poor quality data and underutilized health information [16–19]. Information on the individual woman meant to allow personalized care throughout pregnancy and childbirth is often neither easily accessed at follow up visits, nor shared between levels of care, or shared with women themselves to improve self-care. When information is shared, it is often not under robust governance to secure privacy and safety (Myhre et al: eRegistries: Governance for maternal and child health registries, submitted). Most public health data collection strategies are inefficient reporting chores, where care providers are viewed only as data collectors, and women only as data points. Not harvesting the data created and registered at the point-of-care, LMIC spend scarce resources on expensive data collection either by duplicate

Frame 1 Definitions

eHealth is the cost-effective and secure use of information and communication technologies in support of health and health-related fields, including healthcare services, health surveillance, health literature, health education, knowledge, and research.[107]

eRegistries are systems using information and communication technologies for the systematic longitudinal collection, storage, retrieval, analysis, and dissemination, of uniform information on health determinants and outcomes of individual persons, to serve healthcare services, health surveillance, health education, knowledge, and research. *Adapted from* [107-109]

Electronic Decision Support is an information system aimed to support clinical decision-making, linking patient-specific information in electronic health records with evidence-based knowledge to generate case-specific guidance messages through a rule- or algorithm-based software.[79]

Frame 1 Definitions [79, 107–109]

data entry from paper files, or undertaking household surveys to collect information from the population, with little and biased information of moderate validity on coverage of health interventions [20, 21, Flenady et al: eRegistries: Indicators for the WHO Essential Interventions for reproductive, maternal, newborn, and child health, submitted].

The UN Global Strategy has not formulated a specific eHealth component to support its activities [6], but such eHealth solutions will have to provide seamless and secure information following individuals across health system levels to serve the uniquely longitudinal focus on continuity and quality of care. It will also need to enable regional and national monitoring of coverage of health interventions delivered at the point-of-care. The *«integrated backbone systems»* [4, 5] that can deliver on both, are electronic health registries – eRegistries (Frame 1). Unlike health information system architectures that manage only aggregate data or clinical health records with unstructured text or forms, eRegistries are based on systematic and uniform data on pre-defined health outcomes and determinants, including care provision. This represents a database that can drive multiple e- and mHealth applications for health systems, individual care providers, and the individual clients and patients.

This eRegistries initiative, led by the Norwegian Institute of Public Health and the WHO Department of Reproductive Health and Research (RHR), with Queensland University, the University of Oxford, and the Health Information Systems Program Vietnam, aimed to develop a common framework of evidence, guidance and technical tools to facilitate the development and country implementation of eRegistries for reproductive, maternal, newborn and child health (RMNCH) in LMIC. eRegistries only have value if they can alleviate health system constraints hampering UHC. In this first paper of the eRegistries Series, we use the WHO frameworks and taxonomy for mHealth and health systems constraints in RMNCH to review what eRegistries, acting as the backbone HIS, can and should contribute to facilitate achievement of UHC of high quality care. We report on a systematic review of scientific literature from registries for RMNCH in LMIC, and on a survey of country readiness to develop eRegistries for RMNCH.

In the second paper (Flenady et al, submitted), we review the current availability of data and indicator gaps for monitoring and evaluation of coverage of the WHO Essential Interventions, Commodities and Guidelines for RMNCH [22]. We present the process and results in the harmonization and development of a suite of process (or coverage) and outcome indicators for use in eRegistries.

In the third paper (Myhre et al, submitted), we report the current status of ethical and legal issues pertaining to eRegistries in LMIC. Given the highly sensitive nature of RMNCH data, we assess existing privacy legislation, access, and data security practices and report on the development of a governance toolkit that outlines best practices for responsible data stewardship.

In the fourth and last paper (Frost et al: eRegistries: Architecture and free open source software for maternal and child health registries, submitted), we draw on the first three papers' findings of identified needs, to report on the formulation of minimum criteria for free and open source software for eRegistries as the integrating backbone for HIS in RMNCH. We review potential systems and their functionalities, and report on the *eRegistries* application - a customizable point-of-care registry using WHO Essential Interventions care algorithms developed in DHIS2, the most commonly nationally deployed free and open source software health management information system [23].

Methods

Framework for eHealth in RMNCH

The WHO RHR, the Johns Hopkins University Global mHealth Initiative, the United Nations Children's Fund, and frog Design jointly developed the "mHealth and ICT [Information and Communication Technologies] Framework" to describe commonly used mHealth applications in RMNCH [24], and subsequently used for systematic review of evidence [25]. We used this framework and the taxonomy for primary health systems constraint categories developed by the WHO mHealth Technical and Evidence Review Group (mTERG) for RMNCH [26] to identify applications to alleviate common health systems constraints that can be supported by an eRegistry (Fig. 1).

Survey of public health officials

Health officials working in any of the 75 LMIC monitored by the Commission on Information and Accountability for Women's and Children's Health, and Palestine, were recruited by emails to RMNCH medical and health organizations, ministries of health, public health institutes, and other relevant government offices (e.g., statistics bureaus, RMNCH departments, etc.). The survey was reviewed and provided with a Letter of Exemption by the Regional Committees for Medical and Health Research Ethics in Norway, confirming that the anonymous survey was not medical research on human subjects, and did not need ethical approval (Reference number: IRB 0000 1870). Launched in November 2013, responses were accepted until February 2015. The sample consisted of 298 individuals from 64 countries. Approximately two-thirds of respondents worked at the national or regional level. The survey included questions on national registry infrastructure, reporting and dissemination practices, and data quality. Issues such as privacy legislation, access by individuals and professionals, and data security are presented in the third paper, as well as additional details on the survey methodology (Myhre et al, submitted).

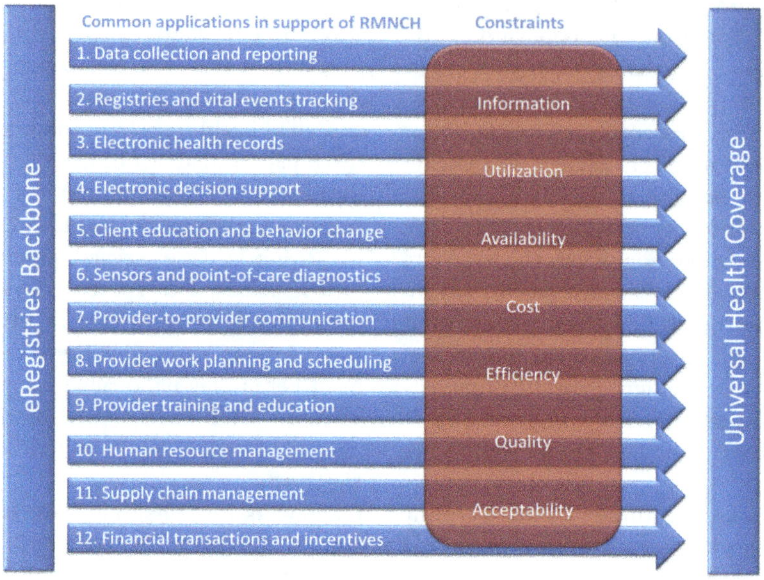

Fig. 1 Framework for eRegistries in support of UHC in RMNCH. eRegistries in support of the 12 common electronic and mobile applications to overcome the seven principal constraints for universal health coverage in RMNCH, adapted from [24, 26]

Country-level values are presented for all results. Decision rules for combining multiple responses into a single country response were adapted for each question; country averages were calculated for continuous data. Generalized linear models (PROC GLIMMIX) were used for confidence intervals around continuous data, while exact confidence intervals were calculated around binary and categorical data using SAS 9.4.

Systematic search of literature

A systematic search of literature was conducted including papers from 2005–March 2015 using Medline, Embase, ISI Web of Science, Cochrane Library and Global Health. The searches used terms indicative of RMNCH registries and were limited to the 76 LMIC as above (Additional file 1). After de-duplication, 4237 articles were identified. We included studies based on longitudinal data collection systems for individual level RMNCH data, and excluded all alternative data collections such as cross sectional surveys and health record document reviews. Two investigators independently scored publications for inclusion and extracted data. We included the following data points (within the categories in parentheses): the country/-ies of operation, the extent of the registry data collection (in facilities only, in community services only, both, or not defined), the scale of the implementation of the registry (national, district, local, or not defined), the specified population captured by the registry data collection (a total population, only subgroups/select population, or not defined), the data collection method used (paper, electronic, both, or not defined), whether the primary data was collected and entered directly into the registry, or if the registry was based on a secondary/duplicate data collection from existing sources (direct, duplicated, or not defined). In cases of conflicting scores/data, consensus was reached after independent scoring by a third investigator. Full text was read for 302 publications with abstracts considered potentially relevant (Additional file 1).

Results and discussion

The systematic and uniform data in eRegistries allows eHealth functionalities that give registries the potential to go far beyond simple registration tools [9, 27], and constitute an entire ecosystem of public health information and communication strategies (Frame 1). We mapped the potential uses of eRegistries in RMNCH onto two mHealth frameworks (Fig. 1): First, a set of 12 applications commonly used in RMNCH reflecting domains of work with empirical evidence of pervasive utility [24], and second, seven primary constraints to UHC for health systems (Frame 2) [26]:

Commonly used mHealth applications within RMNCH

Data collection and reporting

Electronic HIS are in widespread use in LMIC to lessen health systems' information constraints (Frame 2). Primary data creation in RMNCH occurs at the point-of-care, where frontline health workers document their clients' health, services provided, and any specific data required for reporting to managers or national health statistics. A well-designed electronic application for systematic data collection and management will correspond intimately to the health workers' needs in care provision

Frame 2 Constraints in health systems for RMNCH

from [26]

Information – is the availability of high quality health-relevant data on clients, populations, health and vital events, where and when it is needed. As a constraint category, items include: the absence of data to enable unique identification of clients or services provided; poor quality of data; the absence or delay in timing of individual or aggregate level data; challenges in communication between health system, providers or clients; and difficulties accessing needed data or information relevant to health service provision or use.

Availability – is having the right type of care available to those who would need it, as well as having the appropriate type of service providers and materials. As a constraint, items in this category focus on barriers that may limit both supply- and user-side availability of health goods and services.

Cost - includes the direct cost of treatment and informal payments, and also indirect costs that deter individuals from seeking treatment. As a constraint, items include direct and indirect financial barriers associated with the provision of, or access to, specific health interventions or behaviours.

Efficiency - accessing or providing appropriate health services in a timely manner and with minimal expenditure of effort. As a constraint category this refers to barriers that impede a person's or a health system's ability to accomplish a given goal, job, or task with minimal time and effort expenditure.

Quality - the technical ability of health services to positively affect people's health. Constraints within this category include barriers that impede a healthcare system from functioning optimally and providing individuals and patient populations with healthcare that improves desired health outcomes.

Acceptability – is the alignment of health services with individual, social and cultural norms, and with expectations of quality. Constraints in this category include: social and cultural barriers to the individual in accessing services or continuing treatment; and factors negatively affecting providers' ability to provide specific types of services, or their ability to provide services to specific categories of people on the basis of their ethnicity, health status, age or sex.

Utilization – Constraints in this category impede an individual's or group's use of a particular health service or treatment – e.g., low demand for services; poor transportation infrastructure or geographic distance to needed health services; poor understanding of the treatment regimen; poor provider skills; financial barriers among patients.

Frame 2 Constraints in health systems for RMNCH

[28, 29]. It can, at the same time, upload all or selected data items to create a registry for use in the care system. Additional electronically derived geographic information systems [30], and linkage of individuals to households [31, 32], can add to outreach utility and potentially link data to non-health data sources. Integrated with the national HIS, it allows managers to safely monitor and assess programs (Frost et al, submitted). This eliminates duplicate data entry for reporting which often consumes large proportion of provider's time in LMIC [28, 33], easing constraints of health systems' costs, availability and efficiency (Frame 2).

In registries in LMIC, real-time health surveillance tools are used for rapid quality improvement cycles [31]. LMIC registries contribute to independent prospective monitoring of trials and interventions [34–36], and large data collections are exploited to study rare conditions [35, 37, 38] and drug exposure [35, 36], or conversely, register rare conditions only [37, 39, 40]. Registries in LMIC follow mothers to study recurrence of pregnancy outcomes [41, 42], link mothers with offspring [29, 43–45] with their subsequent newborn health records [46], and link children with siblings [47–49]; in some cases registries study long-term and family-based health determinants and recurrence [41, 42] or undertaking twin studies [48, 49].

The ease of electronic feedback of data to providers is associated with improved quality of data [16]. eRegistry forms improve data quality with functionalities such as logical checks and limitations, warning prompts for improbable or missing data entries [29, 50, Frost et al, submitted], or pre-defined algorithms to improve correct categorizations, e.g. for causes of death [31]. Prospective and longitudinal data collection in eRegistries can reduce reporting bias on intervention coverage. For example, an adverse outcome can bias any retrospective registration of health determinants and care provision, i.e. what risks and health conditions she experienced in pregnancy and what was done to identify and manage them. This bias can make real-life estimations of effect of intervention coverage unhelpful.

Registries and vital events tracking

Recognizing the critical position of civil registration and vital statistics (CRVS) data in alleviating information constraints (Frame 2), the poor quality and coverage in LMIC, and the modest progress over the last 30 years, universal coverage of CRVS systems is a key goal for the post-2015 agenda [4, 51–53]. Well-functioning CRVS are independently associated with improved health, in particular lower child mortality [54]. Electronic and mobile applications are in widespread use for CRVS in LMIC. In settings with high proportions of home deliveries, mobile phones can extend the infrastructure by engaging frontline health workers to register births in communities [55, 56].

Being born is an essential health determinant, and dying likewise an essential outcome. CRVS systems thus share many characteristics and data with eRegistries for RMNCH that track individuals with unique identifiers (i.e. personal identification numbers (PIN)), or if lacking, issue such identifiers for care provision [57, 58]. Both in sentinel sites and total populations, several LMIC have created seamless integration of CRVS and HIS to benefit both enumeration of the population and support care provision, health monitoring, identify service delivery gaps and inequities, and improve accountability [38, 59]. Lack of such information can add to constraints of cost, acceptability and utilization of services by restricting eligibility (Frame 2).

The voluntary registration of all pregnancies can improve accountability and quality of vital events tracking related to RMNCH in LMIC [27, 60]. As pregnancy and date of birth are key in defining maternal mortality, eRegistries of pregnancies and births can facilitate correct classification when integrated with a CRVS registering deaths of women in fertile age. Stillbirths and neonatal deaths are poorly registered in many settings with a high percentage of home deliveries, stigma, and a lack of incentives to register a dead baby, for either care professionals, or for parents. The magnitude of the issue can be unmasked by counting third trimester pregnancies registered in eRegistries with no subsequent report of a live infant, civil registration, vaccination or other incentivizing benefits that can be integrated or linked to the registry.

Electronic health records

As stated in MA4Health, quality, cost and efficiency constraints cannot be overcome without patient data being shared across sites and levels of care (Frame 2) [5]. RMNCH has a long tradition of using simplified client-held paper records of systematic and uniform data for communication along the continuity of care and to facilitate self-care [61]. This tradition makes RMNCH particularly fitting for the use of eRegistries where systematic and uniform data are the key to functionality, including the ability to manage data items such as unstructured text notes and narratives as in health records. Conversely, electronic health records built on an architecture of unstructured text and forms as data items can not support the functionalities of an eRegistry. In LMIC, the traditional maternity, child health and vaccination cards are valued, and while loss of records by women is not typically reported as a major problem, the communication flow can be broken as they are often not brought to care visits, and confidentiality has been questioned [61]. The value of information following the woman is evident in societies with traditions wherein women travel to their parental home to deliver. In such settings, single facility based or local electronic systems can not only be expensive and hard to maintain [62], but represents an inferior tool for information management – although some projects have provided women with printed versions [32] or uploaded records to a server for women themselves to have electronic access [58].

Even in settings of less mobility in care seeking, a backbone registry accessible across its regional or national jurisdiction supports continuity of health records at all levels of care, with secure governance and storage preventing irreversible loss or damage to facility or client-held paper records. An electronic version adds to patient safety by also making information available in emergencies when a paper card may be unavailable. Mobile units enable entries and access to health records from community and outreach activities. In LMIC, research based on registries often extract their data from electronic health records (Additional file 1). Some also link individuals' records to biobanks and lab tests [49].

Electronic decision support

Best practice guidelines are well-established in RMNCH, and achieving effective coverage of interventions, i.e. high quality of care, is key in the post-2015 agenda [63–65]. Guidelines may appear straightforward, but are seldom followed in the correct and complete sequence. This know-do gap constrains quality of care services (Frame 2) [66, 67]. A commonly cited hindering factor is unavailability of guidelines in a user-friendly, readily accessible manner at the point-of-care [68, 69].

Checklists are informational job aids extracting vital elements of guidelines for clinical care to simplify the presentation and highlight actions required. They are in common use to reduce variation in performance and assist in improving quality of care in LMIC [69–71].

Corresponding intimately to the systematic and uniform approach to data in eRegistries, data entry at the point-of-care in eRegistries can be designed as interactive checklists, which integrate decision support for diagnosis, treatment and referral algorithms (Frame 1) [32, 69, Frost et al, submitted].

Integrated decision support and reminders for guideline adherence in preventive care are shown to strengthen health systems and link HIS to improved quality coverage of care [72–75]. Such tools are generally associated with high user satisfaction, but require training for use, and developing comprehensive tools for all essential interventions and guidelines in RMNCH requires substantial preparations to ensure that they reflect the actual work flow of providers [69, 76, 77, Frost et al, submitted]. However, most studies exploring these effects have been conducted in facility settings, and better evidence is needed to enhance community based RMNCH care in LMIC [78–80].

Client education and behavior change communication

Feeding back the registered information to individuals contributes by informing the public about the objectives and values of registration, as the UN recommends for CRVS. But the underutilization of data to empower women and communities has largely been overlooked. The use of registry data for community and client education and behavior change communication, has the potential to impact utilization and acceptability constraints, as well as empower women to demand improvements in health system quality, accessibility, cost and efficiency (Frame 2).

Women are principal stakeholders for their own information, and communicating it back to them should be personalized, timely and actionable. General pregnancy information can be of variable interest to the individual woman if not tailored to her needs, and mHealth solutions to communicate with her may not help much unless personalized [77]. Therefore, efforts have been made in LMIC to register women and children to deliver pregnancy stage and age appropriate messaging [81–83]. mHealth solutions building on eRegistries can communicate to her mobile phone or web-applications with personalized and culturally sensitive information according to the data registered about her. eRegistries can automate provision of information directly to women, or as a prompt to her care provider to send the information, to complement in-person approaches and assist in bridging communication barriers with multi-language support for messaging. For example, gestational age data can ensure timely advice for birth preparation, while risk or complication data can tailor information for high risk pregnancies, services or treatment data can prompt reminders of medications or appointments, and vaccination data and residential address can be used to inform of available outreach vaccination services. Such information on the importance and availability of services can empower the demand for services and improve health care utilization and acceptability (Frame 2). One of the most established applications of mHealth in LMIC is messaging of reminders for appointments and treatments, to improve care utilization and efficiency [80].

Crucially, reliance on mobile phone access for communication frequently raises questions about equity [25]. Not having access to a mobile phone is a significant marker of risk for poor outcomes that should be registered, and alternative communication methods should be provided [84].

Sensors and point-of-care diagnostics

The restriction of diagnostics to fixed site laboratories adds constraints of availability, cost, acceptability and utilization (Frame 2). Miniaturized point-of-care diagnostic tests and sensors combined with the computing, storage and communication power of mobile phones and tablets have led to a rapidly expanding range of mHealth innovations for diagnostic tests in communities [85]. Standard tests in RMNCH from blood and urine, and external sensors for fetal Doppler and blood pressure exist in low-cost mobile units for LMIC settings. The results of such tests is key information both for RMNCH care provision and health surveillance, and should be integrated in the backbone HIS. An example of such successful integration in LMIC is the implementation of Swasthya Slate, linking a small independent diagnostic unit to a tablet used by frontline community health workers to upload individual results to a cloud-based eRegistry available to care professionals, clients, and program managers [58].

Provider-to-provider communication

Insufficient communication at hand-offs and referrals significantly constrains quality and efficiency (Frame 2). An integrating backbone HIS for seamless information-sharing across multiple providers and levels of care is a key element in MA4Health's global roadmap. Where disconnected cadres of providers interact with the same client, duplicating care, information and reporting efforts, shared health records implicitly constitute a key type of provider-to-provider communication. Within functioning health systems, shared information can cut delays and time spent in hand-offs and referrals to other providers—whether simplifying a traditional referral, or in the simplest form reduced to an automated transfer from one provider's electronic work schedule to another's. Mobile solutions can extend the reach of real-time information sharing e.g. of results from laboratories to frontline health workers.

Paper records are not only logistically difficult to share, but are reputed for illegibility and incompleteness [28]. From a client-held antenatal care paper record, it can be difficult to identify the care providers managing a woman, hampering their ability to communicate. For providers to be accredited as users in eRegistries, a unique user identification is created, and every entry of information logged to the individual provider (Frost et al, submitted). Their contact information can be available to others engaged in providing services to the client, and to the clients themselves, facilitating communication and identifying unwarranted "shopping" of services across providers.

Provider work planning and scheduling

Shortage of care providers in LMIC severely constrains availability, quality and efficiency of RMNCH services (Frame 2). Resources are wasted not only by underutilizing the time-saving benefits of electronic applications discussed here, but also by inefficiencies such as clients missing scheduled appointments or unneeded variation in daily work-load [80]. Likewise, systems become inefficient in providing adequate care when they are unaware of the time and location at which clients will require care. Optimizing the efficiency of the work force has therefore been a key element in many deployments of e- and mHealth programs in LMIC, including functionalities ranging from simple electronic scheduling, or household visit support with geographic information systems, to integration of messaging services to create mobile phone reminders about upcoming antenatal care visits, missed scheduled appointments, new deliveries and newborns eligible for postpartum and newborn care [31, 32, 86].

Provider training and education

Poorly performing providers cause quality, cost, efficiency, utilization and acceptability constraints (Frame 2). Interactive mHealth solutions are used for continued medical education and training support in LMIC—mostly in generic forms applied to a cadre of health workers. A standard course may not be professionally motivating for providers at different levels of performance. eRegistries create inherent accountability with data on the client population, care performance and outcomes, which facilitate individually targeted training, including the potential for automated audit and feedback [69, 87].

The variability in the approaches and results of audit and feedback interventions, including those specifically using registry data, might be explained by limited consensus and use of theories underlying multiple causal pathways [88–93]. Reviews in the framework of Feedback Intervention Theory have identified that verbal, discouraging, praising or self-esteem-affecting feedback attenuates beneficial effects on performance, while task-oriented computerized feedback augments it [94, 95]. Frequent, swift, and correct solution feedback, including a goal setting action plan, also augment effects. Effects are stronger for familiar memory tasks and weaker for following rules and completing complex tasks [94, 95]. The Model of Actionable Feedback further proposes that in order to be actionable, feedback must be timely, individualized, non-punitive and meaningful [96, 97]. These findings fit well with systematic reviews of feedback to healthcare providers that also identified larger effects if it was delivered to non-physicians by a supervisor or trustworthy colleague, in a domain where the recipient was underperforming [91, 92].

There is evident potential of eRegistries to deliver computerized, individualized, trustworthy, non-punitively neutral, timely, frequent and task-oriented feedback to health workers to focus attention to the largest quality gaps. However, stronger evidence is needed. Few studies have evaluated the effect of feedback on improving RMNCH, and studies from LMIC are lacking [91, 92, 98].

Human resource management

Closely linked to applications for work planning and scheduling, as well as those improving working conditions and satisfaction, better human resource management is needed to meet workforce constraints. Population-based data on health, health determinants and effective coverage of services is necessary for better and more targeted distribution of health workers. This is a critical issue in many LMIC settings where extremely low provider to client ratios remain a long-term problem. Monitoring and management of public health providers in LMIC is made more complex by prevalent dual practice—individual professionals providing services both privately and in the public health system—which in poorly regulated settings can add constraints to accessibility, cost, efficiency, quality, as well as equity (Frame 2) [99]. Information on actual performance of the workforce is therefore needed. As providers accessing individual patient data have unique user identities, eRegistries also represent provider registries, where their service provision is logged. Just as client data can be aggregated or disaggregated from national to individual level, so can provider data, joined with client data to support allocation of human resources needed to deliver services based on the number of beneficiaries [32]. Supportive supervision can enable program managers to identify lower quality of services than expected given the resources invested, and the real-time registration of services provided, can contribute in addressing absenteeism and enabling substitution when critical services are not provided.

Supply chain management

mHealth applications in Logistics Management Information Systems (LMIS) are widespread in LMIC to improve data visibility, enhance decision making, and address availability and cost constraints of health systems (Frame 2) [100]. Paper LMIS have low reporting rates in LMIC, due to e.g. unreliable postal systems, poor transport infrastructure, and a heavy workload among store managers. Electronic and mobile LMIS address these constraints, improving reporting rates, data visibility, and use [101].

eRegistries contain key data to combine with LMIS for improved quantification, forecasting and distribution of health commodities, including dispensed-to-users data, provider and client needs and preferences, and seasonality. The rich patient data available from eRegistries can also improve prediction of future needs, using better-quality information about population risk and demographics. Integration of HIS and LMIS is rarely seen [32], typically operating as isolated silos, but is recommended by the UN Commission on Life-Saving Commodities for Women and Children [102]. Combining eRegistry and LMIS data can provide another tool for transparency and accountability, comparing numbers of commodities issued from storage with those dispensed to users to identify potential theft/leakage.

Financial transactions and incentives

The use of mobile payments in LMIC bring financial services within reach of previously unbanked populations. Throughout LMIC, 60 % now have coverage of mobile financial services, and sub-Saharan Africa is leading other regions in the number of deployments [103]. This can assist in alleviating accessibility, acceptability and utilization constraints (Frame 2), and eRegistries in RMNCH can facilitate the use of such transactions and incentives. This includes making information available at point-of-care on eligibility for universal health insurance schemes, data on service delivery for performance based incentives, on registered conditions eligible for financial support such as transportation for institutional delivery, or incentives for child vaccination.

Country capacity for electronic health registries in RMNCH

While the potential of eRegistries are clear, the perceived needs and capacities in LMIC to deploy them are not. Unique identifier systems issuing PINs are a requirement for any population registry, enabling detection and elimination of duplicate records, or fraudulent identities. It also enables linkages through integrated backbone systems for multiple data entries and uses as in eRegistries.

According to the public health officials surveyed, 60 % (95 % confidence interval: 47–72) of LMIC issue PINs for both permanent and temporary residents while 17 % (9–29) of countries issue them to permanent residents only. A small percent (3 % (0–11)) indicated that the system was in an initial stage and one sixth indicated that they did not issue PINs; three percent did not know. Eight out of ten LMIC indicating that they do not issue PINs were located in the African region. In the vast majority of countries with PINs, the use was reported to be proof of citizenship (94 % (84–99)), or needed for access to education (57 % (42–71)), health services (51 % (36–65)), financial services (53 % (38–67)), and for taxation (45 % (31–60)). Few offer automatic registration at birth. Barriers to birth registration indicate that home delivery, cultural mores, societal taboos, and religious traditions all contribute to low registration practices at birth [104]. Adult applications are the most common method for acquiring a PIN. Half of countries offer only one option to obtain a PIN whereas 51 % (37–65) offer multiple options (Table 1).

The latest 2013 UNICEF report on birth registration, based on informants from household surveys with data on average from 2010, reported that about four in ten children under five were registered in CRVS in LMIC. A higher proportion of countries report in our survey that they do at least register births. Nearly half of countries report coverage greater than 90 % for registering birth, pregnancy and child health, but many regions still experience very low coverage, and a recorded birth does not translate to formal birth registration to acquire a PIN. Closer integration with birth registration in health systems may facilitate the registration process [104]. Cause of death registries are of notoriously poor coverage and quality in many regions (Table 2) [105].

Table 1 Unique identity systems' administrative oversight and acquisition

Agency in charge	Frequency	Percent[a]
Ministry of Health	7	14 % (6–26)
All other Ministry offices	41	80 % (67–90)
National office/agencies	34	67 % (52–79)
Local level offices/agencies	13	25 % (14–40)
Acquisition		
Application required at birth	27	53 % (38–67)
Automatically issued at birth	11	22 % (11–35)
Application required as an adult[b]	30	59 % (44–72)
Automatically issued as an adult[b]	6	12 % (4–24)
Other	8	16 % (7–29)

[a]Percent column does not add up to 100 % as the question asked respondents to check all that apply
[b]Adult was considered 16 years or older. 95 % confidence intervals in parentheses

Table 2 Coverage of vital and health statistics in national registries

Registry (Countries)	>90 % coverage	50–89 % coverage	<50 % coverage	I don't know	No national registry
Birth (*N* = 62)	55 % (42–68)	27 % (17–40)	10 % (4–20)	6 % (2–16)	2 % (0–9)
Cause of death (*N* = 61)	38 % (26–51)	21 % (12–34)	20 % (11–32)	16 % (8–28)	5 % (1–14)
Pregnancy (*N* = 61)	43 % (30–56)	34 % (23–48)	11 % (5–22)	10 % (4–20)	2 % (0–9)
Child (*N* = 62)	45 % (32–58)	26 % (16–39)	15 % (7–26)	11 % (5–22)	3 % (0–11)

95 % confidence intervals in parentheses

Overall, the responding public health officials in LMIC rate the quality of their national health data quite modestly on a scale from 5 (excellent) to 1 (poor): A quarter of countries have health data scored as poor by their officials in terms of timeliness and security, one fifth as poor on completeness and update status, and across all domains of data quality (accuracy, completeness, integrity, access, security, timeliness, update status and utilization) average scores range from 2.3 to 2.5 ((95 % confidence interval: 2.1–2.6). Nonetheless, on a range from 5 (very influential) to 1 (not influential at all), public health officials generally score the influence of national data reports on public health decision-making highly. Data had the highest influence on planning public health programs and monitoring of the Millennium Development Goals (average score 4.3 (4.1–4.4)), somewhat less on monitoring, evaluation and improvement of health programs (3.9–4.1 (3.6–4.3)), and the least influence on budget allocations (3.4 (3.2–3.6)) and research (3.7 (3.4–3.9)). For other use of data for feedback to the health system, respondents generally score the quality as low as the quality of the data (same scale): The highest quality of feedback for effective coverage of antenatal care (2.7 (2.5–2.9)), and the lowest for quality of care in facilities (2.3 (2.1–2.5)).

Most LMICs are in a phase of transition from paper to mixed paper and electronic formats, and only a low percentage report using fully electronic registries (Table 3). With the tardiness of paper registrations, approximately half the countries have mortality figures updated annually, while one in five report a time lag from data collection to publicly available reports of more than three years on average. Data on intervention coverage in antenatal, delivery, postpartum and newborn care collected by health professionals fare similarly with two of three countries reporting having this publicly available within one year of data collection.

Scientific capacity for electronic health registries in RMNCH

Capacity to operate eRegistries of high scientific quality in LMIC should be expected to be an important constraint given the slow emergence of such registries and the current status of data. From 2005 to 2015, we identified 66 publications from 32 health registries in 24 LMIC—from a broad search in LMIC literature in the field of RMNCH resulting in 4237 abstracts screened and 302 papers read in full. The registries identified are presented in Table 4.

The majority of health registries in RMNCH that have reached the mature stage of authoring scientific publications, operate at a scaled regional or national level, and they have come further in the transition from paper to electronic data capture than the national registration systems reported from national levels in the survey. Countries such as Kenya, Zambia, Burkina Faso, Ghana and Tanzania have all published research based on primary data entry in fully electronic registries at national or regional levels. While data collection format and the source of primary data is often poorly described in publications, it appears that in most countries, undertaking research in registry methodology still represents duplicate data collection efforts to transfer data from paper forms to an electronic database.

Conclusions

We find that purposefully designed eRegistries, acting as an integrating backbone HIS, can be the operative

Table 3 Data transmission format from health facilities to central data collection for registries

Registry (Countries)	Electronic	Paper & Electronic	Paper	No national registry	I don't know
Birth (*N* = 62)	5 % (1–14)	69 % (56–80)	18 % (9–30)	3 % (0–11)	5 % (1–14)
Cause of death (*N* = 59)	3 % (0–12)	61 % (47–73)	19 % (10–31)	7 % (2–16)	10 % (4–21)
Pregnancy (*N* = 61)	3 % (0–11)	61 % (47–73)	25 % (15–37)	5 % (1–14)	7 % (2–16)
Child (*N* = 61)	3 % (0–11)	66 % (52–77)	18 % (9–30)	7 % (2–16)	7 % (2–16)

95 % confidence intervals in parentheses

Table 4 RMNCH Registries with scientific publications

Countries	Registry scope	Registry scale	Population	Data collection format	Data entry source	Health focus[a]	Registry name and operation[b]
Brazil	Community	National	Total	E & Paper	Duplicate	A + CRVS	Brazilian National Birth Registry (SINASC) - N
Peru	Facility	National	Total	Electronic	Primary	B + CRVS	Online Registration of Certificates of Live Births - N
China	Facility	National	Sample	E & Paper	Duplicate	B + Birth defects	Birth Defects Monitoring Network - I
Egypt	Community	National	Total	E & Paper	Duplicate	A + IVF	Egyptian IVF registry - N
Peru	Community	National	N/A	Electronic	Primary	ABC	Peruvian Perinatal Information System (SIP) -I
Ghana	Both C & F	Regional	Total	E & Paper	Duplicate	ABCD	Navrongo Health and Demographic Surveillance System-NI
Kenya	Community	Regional	Total	Electronic	Primary	ABD	KEMRI Centers for Disease Control & Prevention-NI
Yemen	Community	Regional	Total	Electronic	Duplicate	C + Cancer	Aden Cancer Registry- N
Kenya	Community	Regional	Total	E & Paper	Duplicate	ABD + Vaccines	Kilifi Health and Demographic Surveillance System -NI
Uganda	Community	Regional	Total	E & Paper	Duplicate	A + HDR	Health and Demographic Surveillance Site (HDSS) -NI
Guinea-Bissau	Facility	Regional	Total	E & Paper	Duplicate	AC + Twins, Vacc.	Bandim Health Project (BHP) - NI
Guinea-Bissau	Facility	Regional	Total	E & Paper	Duplicate	AC + Twins, Vacc.	Guinea-Bissau Twin Registry-NI
China	Community	Regional	Sample	Electronic	Primary	C + Vaccines	Zhejiang Immunization Information System (ZJIIS) - N
Bangladesh	Community	Regional	Sample	Paper	Duplicate	AB	A registry for the JiVitA 1 project - NI
Zambia	Facility	Regional	Sample	Electronic	Primary	AB	Zambia Electronic Perinatal Record System NI
Burkina Faso, Ghana, Tanzania	Facility	Regional	Sample	Electronic	Primary	AB	Quality of Prenatal & Maternal Care Clinical Decision Support (QUALMAT) - NI
Tanzania	Facility	Regional	Sample	Paper	Duplicate	ABC	KCMC Medical Birth Registry - NI
Chile	Facility	Regional	Sample	Electronic	Duplicate	A + ART	Latin American Registry (RLA) of assisted reprod. tech. - NI
Senegal	Community	Regional	Sample	E & Paper	Duplicate	ABD	Millennium Villages Project information system- NI
Indonesia	Community	Local	Total	E & Paper	Duplicate	ABC + Malaria	Sistem Informasi Kesehatan Daerah (SIKDA)- NI
China	Community	Local	Total	E & Paper	Duplicate	ABC	Gongcheng Maternal, Newborn and Child Health Information System - NI
Bangladesh	Both C & F	Local	Sample	E & Paper	Duplicate	A	Projahnmo-II Project - Pregnancy Registration - NI
Kenya, Pakist., Guatem., Zambia, India, Argent.	Both C & F	Local	Sample	E & Paper	Duplicate	ABC	Global Network Maternal and Newborn Health Registry - NI
Nigeria	Facility	Local	Sample	E & Paper	Duplicate	AC + Vaccines	OpenMRS for the Family Health Unit - NI
Kenya	Facility	Local	Sample	E & Paper	Duplicate	AB + HIV	Academic Model Providing Access to Healthcare (AMPATH)- NI
Cameroon	Facility	Local	Sample	E & Paper	Duplicate	AB	Obstetric health information system -NI
Nepal	Facility	Local	Sample	E & Paper	Primary	A + CVD	Prospective single-centre registry - NI

Table 4 RMNCH Registries with scientific publications *(Continued)*

Brazil, Ghana, Kenya, Uganda, Tanzania	Community	Local	Total	E & Paper	Duplicate	A + Drug expo.	WHO Pregnancy Registry of drug exposures using OpenClinica - NI
Brazil	Facility	Local	Total	E & Paper	Primary	B + Vaccines	Quality-Health Card/Electronic Immunisation Registry-N
India	Facility	Local	Sample	E & Paper	Duplicate	ABC + Epilepsy	Indian Registry of Epilepsy and Pregnancy (IREP) -N

[a] *A* Pregnancy, *B* Childbirth, *C* Infant/child, *D* Deaths
[b] *N* Operated nationally, *I* Operated by international organizations, *NI* Operated in collaboration between national and international organizations. *N/A* Not available information in publications. References in Additional file 1

infrastructure for several commonly deployed applications to strengthen RMNCH, and offer crucial data and support for all. Collectively, they have the potential to alleviate the principal constraints of health systems for UHC in RMNCH. Yet, although many examples exist of successful implementation of individual applications based on registry functionalities, none have integrated more than a few within one single backbone system. While electronic solutions with registry functionalities are widely used in LMIC for data collection, reporting, CRVS, health records and clinical decision support, planning and scheduling, and inherently for communication of health information between providers, they appear underutilized for client behavior change communication, provider audit and feedback, and management of human resources, supply chains and financial incentives.

Almost all countries are investing resources into systems to support registration of births and vital events in RMNCH, and the majority are currently in transition from paper to a future of electronic HIS where eRegistries could become an integrating backbone and contribute to relieve the constraints they experience in data collection, management, analysis and dissemination. Public health officials in LMICs convey a strong message of the importance their national RMNCH-related data for country policies and program management, despite the many times mediocre coverage and quality, and long delays and suboptimal quality of feedback of data to the health system. The MA4Health post-2015 roadmap and action plan should further galvanize national investment and commitments to support the transition to electronic solutions [4, 106].

There is accumulating experience on operating health registries in LMIC to draw lessons from, and eRegistries are emerging at regional and national scale. While the finding for infrastructure capacities is encouraging for future emergence of eRegistries in RMNCH, the scientific activity is limited.

Capacity building and support for eRegistries is crucial to achieve the goals set for the post-2015 agenda reflected in the MA4Health roadmap. In this series, we offer tools and frameworks to achieve that end, including key considerations in the selection of data items and indicators, architectural standards and interoperability, and ethics and governance.

Abbreviations

CRVS: civil registration and vital statistics; eHealth: (See Frame 1); eRegistries: (See Frame 1); HIS: Health information systems; LMIC: Low- and middle-income countries; LMIS: Logistics management information systems; MA4Health: World Bank/WHO/USAID measurement and accountability for results in health: a common agenda for the post 2015 era; mHealth: Mobile eHealth (See Frame 1); PIN: Personal identification numbers; RMNCH: Reproductive, maternal, newborn and child health; UHC: Universal health coverage; UN Global Strategy: United Nations: Survive, Thrive, Transform. The Global Strategy for Women's, Children's and Adolescents' Health; WHO: World Health Organization.

Competing interests

The authors have no conflicts of interest to declare.

Authors' contributions

JFF conceptualized and led the eRegistries initiative and drafting of the manuscript. SLM led the survey and drafted the report with IKF, JVJ and JFF. LN, HS and SLM undertook the systematic review and drafted the report with JFF. KM and MV reviewed literature and drafted reports on audit and feedback, and checklists and decision support, respectively. All authors contributed to the content of the paper, read, and approved the final version.

Acknowledgements

We thank Ameha Wudie Dammena, Elin Wyller, and staff members of Statistics Norway and the Norwegian Institute of Public Health for their technical support and advice, colleagues participating in consultation workshops in Thailand and Vietnam for their guidance, and survey respondents for their time and efforts.
The views expressed in this article do not necessarily represent the decisions, policy, or views of the authors' affiliations.

Funding

The Norwegian Agency for Development Cooperation (Norad) funded the harmonized Reproductive Health Registries project (GLO-4279 QZA 12/0355 harmonized Reproductive Health Registries) that led to the eRegistries Initiative (QZA-14/0022 Every Mother and Child Counts). This was led in partnership by the Norwegian Institute of Public Health and the WHO Department for Reproductive Health and Research, with Queensland University (Australia), the University of Oxford (UK), and the Health Information Systems Program (Vietnam).

The contribution by JFF, JVJ and VN was supported in part by the Centre for Intervention Science in Maternal and Child Health (CISMAC; project number 223269), which is funded by the Research Council of Norway through its Centers of Excellence scheme and the University of Bergen, Norway.

Author details

[1]Department of International Public Health, Norwegian Institute of Public Health, Pb 4404 Nydalen, N-0403 Oslo, Norway. [2]Centre for Intervention Science in Maternal and Child Health (CISMAC), University of Bergen, Bergen, Norway. [3]John Snow, Inc., Boston, MA, USA. [4]Department of Reproductive Health and Research, World Health Organization, Geneva, Switzerland. [5]Faculty of Medicine, University of Oslo, Oslo, Norway. [6]HeLEX - Centre for Health, Law and Emerging Technologies, Nuffield Department of Population Health, University of Oxford, Oxford, UK. [7]Health Information System Programme (HISP) Vietnam, Ho Chí Minh, Vietnam. [8]Department of Informatics, University of Oslo, Oslo, Norway. [9]Department of Epidemiology and Biostatics, School of Public Health, College of Health Sciences, Makerere University, Kampala, Uganda. [10]Mater Research Institute, The University of Queensland, Brisbane, Australia. [11]International Stillbirth Alliance, Millburn, NJ, USA.

References

1. Wilson K, Gertz B, Arenth B, Salisbury N. The journey to scale: moving together past digital health pilots. Seattle: PATH; 2014.
2. WHO. Accountability for women's and children's health: report on progress to May 2014. Geneva: World Health Organization; 2014.
3. Principles for digital development [http://digitalprinciples.org]. Accessed 15 Sept 2015.
4. World Bank, USAID and WHO. The Roadmap for Health Measurement and Accountability. Washington, DC: MA4Health; 2015.
5. Haazen DS, Slote (USAID/Global Health), Al-Shorbaji N, D'Adamo M. eHealth Technical Paper for MA4Health - Measurement and Accountability for Results in Health: A Common Agenda for the Post 2015 Era. Washington, DC: MA4Health; 2015.
6. United Nations. Survive, Thrive, Transform. The Global Strategy for Women's, Children's and Adolescents' Health. New York: United Nations; 2015.
7. WHO. Strategies toward ending preventable maternal mortality (EPMM). Geneva: World Health Organization; 2015.
8. WHO and UNICEF. Every Newborn: an action plan to end preventable deaths. Geneva: World Health Organization; 2014.
9. Mehl G, Labrique A. Prioritizing integrated mHealth strategies for universal health coverage. Science. 2014;345(6202):1284–7.
10. Kendall T. Critical maternal health knowledge gaps in low- and middle-income countries for post-2015: Researchers' perspectives. Boston, MA: Harvard T.H. Chan School of Public Health; 2015.
11. Marchant T, Tilley-Gyado RD, Tessema T, Singh K, Gautham M, Umar N, et al. Adding content to contacts: measurement of high quality contacts for maternal and newborn health in Ethiopia, North East Nigeria, and Uttar Pradesh, India. PLoS One. 2015;10(5):e0126840.
12. Hodgins S, D'Agostino A. The quality–coverage gap in antenatal care: toward better measurement of effective coverage. Glob Health Sci Pract. 2014;2(2):173–81.
13. World Health Organization and World Bank Group. Monitoring progress towards universal health coverage at country and global levels. Framework, measures and targets. Geneva: World Health Organization; 2014.
14. Boerma T, AbouZahr C, Evans D, Evans T. Monitoring intervention coverage in the context of universal health coverage. PLoS Med. 2014;11(9):e1001728.
15. Boerma T, Eozenou P, Evans D, Evans T, Kieny MP, Wagstaff A. Monitoring progress towards universal health coverage at country and global levels. PLoS Med. 2014;11(9):e1001731.
16. Ndabarora E, Chipps JA, Uys L. Systematic review of health data quality management and best practices at community and district levels in LMIC. Inform Dev. 2014;30(2):103–20.
17. Lium JT, Tjora A, Faxvaag A. No paper, but the same routines: a qualitative exploration of experiences in two Norwegian hospitals deprived of the paper based medical record. BMC Med Inform Decis Mak. 2008;8:2.
18. Corrao S, Arcoraci V, Arnone S, Calvo L, Scaglione R, Di Bernardo C, et al. Evidence-Based Knowledge Management: an approach to effectively promote good health-care decision-making in the Information Era. Intern Emerg Med. 2009;4(2):99–106.
19. George A. 'By papers and pens, you can only do so much': views about accountability and human resource management from Indian government health administrators and workers. Int J Health Plann Manage. 2009;24(3): 205–24.
20. Mbondji PE, Kebede D, Soumbey-Alley EW, Zielinski C, Kouvividila W, Lusamba-Dikassa P-S. Health information systems in Africa: descriptive analysis of data sources, information products and health statistics. J R Soc Med. 2014;107(1 suppl):34–45.
21. Liu L, Li M, Yang L, Ju L, Tan B, Walker N, et al. Measuring coverage in MNCH: a validation study linking population survey derived coverage to maternal, newborn, and child health care records in rural China. PLoS One. 2013;8(5):e60762.
22. WHO. Essential Interventions, Commodities and Guidelines for Reproductive, Maternal, Newborn and Child Health. Geneva: World Health Organization; 2012.
23. Health Information Systems Programme (HISP). DHIS 2 [https://www.dhis2.org/]. Accessed 15 Sept 2015.
24. Labrique AB, Vasudevan L, Kochi E, Fabricant R, Mehl G. mHealth innovations as health system strengthening tools: 12 common applications and a visual framework. Glob Health Sci Pract. 2013;1(2):160–71.
25. Hall CS, Fottrell E, Wilkinson S, Byass P. Assessing the impact of mHealth interventions in low- and middle-income countries – what has been shown to work? Global Health Action. 2014;7:25606. doi:10.3402/gha.v3407.25606.
26. Mehl G, Vasudevan L, Gonsalves L, Berg M, Seimon T, Temmerman M, et al. Harnessing mHealth in low-resource settings to overcome health system constraints and achieve universal access to healthcare. In: Marsch LA, Lord SE, Dallery J, editors. Behavioral Healthcare and Technology Using Science-Based Innovations to Transform Practice. Oxford, UK: Oxford University Press; 2014.
27. Labrique AB, Pereira S, Christian P, Murthy N, Bartlett L, Mehl G. Pregnancy registration systems can enhance health systems, increase accountability and reduce mortality. Reprod Health Matters. 2012;20(39):113–7.
28. Thompson A, Castle E, Lubeck P, Makarfi PS. Experience implementing OpenMRS to support maternal and reproductive health in Northern Nigeria. Stud Health Technol Inform. 2010;160(PART 1):332–6.
29. Chi BH, Vwalika B, Killam WP, Wamalume C, Giganti MJ, Mbewe R, et al. Implementation of the Zambia Electronic Perinatal Record System for comprehensive prenatal and delivery care. Int J Gynecol Obstet. 2011; 113(2):131–6.
30. Ebener S, Guerra-Arias M, Campbell J, Tatem AJ, Moran AC, Amoako Johnson F, et al. The geography of maternal and newborn health: the state of the art. Int J Health Geogr. 2015;14:19.
31. Moshabela M, Sene M, Nanne I, Tankoano Y, Schaefer J, Niang O, et al. Early detection of maternal deaths in Senegal through household-based death notification integrating verbal and social autopsy: a community-level case study. BMC Health Serv Res. 2015;15:9.
32. Siika AM, Rotich JK, Simiyu CJ, Kigotho EM, Smith FE, Sidle JE, et al. An electronic medical record system for ambulatory care of HIV-infected patients in Kenya. Int J Med Inform. 2005;74(5):345–55.
33. Ngana FR, Myers BA, Belton S. Health reporting system in two subdistricts in Eastern Indonesia: Highlighting the role of village midwives. Midwifery. 2012;28(6):809–15.
34. Bang A, Bellad R, Gisore P, Hibberd P, Patel A, Goudar S, et al. Implementation and evaluation of the Helping Babies Breathe curriculum in three resource limited settings: does Helping Babies Breathe save lives? A study protocol. BMC Pregnancy Childbirth. 2014;14:116.
35. Odhiambo FO, Laserson KF, Sewe M, Hamel MJ, Feikin DR, Adazu K, et al. Profile: The KEMRI/CDC health and demographic surveillance system-Western Kenya. Int J Epidemiol. 2012;41(4):977–87.
36. Mehta U, Clerk C, Allen E, Yore M, Sevene E, Singlovic J, et al. Protocol for a drugs exposure pregnancy registry for implementation in resource-limited settings. BMC Pregnancy Childbirth. 2012;12:89.
37. Ba-Saddik IA. Childhood cancer in Aden, Yemen. Cancer Epidemiol. 2013; 37(6):803–6.
38. Nhoncanse GC, Melo DG. Reliability of birth certificates as a source of information on congenital defects in the City of Sao Carlos, Sao Paulo, Brazil. Cien Saude Colet. 2012;17(4):955–63.
39. Li X, Zhu J, Wang Y, Mu D, Dai L, Zhou G, et al. Geographic and urban-rural disparities in the total prevalence of neural tube defects and their subtypes

during 2006-2008 in China: a study using the hospital-based birth defects surveillance system. BMC Public Health. 2013;13:161.
40. Chhetri S, Shrestha NR, Pilgrim T. Pregnancy complicated by heart disease in Nepal. Heart Asia. 2014;6(1):26–9.
41. Mahande MJ, Daltveit AK, Mmbaga BT, Obure J, Masenga G, Manongi R, et al. Recurrence of perinatal death in Northern Tanzania: a registry based cohort study. BMC Pregnancy Childbirth. 2013;13:166.
42. Mahande MJ, Daltveit AK, Obure J, Mmbaga BT, Masenga G, Manongi R, et al. Recurrence of preterm birth and perinatal mortality in northern Tanzania: registry-based cohort study. Trop Med Int Health. 2013;18(8):962–7.
43. Welaga P, Moyer CA, Aborigo R, Adongo P, Williams J, Hodgson A, et al. Why are babies dying in the first month after birth? A 7-year study of neonatal mortality in northern Ghana. PLoS One. 2013;8(3):e58924.
44. Bergsjo P, Mlay J, Lie RT, Lie-Nielsen E, Shao JF. A medical birth registry at Kilimanjaro Christian Medical Centre. East Afr J Public Health. 2007;4(1):1–4.
45. Abu Habib N, Wilcox AJ, Daltveit AK, Basso O, Shao J, Oneko O, et al. Birthweight, preterm birth and perinatal mortality: a comparison of black babies in Tanzania and the USA. Acta Obstet Gynecol Scand. 2011;90(10):1100–6.
46. Mmbaga BT, Lie RT, Olomi R, Mahande MJ, Kvale G, Daltveit AK. Cause-specific neonatal mortality in a neonatal care unit in Northern Tanzania: a registry based cohort study. BMC Pediatr. 2012;12:116.
47. Chiwanga ES, Massenga G, Mlay P, Obure J, Mahande MJ. Maternal outcome in multiple versus singleton pregnancies in Northern Tanzania: a registry-based case control study. Asian Pac J Reprod. 2014;3(1):46–52.
48. Bjerregaard-Andersen M, Biering-Sorensen S, Gomes GM, Bidonga A, Jensen DM, Rodrigues A, et al. Infant twin mortality and hospitalisations after the perinatal period - a prospective cohort study from Guinea-Bissau. Trop Med Int Health. 2014;19(12):1477–87.
49. Bjerregaard-Andersen M, Gomes MA, Joaquim LC, Rodrigues A, Jensen DM, Christensen K, et al. Establishing a twin registry in Guinea-Bissau. Twin Res Hum Genet. 2013;16(1):179–84.
50. Haskew J, Ro G, Saito K, Turner K, Odhiambo G, Wamae A, et al. Implementation of a cloud-based electronic medical record for maternal and child health in rural Kenya. Int J Med Inform. 2015;84(5):349–54.
51. Okoko L: Mapping HIS software platforms in West Africa - Real Time Data For Ebola Response. In USAID Google Docs. Retrieved 15 Sept 2015 from https://docs.google.com/spreadsheets/d/1CUA2aiSC4D-Q6ePN1RBm848Ux9KTi=Tadr8GKV5le8/edit?pli=1#gid=45737138.
52. AbouZahr C, de Savigny D, Mikkelsen L, Setel PW, Lozano R, Lopez AD. Towards universal civil registration and vital statistics systems: the time is now. Lancet. 2015;386(10001):1407–18.
53. Mikkelsen L, Phillips DE, AbouZahr C, Setel PW, de Savigny D, Lozano R, et al. A global assessment of civil registration and vital statistics systems: monitoring data quality and progress. Lancet. 2015;386(10001):1395–406.
54. Phillips DE, AbouZahr C, Lopez AD, Mikkelsen L, de Savigny D, Lozano R, et al. Are well functioning civil registration and vital statistics systems associated with better health outcomes? Lancet. 2015;386(10001):1386–94.
55. Kabadi GS, Mwanyika H, de Savigny D. Innovations in monitoring vital events: a scalable intervention using mobile phone messaging (SMS) support for vital registration coverage. Lancet. 2013;381:S69.
56. Oomman N, Mehl G, Berg M, Silverman R. Modernising vital registration systems: why now? Lancet. 2013;381(9875):1336–7.
57. Li Q, Hu Y, Zhong YP, Chen YP, Tang XW, Guo J, et al. Using the immunization information system to determine vaccination coverage rates among children aged 1-7 years: a report from Zhejiang Province, China. Int J Environ Res Public Health. 2014;11(3):2713–28.
58. Swasthya Slate [http://www.swasthyaslate.org/]. Accessed 15 Sept 2015.
59. Curioso WH, Pardo K, Loayza M. Transforming the Peruvian birth information system. Rev Peru Med Exp Salud Publica. 2013;30(2):303–7.
60. Goudar SS, Carlo WA, McClure EM, Pasha O, Patel A, Esamai F, et al. The maternal and newborn health registry study of the global network for Women's and children's health research. Int J Gynaecol Obstet. 2012;118(3):190–3.
61. Turner KE, Fuller S: Patient-Held Maternal and/or Child Health Records: Meeting the Information Needs of Patients and Healthcare Providers in Developing Countries? Online J Public Health Inform. 2011;3(2). doi:10.5210/ojphi.v3i2.3631.
62. Kihuba E, Gathara D, Mwinga S, Mulaku M, Kosgei R, Mogoa W, et al. Assessing the ability of health information systems in hospitals to support evidence-informed decisions in Kenya. Global Health Action. 2014;7:24859. doi:10.3402/gha.v3407.24859.
63. Requejo JH, Bhutta ZA. The post-2015 agenda: staying the course in maternal and child survival. Arch Dis Child. 2015;100 Suppl 1:S76–81.
64. WHO. Global Strategy for Women's, Children's and Adolescents' Health. Zero draft for consultation. Geneva: World Health Organization; 2015.
65. Bryce J, Arnold F, Blanc A, Hancioglu A, Newby H, Requejo J, et al. Measuring coverage in MNCH: new findings, new strategies, and recommendations for action. PLoS Med. 2013;10(5):e1001423.
66. World Health Organization. Bridging the "Know–Do" Gap, Meeting on Knowledge Translation in Global Health. Geneva: World Health Organization; 2005.
67. Pablos-Mendez A, Shademani R. Knowledge translation in global health. J Contin Educ Health Prof. 2006;26(1):81–6.
68. Francke AL, Smit MC, de Veer AJ, Mistiaen P. Factors influencing the implementation of clinical guidelines for health care professionals: a systematic meta-review. BMC Med Inform Decis Mak. 2008;8:38.
69. Blank A, Prytherch H, Kaltschmidt J, Krings A, Sukums F, Mensah N, et al. "Quality of prenatal and maternal care: bridging the know-do gap" (QUALMAT study): an electronic clinical decision support system for rural Sub-Saharan Africa. BMC Med Inform Decis Mak. 2013;13:44.
70. Necochea E, Tripathi V, Kim Y-M, Akram N, Hyjazi Y, da Luz Vaz M, et al. Implementation of the Standards-Based Management and Recognition approach to quality improvement in maternal, newborn, and child health programs in low-resource countries. Int J Gynecol Obstet. 2015; 130(Supplement 2):S17–24.
71. Braham DL, Richardson AL, Malik IS. Application of the WHO surgical safety checklist outside the operating theatre: medicine can learn from surgery. Clin Med. 2014;14(5):468–74.
72. Lau F, Kuziemsky C, Price M, Gardner J. A review on systematic reviews of health information system studies. J Am Med Inform Assoc. 2010;17(6):637–45.
73. Main EK, Bingham D. Quality improvement in maternity care: promising approaches from the medical and public health perspectives. Curr Opin Obstet Gynecol. 2008;20(6):574–80. doi:10.1097/GCO.1090b1013e3283184040.
74. Osheroff JA, Teich JM, Middleton B, Steen EB, Wright A, Detmer DE. A roadmap for national action on clinical decision support. J Am Med Inform Assoc. 2007;14(2):141–5.
75. Kawamoto, K, Houlihan, CA, Balas, EA, Lobach, DF. Improving clinical practice using clinical decision support systems: review of trials to identify features critical to success. BMJ (Clinical research ed). 2005;330(7494):765.
76. Zakane SA, Gustafsson LL, Tomson G, Loukanova S, Sié A, Nasiell J, et al. Guidelines for maternal and neonatal "point of care": Needs of and attitudes towards a computerized clinical decision support system in rural Burkina Faso. Int J Med Inform. 2014;83(6):459–69.
77. Nair M, Yoshida S, Lambrechts T, Boschi-Pinto C, Bose K, Mason EM, et al. Facilitators and barriers to quality of care in maternal, newborn and child health: a global situational analysis through meta-review. BMJ Open. 2014; 4(5):e004749.
78. Fausett MB, Propst A, Van Doren K, Clark BT. How to develop an effective obstetric checklist. Am J Obstet Gynecol. 2011;205(3):165–70.
79. Moja L, Kwag KH, Lytras T, Bertizzolo L, Brandt L, Pecoraro V, et al. Effectiveness of computerized decision support systems linked to electronic health records: a systematic review and meta-analysis. Am J Public Health. 2014;104(12):e12–22.
80. Free C, Phillips G, Watson L, Galli L, Felix L, Edwards P, et al. The effectiveness of mobile-health technologies to improve health care service delivery processes: a systematic review and meta-analysis. PLoS Med. 2013;10(1):e1001363.
81. MacLeod B, Phillips J, Stone AE, Walji A, Awoonor-Williams JK: The Architecture of a Software System for Supporting Community-based Primary Health Care with Mobile Technology: The Mobile Technology for Community Health (MoTeCH) Initiative in Ghana. Online J Public Health Inform. 2012; 4(1). doi:10.5210/ojphi.v4i1.3910.
82. Crawford J, Larsen-Cooper E, Jezman Z, Cunningham SC, Bancroft E. SMS versus voice messaging to deliver MNCH communication in rural Malawi: assessment of delivery success and user experience. Glob Health Sci Pract. 2014;2(1):35–46.
83. The power of health in every mama's hand [http://www.mobilemamaalliance.org/]. Accessed 15 Sept 2015.
84. Jennings L, Omoni A, Akerele A, Ibrahim Y, Ekanem E. Disparities in mobile phone access and maternal health service utilization in Nigeria: a population-based survey. Int J Med Inform. 2015;84(5):341–8.

85. Vashist SK, Mudanyali O, Schneider E, Zengerle R, Ozcan A. Cellphone-based devices for bioanalytical sciences. Anal Bioanal Chem. 2014;406(14):3263–77.
86. Luhm KR, Cardoso MRA, Waldman EA. Vaccination coverage among children under two years of age based on electronic immunization registry in Southern Brazil. Rev Saude Publica. 2011;45(1):90–8.
87. Jamtvedt G, Young JM, Kristoffersen DT, O'Brien MA, Oxman AD. Audit and feedback: effects on professional practice and health care outcomes. Cochrane Database Syst Rev (Online). 2006;2:Cd000259.
88. Colquhoun HL, Brehaut JC, Sales A, Ivers N, Grimshaw J, Michie S, et al. A systematic review of the use of theory in randomized controlled trials of audit and feedback. Implement Sci. 2013;8:66.
89. Larson EL, Patel SJ, Evans D, Saiman L. Feedback as a strategy to change behaviour: the devil is in the details. J Eval Clin Pract. 2013;19(2):230–4.
90. Ivers NM, Sales A, Colquhoun H, Michie S, Foy R, Francis JJ, et al. No more 'business as usual' with audit and feedback interventions: towards an agenda for a reinvigorated intervention. Implement Sci. 2014;9:14.
91. Ivers N, Jamtvedt G, Flottorp S, Young JM, Odgaard-Jensen J, French SD, et al. Audit and feedback: effects on professional practice and healthcare outcomes. Cochrane Database Syst Rev (Online). 2012;6:Cd000259.
92. Ivers NM, Grimshaw JM, Jamtvedt G, Flottorp S, O'Brien MA, French SD, et al. Growing literature, stagnant science? Systematic review, meta-regression and cumulative analysis of audit and feedback interventions in health care. J Gen Intern Med. 2014;29(11):1534–41.
93. van der Veer SN, de Keizer NF, Ravelli ACJ, Tenkink S, Jager KJ. Improving quality of care. A systematic review on how medical registries provide information feedback to health care providers. Int J Med Inform. 2010;79(5): 305–23.
94. Carver CS, Scheier MF. Control theory: a useful conceptual framework for personality-social, clinical, and health psychology. Psychol Bull. 1982;92(1): 111–35.
95. Kluger AN, DeNisi A. The effects of feedback interventions on performance: A historical review, a meta-analysis, and a preliminary feedback intervention theory. Psychol Bull. 1996;119(2):254–84.
96. Hysong SJ, Best RG, Pugh JA. Audit and feedback and clinical practice guideline adherence: making feedback actionable. Implement Sci. 2006;1:9.
97. Hysong SJ, Teal CR, Khan MJ, Haidet P. Improving quality of care through improved audit and feedback. Implement Sci. 2012;7:45.
98. Salam RA, Lassi ZS, Das JK, Bhutta ZA. Evidence from district level inputs to improve quality of care for maternal and newborn health: interventions and findings. Reprod Health. 2014;11 Suppl 2:S3.
99. Hipgrave DB, Hort K. Dual practice by doctors working in South and East Asia: a review of its origins, scope and impact, and the options for regulation. Health Policy Plan. 2013;29(6):703–16.
100. Mendoza G, Okoko L, Konopka S, Jonas E. mHealth Compendium, vol. 3. Arlington: African Strategies for Health project, Management Sciences for Health; 2013.
101. Shieshia M, Noel M, Andersson S, Felling B, Alva S, Agarwal S, et al. Strengthening community health supply chain performance through an integrated approach: Using mHealth technology and multilevel teams in Malawi. J Glob Health. 2014;4(2):020406.
102. Management Sciences for Health. Systems for Improved Access to Pharmaceuticals and Services (SIAPS) Program. Considerations for the Integration of HMIS and LMIS. Arlington: Management Sciences for Health; 2014.
103. GSMA. Mobile Financial Services for the Unbanked. State of the Industry 2014. London: GSMA; 2014.
104. Muzzi M. UNICEF Good Practices in Integrating Birth Registration into Health Systems (2000–2009); Case Studies: Bangladesh, Brazil, the Gambia and Delhi, India. New York: UNICEF; 2009.
105. Phillips DE, Lozano R, Naghavi M, Atkinson C, Gonzalez-Medina D, Mikkelsen L, et al. A composite metric for assessing data on mortality and causes of death: the vital statistics performance index. Popul Health Metr. 2014;12:14.
106. World Bank, USAID and WHO. Health Measurement and Accountability Post 2015: Five-Point Call to Action. Washington, DC: MA4Health; 2015.
107. WHO. World Health Assembly Resolution 58.28: eHealth. Geneva: World Health Organization; 2005.
108. Brooke EM. The current and future use of registers in health information systems. Geneva: World Health Organization; 1974.
109. Agency for Healthcare Research and Quality. Registries for Evaluating Patient Outcomes: A User's Guide. 3rd ed. Rockville: Agency for Healthcare Research and Quality; 2014.

Permissions

All chapters in this book were first published in P&C, by BioMed Central; hereby published with permission under the Creative Commons Attribution License or equivalent. Every chapter published in this book has been scrutinized by our experts. Their significance has been extensively debated. The topics covered herein carry significant findings which will fuel the growth of the discipline. They may even be implemented as practical applications or may be referred to as a beginning point for another development.

The contributors of this book come from diverse backgrounds, making this book a truly international effort. This book will bring forth new frontiers with its revolutionizing research information and detailed analysis of the nascent developments around the world.

We would like to thank all the contributing authors for lending their expertise to make the book truly unique. They have played a crucial role in the development of this book. Without their invaluable contributions this book wouldn't have been possible. They have made vital efforts to compile up to date information on the varied aspects of this subject to make this book a valuable addition to the collection of many professionals and students.

This book was conceptualized with the vision of imparting up-to-date information and advanced data in this field. To ensure the same, a matchless editorial board was set up. Every individual on the board went through rigorous rounds of assessment to prove their worth. After which they invested a large part of their time researching and compiling the most relevant data for our readers.

The editorial board has been involved in producing this book since its inception. They have spent rigorous hours researching and exploring the diverse topics which have resulted in the successful publishing of this book. They have passed on their knowledge of decades through this book. To expedite this challenging task, the publisher supported the team at every step. A small team of assistant editors was also appointed to further simplify the editing procedure and attain best results for the readers.

Apart from the editorial board, the designing team has also invested a significant amount of their time in understanding the subject and creating the most relevant covers. They scrutinized every image to scout for the most suitable representation of the subject and create an appropriate cover for the book.

The publishing team has been an ardent support to the editorial, designing and production team. Their endless efforts to recruit the best for this project, has resulted in the accomplishment of this book. They are a veteran in the field of academics and their pool of knowledge is as vast as their experience in printing. Their expertise and guidance has proved useful at every step. Their uncompromising quality standards have made this book an exceptional effort. Their encouragement from time to time has been an inspiration for everyone.

The publisher and the editorial board hope that this book will prove to be a valuable piece of knowledge for researchers, students, practitioners and scholars across the globe.

List of Contributors

Chi Zhou, Baodan Zhang, Hao Chen, Weijue Wang, Liu Huang, Liangwen Xu and Lei Yang
Medical School, Hangzhou Normal University, 16 Xuelin Rd., Xiasha District, Hangzhou 310036, China

Weijun Zheng
School of Basic Medical Science, Zhejiang Chinese Medical University, Hangzhou 310053, China

Qi Yuan
Research Division, Institute of Mental Health, Singapore 539747, Singapore

Benjamin M. Hunter and Susan F. Murray
King's College London, Department of International Development, The Strand, London WC2R 2LS, UK

Mahua Mandal
MEASURE Evaluation, Carolina Population Center, University of North Carolina at Chapel Hill, Chapel Hill, NC, USA

Arundati Muralidharan
WaterAid India, New Delhi, India

Sara Pappa
Health Policy Plus (HP+), Palladium, Washington, DC, USA

Lucinda Manda-Taylor, Daniel Mwale, Tamara Phiri and Victor Mwapasa
University of Malawi, College of Medicine, Blantyre, Malawi

Aisling Walsh, Ruairi Brugha and Elaine Byrne
Royal College of Surgeons in Ireland, Dublin, Ireland

Anne Matthews
Dublin City University, Dublin, Ireland

Alexandre Archanjo Ferraro and Sandra Josefina Ferraz Ellero Grisi
Department of Pediatrics, School of Medicine, Universidade de Sao Paulo, Av Dr Eneas Carvalho Aguiar, 647, Sao Paulo 05403-900, Brazil

Guilherme Vanoni Polanczyk, Adriana Argeu, Euripides Constantino Miguel and Bacy Fleitlich-Bilyk
Department of Psychiatry, School of Medicine, Universidade de Sao Paulo, Sao Paulo, Brazil

Luis Augusto Rohde
Department of Psychiatry, School of Medicine, Universidade de Sao Paulo, Sao Paulo, Brazil
Department of Psychiatry and Legal Medicine, School of Medicine, Universidade Federal do Rio Grande do Sul, Porto Alegre, Brazil

Daniel D. Reidpath and Pascale Allotey
Global Public Health and SEACO, JC School of Medicine and Health Sciences, Monash University, Subang Jaya, Malaysia

Abraham R. Oduro
Navrongo Health Research Centre, Navrongo, Ghana

Raymond A. Aborigo
Global Public Health and SEACO, JC School of Medicine and Health Sciences, Monash University, Subang Jaya, Malaysia
Navrongo Health Research Centre, Navrongo, Ghana

Shabir A. Madhi
Medical Research Council: Respiratory and Meningeal Pathogens Research Unit, University of the Witwatersrand, Johannesburg, South Africa
Department of Science and Technology/National Research Foundation: Vaccine Preventable Diseases, University of the Witwatersrand, Johannesburg, South Africa
National Institute for Communicable Diseases: a division of National Health Laboratory Service, Centre for Vaccines and Immunology, Johannesburg, South Africa

Luis M. Rivera
Hospital Universitario Maternidad Nuestra Señora De La Altagracia Perinatology Department, Gazcue, Santo Domingo, Dominican Republic

Xavier Sáez-Llorens
Hospital del Niño "Dr. José Renán Esquivel", Infectious Disease Department, Panama City, Panama
National System of Investigators (SNI), National Research of the National Secretariat for Science, Technology and Innovation of Panama (SENACYT), Panama City, Panama

Clara Menéndez
Barcelona Institute of Global Health (ISGlobal), Hospital Clinic of Barcelona, Universitat de Barcelona, Barcelona, Spain
Manhiça Health Research Center (CISM), Manhiça, Mozambique

Nazira Carrim-Ganey
Setshaba Research Centre, Soshanguve, South Africa

Mark F. Cotton
Department of Paediatrics and Child Health, Stellenbosch University and Tygerberg Children's Hospital, Cape Town, South Africa

Darren Katzman and Mariëtha M. Luttig
GSK, Bryanston, South Africa

Rosalba Candelario, Sherryl Baker and Mahua Roychoudhury
GSK (formerly employee of Novartis Vaccines Division), Cambridge, MA, USA

Chol Chol
School of Public Health, The University of Sydney, Sydney, Australia

Cynthia Hunter
Senior Lecturer, School of Public Health, The University of Sydney, Sydney, Australia

Berhane Debru
Director General of Research and Human Resource Development, Ministry of Health, Asmara, Eritrea

Berhana Haile
Director of Family and Community Health, Ministry of Health, Asmara, Eritrea

Joel Negin
School of Public Health, The University of Sydney, Sydney, Australia

Robert G. Cumming
School of Public Health, The University of Sydney, Sydney, Australia

Gershom Chongwe, Choolwe Jacobs, Jessy Zgambo and Charles Michelo
Department of Epidemiology and Biostatistics, School of Public Health, University of Zambia, Lusaka, Zambia

Helen Chipukuma
Department of Health Policy and Management, School of Public Health, University of Zambia, Lusaka, Zambia

Steven Chifundo Azizi
Department of Epidemiology and Biostatistics, School of Public Health, University of Zambia, Lusaka, Zambia
Malawi Defence Force, Malawi Military Health Services, Kamuzu Barracks, Private Bag 43, Lilongwe, Malawi

Helen Chipukuma
Department of Health Policy and Management, School of Public Health, University of Zambia, Lusaka, Zambia

Tonya MacDonald
School of Midwifery, Health Sciences Building, Laurentian University, 935 Ramsey Lake Road, Sudbury, ON P3E 2C6, Canada

Suzanne Jackson
Dalla Lana School of Public Health, Health Sciences Building, University of Toronto, 155 College Street, Suite 526, Toronto, ON M5T 3M7, Canada

Marie-Carmèle Charles
Cégep du Vieux Montréal, Montreal, Canada

Marius Periel, Marie-Véna Jean-Baptiste, Alex Salomon and Éveillard Premilus
Hôpital Albert Schweitzer, Deschapelles, Haiti

Malalai Naziri and Karen M. Edmond
UNICEF Afghanistan, Kabul, Afghanistan

Jane Burke and Sediq Seddiqi
ATR Consulting Afghanistan, Kabul, Afghanistan

Abo Ismael Foshanji and Farhad Farewar
Afghanistan Ministry of Public Health, Kabul, Afghanistan

Ariel Higgins-Steele
UNICEF Afghanistan, Kabul, Afghanistan
United Nations Office Complex in Afghanistan (UNOCA), Jalalabad Road, Kabul, Afghanistan

Debbie Booth
The University of Newcastle, Callaghan, Australia

Binod Bindu Sharma
Mothers and Babies Research Centre, Hunter Medical Research Institute, Lookout Rd, New Lambton Heights, NSW 2305, Australia
The University of Newcastle, Callaghan, Australia

Lisa Jones
Department of Neonatology, John Hunter Hospital, Lookout Rd, New Lambton Heights, NSW 2305, Australia
Department of Obstetrics and Gynaecology, Sydney Medical School, University of Sydney, Camperdown, Australia

Deborah Joanne Loxton
Priority Research Centre for Generational Health and Ageing, The University of Newcastle, Callaghan, Australia
Hunter Medical Research Institute, Lot 1 Kookaburra Circuit, New Lambton Heights, NSW 2305, Australia

Roger Smith
Mothers and Babies Research Centre, Hunter Medical Research Institute, Lot 1 Kookaburra Circuit, New Lambton Heights, NSW 2305, Australia
Department of Endocrinology, John Hunter Hospital, Lookout Rd, New Lambton Heights, NSW 2305, Australia
Priority Research Centre for Reproductive Science, The University of Newcastle, Callaghan, Australia

Ali Mehryar Karim, Nebreed Fesseha Zemichael, Tesfaye Shigute, Dessalew Emaway Altaye, Selamawit Dagnew, Firew Solomon, Mulu Hailu, Gizachew Tadele, Bantalem Yihun and Wuleta Betemariam
The Last Ten Kilometers Project (L10K) 2020, JSI Research & Training Institute, Inc, Bole Sub-City, Kebele 03/05, Hs # 2111, Addis Ababa, Ethiopia

Nebiyu Getachew
Ethiopia Performance Monitoring and Evaluation Service (EPMES), Social Impact, Bole Sub-City, Woreda 13, House # 478, Addis Ababa, Ethiopia

Christianne J. M. de Groot
Department of Obstetrics and Gynaecology, VU University Medical Center, De Boelelaan 1118, 1081, HZ, Amsterdam, The Netherlands

Jorine de Haan
Department of Obstetrics and Gynaecology, VU University Medical Center, De Boelelaan 1118, 1081, HZ, Amsterdam, The Netherlands
Department of Oncology, KU Leuven, Herestraat 49, 3000 Leuven, Belgium

Christianne A. R. Lok
Department of Gynaecologic Oncology, Center for Gynaecologic Oncology Amsterdam, Amsterdam, The Netherlands

Joke S. Schutte
Department of Obstetrics and Gynaecology, Isala Clinics, Zwolle, the Netherlands

Lia van Zuylen
Department of Medical Oncology, Erasmus MC Cancer Institute, Rotterdam, the Netherlands

Fay F. Warnock
Developmental Neurosciences, Child and Family Research Institute, L408, 4480 Oak Street, Vancouver, BC, Canada
University of British Columbia (BC), School of Nursing, Vancouver, BC, Canada

Kenneth D. Craig
Department of Psychology, University of British Columbia (BC), Vancouver, BC, Canada

Roger Bakeman
Georgia State University, Atlanta, Georgia 30303, USA

Thaila Castral
University of Goiás Faculty of Nursing, Goiânia, GO, Brazil

Jila Mirlashari
School of Nursing and Midwifery, Tehran University of Medical Sciences, Tehran, Iran

Ann K. Blanc and Katharine J. McCarthy
Population Council, New York, NY, USA

Karla Berdichevsky and Claudia Diaz
Population Council, Mexico City, Mexico

Abbey Byrne, Tanya Caulfield, Alison Morgan and Michelle Kermode
Nossal Institute for Global Health, University of Melbourne, 161 Barry St, Carlton, VIC 3010, Australia

Pamela Onyo, Josephat Nyagero and John Nduba
Amref Health Africa, Nairobi, Kenya

Collins O. F. Zamawe
Parent and Child Health Initiative (PACHI), Research Centre, Amina house, Off Chilambula Road, Capital City, Lilongwe 3, Malawi
The Ministry of Health, Lilongwe, Malawi

Masford Banda
MaiMwana Project, Mchinji, Malawi

Albert N. Dube
Parent and Child Health Initiative (PACHI), Research Centre, Amina house, Off Chilambula Road, Capital City, Lilongwe 3, Malawi
The University of Malawi, College of Medicine, School of Public Health, Blantyre, Malawi

Sonja L. Myhre, Ane Lunde, Kjersti Mørkrid, Ingrid K. Friberg and Steve French
Department of International Public Health, Norwegian Institute of Public Health, Pb 4404 Nydalen, N-0403 Oslo, Norway

J. Frederik Frøen and Mahima Venkateswaran
Department of International Public Health, Norwegian Institute of Public Health, Pb 4404 Nydalen, N-0403 Oslo, Norway
Centre for Intervention Science in Maternal and Child Health (CISMAC), University of Bergen, Bergen, Norway

Marleen Temmerman
John Snow, Inc., Boston, MA, USA

Michael J. Frost
Department of International Public Health, Norwegian Institute of Public Health, Pb 4404 Nydalen, N-0403 Oslo, Norway
John Snow, Inc., Boston, MA, USA

Doris Chou and Garrett Mehl
Department of Reproductive Health and Research, World Health Organization, Geneva, Switzerland

Jane Kaye
HeLEX - Centre for Health, Law and Emerging Technologies, Nuffield Department of Population Health, University of Oxford, Oxford, UK

John Lewis
Health Information System Programme (HISP) Vietnam, Ho Chí Minh, Vietnam
Department of Informatics, University of Oslo, Oslo, Norway

Aleena M. Wojcieszek and Vicki J. Flenady
Mater Research Institute, The University of Queensland, Brisbane, Australia
International Stillbirth Alliance, Millburn, NJ, USA

Index

www.ingramcontent.com/pod-product-compliance
Lightning Source LLC
LaVergne TN
LVHW080737210926
848485LV00003B/570